The Really Useful

BOOK ON

INTENSIVE CARE

Two quotations from the first century AD

If I thought it sufficient to follow traditional rules, I should regard it adequate treatment of this investigation to omit nothing that I have read or been taught, provided that it be reasonably sound. But my design is to bring to light the secret principles of this art, and to open the inmost recesses of the subject, giving the result not of teaching received from others, but of my own experience and the guidance of nature herself.

Quintilian Institutio Ontaria, 6,25.

We trained hard – but it seemed that every time we were beginning to form into teams, we would be re-organized. I was to learn later in life that we tend to meet any new situation by re-organizing and a wonderful method it can be for creating the illusion of progress while producing confusion, inefficiency and demoralization.

Gaius Petronius

The Really Useful
BOOK ON
INTENSIVE CARE

ERIC SHERWOOD JONES PhD, FRCP
Formerly Staff Specialist, Whiston and St. Helens Hospitals
Merseyside

DAVID B. McWILLIAM MB, BS, MCog.Sci, FRACP
Director of Intensive Care, Royal Prince Alfred Hospital,
Sydney, Australia

JOHN COAKLEY, MD, FRCP
Staff Specialist, St. Bartholomew's Hospital, London

Illustrated by STELLA LAVELLE, SRN

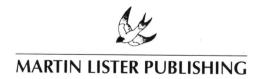

MARTIN LISTER PUBLISHING

This textbook is dedicated to a group of intensive care nurses affectionately known as the Golden Oldies, who taught us almost as much as did the patients.

Published and distributed by
Martin Lister Publishing
24 Pinewood Avenue
Bolton-le-Sands
Carnforth, Lancs. LA5 8AR
UK

ISBN 0 9533396 0 2

British Library Cataloguing-in-Publication Data

A catalogue record for this book is available from the British Library

Typeset by Martin Lister Publishing Services, Carnforth, Lancs., UK

Printed by Arrowhead Books Ltd, Portman Road, Reading, Berks., UK

Contents

SECTION THREE: PRINCIPLES OF THERAPY

Contributors

Francis Beach, MD, FRCP
Staff Specialist, Yeovil District
Hospital, Yeovil (Chapter 5)

Ian Gordon, MB, MRCP
Physician in occupational medicine, Merseyside
(Corrections and amendments to the text)

Andrew Luksza, MB, FRCP
Staff Specialist, District General Hospital, Barrow-in-Furness, Cumbria.
(Flow charts, algorithms and some tables)

Preface

This is a book for beginners; students and hospital staff starting to train in intensive care and the larger numbers who work outside the unit but who need to know the principles involved. The resulting aim of the book will then be achieved; the right patient treated by the right methods at the right time. Put into more eloquent words by Professor Bryan Jennett, the benefits exceed the burdens. The contributors write from the bedside and their experience of intensive care adds up to a hundred years.

The first of the three sections describes the unchanging recipes for success; the right numbers of appropriately trained staff; an adherence to really useful methods of investigation and treatment; the unit itself; the selection of patients most likely to benefit.

The information in the second section is common to all hospital practice and can therefore be found in many texts; it is included for the convenience of the reader. To facilitate description the failure of one body system or organ is described in isolation, but the apprentice will quickly learn that when one system fails, so do the others. For beginners – and ourselves – we have kept to the really useful basics which may appear dated. But then, in the terrestrial mammals the composition of the extracellular fluid has remained unchanged for thirty million years!

The therapy can only be learnt by apprenticeship at the bedside but the background information given in the third section will help the beginner to plan and administer rational treatments and also understand the mechanics and physiology.

To avoid deception, we declare those topics which are deliberately omitted. These fall into two groups: treatments of no value or those which are experimental. In the latter group we have omitted prolonged extracorporeal gas exchange, monoclonal antibodies and advanced theories of ethics because we do not use them.

I take responsibility for any errors or omissions incurred during the editing.

E. S. J.

Acknowledgements

Thanks to Janice Norton for typing the manuscript; my former colleague Malcolm Wright, FRCP, FRCA, for imparting knowledge gained during 25 years of intensive care – an *ex officio* contributor; Brian Sherwood Jones who persuaded us to utilize the algorithm and flow chart and taught us the importance of design for instruction; the librarians of the Liverpool Medical Institution.

Permission was given to reproduce data as follows: Tables and figures – as indicated in the text – from *Essential Intensive Care*, 1978 (Kluwer Academic Publishers); Tables 7.7 and 17.7 and Figure 7.7 (Blackwell Scientific Publications; Table 10.2 (*Lancet*); Table 10.3 and Figures 26.2 and 26.3 (*British Medical Journal*); Figure 17.2 and Table 27.2 (*Intensive Care Medicine*); Tables 19.16 and 29.8 (Churchill-Livingstone); Figures 21.2 and 21.3 (UK Resuscitation Council); Table 27.17 (*Thorax*)

I am especially indebted to Martin Lister for transforming a chaotic typescript into an attractive textbook.

Publication of this book was made possible by a legacy from Amos John Cooke CMG (1885 to 1961)

Some commonly used abbreviations

Mass in grams	g
Length in metres	m
Volume in litres	l
Concentration in millimoles per litre	mmol/l
Time in hours	h
Time in minutes	min
Arterial blood pressure	BP
Central venous pressure	CVP
Pulmonary artery wedge pressure	PAWP
Pressure in liquid or gas in millimetres of mercury	mmHg
Pressure in liquid or gas in kilo Pascal	kPa
Temperature in degrees Celsius	°C
Forced vital capacity (litres)	FVC
Forced expiratory volume in the first second (litres)	FEV_1
Peak expiratory flow in litres per minute	PEF
Tidal volume	V_T
Minute volume ventilation (expired, litres per min)	$\dot{V}_E$
Alveolar ventilation (litres per minute)	$\dot{V}_A$
Alveolar oxygen tension	PAO_2
Arterial oxygen tension	PaO_2
Alveolar CO_2 tension	$PACO_2$
Arterial CO_2 tension	$PaCO_2$
Plasma electrolytes	Nap, Kp, etc.
Kilo calorie	kcal
Kilo joule	kJ
Extracellular fluid	ECF
Intracellular fluid	ICF
Adult respiratory distress syndrome	ARDS
Disseminated intravascular coagulation	DIC

SECTION ONE
PRINCIPLES

1
Raison d'être

'As for the future your task is not to foresee, but to enable it.'

Saint Exupéry

'Human life ... may be reduced to a form of mechanization in which
the incomparable grandeur of the human spirit, the genius of the
human mind and the noblest virtues of the human heart are
asphyxiated in the exhaust fumes of our technological wonders.'

Immanuel Jakobovits

'The feasibility of an operation is not the best justification of its
performance.'

Henry Cohen

I INTRODUCTION
II EVOLUTION OF INTENSIVE CARE
III CODES OF PRACTICE
IV RESULTS
V AUDIT

I INTRODUCTION

Like Topsy our health services have grown and grown since 1946. There is
more and more money for manpower* and new capital programmes but do
we get value for money? Only in recent years has this question been taken
seriously and there is no reason why intensive care should escape scrutiny.
For an extensive analysis of the benefits and burdens of high technology
medicine the interested are referred to the clear and logical monograph by
Jennett (1986). Here we have a potted history and then a short account of
the aims of general intensive care. It seems reasonable to start off with some
definitions of intensive care.

Definitions of intensive care are numerous, inadequate but fortunately
also largely unnecessary. At one time the author (ESJ) attempted (WHO,
1971) to separate intensive care from therapy but the two labels are now
used interchangeably. The British Medical Association (1967) definitions
were adopted by the English National Board for Nursing, Midwifery and
Health Visitors (ENB) and have also stood the test of time.

---

* Sexist! We use male for doctor (70% correct) and female for nurse (90% correct)

3

The care of patients who are deemed recoverable but who need continuous supervision and need or are likely to need prompt use of specialized techniques by skilled personnel.

We have defined an ICU as a special unit providing the following (1) A facility available to all medical staff giving more space, staff and equipment for the care of the patient than can be provided in the ordinary wards. (2) A service which provides continuous observation of the vital functions and can support these functions more promptly and efficiently than can be done elsewhere in the hospital. Both the facility and the service can be developed within a specialist division or ward, but the essence of the ICU is that, like most operating theatres, it is communal.

The newcomer to intensive care must clearly understand how this differs from specialized intensive care and from high-dependency care.

II EVOLUTION

The centralized care of patients with particular diseases is very old, going back to the mid-1800s. The aim, initially at least, was to prevent the spread of the disease such as smallpox or typhoid.

The various practices of the infectious diseases hospital, the design of the wards, basic nursing and so on, were applied, often inadequately, to general hospitals and are very important to intensive care. The reason for this is that the patient in the ICU is susceptible to infection from other patients and the staff, and this secondary or cross infection can only be eliminated by the application of these principles taken from the infectious diseases unit. The therapy given in the infectious diseases unit was non-specific, e.g. tracheostomy for diphtheria, and intravenous fluid therapy, until the advent of serum therapy, chemotherapy and antibiotics. It was many years before centres were established to give specialized therapy to patients with poliomyelitis and tetanus, to quote two examples. Such units served large populations or regions and their experience clearly demonstrated the advantages of such specialized intensive care. The lessons learned included the role of specifically trained nursing teams and the standardization of the methods. We shall see that these principles are equally important to general intensive care. During the same period (1940–1950) other units for specialized cardiothoracic care were established, namely those for cardiothoracic surgery, neurosurgery and the many others listed in Table 1.1; coronary care was the last to join the list. Each of

Table 1.1 Units for intensive care (From
Essential Intensive Care, with permission)

Regional units
    Neonatal
    Surgery
    Paediatric
    Medicine
    Surgery
    Poisoning
    Renal
    Respiratory
    Cardiothoracic surgery
    Neurosurgery
    Spinal injuries
    Burns
    Neuropsychiatric
Local hospital units
    Neonatal – within a maternity unit
    General internal medicine
    Coronary
    General surgery
    Accident
Related therapeutic services
    Recovery room
    Resuscitation
    Arrest team
    Mobile services
    Maternity
    Accident

---

these specialized units, with the notable exception of coronary care, were able to serve large populations and the units were financed on a regional basis. Because ischaemic heart disease is epidemic, coronary care was set up in all sizeable hospitals. Many of the principles, and some of the technology of these specialized units is used in a newer and quite different organization, general intensive care or therapy.

The idea of segregation of severely ill patients within a ward is as old as organized nursing. An experienced ward sister would move such patients to a point in the ward where they might be under intensive observation, at least during the day. Alternatively, one or two patients were put in a side-ward or in cubicles and 'specialed'. This term means that one or more nurses were allocated to the patient to provide more care and preserve continuity of care. There is no doubt that many patients owe their lives to this system, although it has many shortcomings. In particular, the junior medical staff had not received formal training in the care of the acute illnesses, and equipment might not be readily available or in proper working order. A more formalized organization was evolved in the United States and the overall concept was termed Progressive Patient Care (PPC). One reason for the reorganization was to try to curtail the rapidly rising cost of medical care from 1945 onwards. PPC comprised the reorganization of in-patients into three compartments, and the individual patients moved from one to another according to their nursing and medical needs. 'The central theme of the progressive patient care concept is the organization of facilities services and staff around the medical and nursing needs of the patient. Patients are grouped according to their degree of illness and need for care, and the staff serving each group of patients is selected and trained to provide the kind of services needed by that group.' (Haldeman, 1959). The three parts of PPC are intensive care, intermediate care and self-care, which is now widely acknowledged, but rarely practised, in hospitals throughout the world. Intermediate care is the equivalent of our acute (short-stay) medical surgical and accident wards. Self-care is a hotel-like accommodation and service for the ambulant patient requiring little nursing or doctoring. As suggested by the title of the concept, PPC patients would move from one unit to another, usually from intensive to intermediate, and then to self-care.

Parallel developments were taking place in Scandinavia and France. An epidemic of poliomyelitis and the advance in thoracic surgery led to the development of specialized forms of intensive care. The problems of poliomyelitis leading to ventilatory failure and retained secretions now read like the dark ages of respiratory care! In France intensive care got off to an early start and quickly led to the segregation of patients according to their needs rather than specific diseases. A few names and dates are given in Table 1.2. In the United Kingdom the first trial of PPC was in 1959 in the mid-Ulster hospital at Magherafelt; the organization of the nursing was largely the inspiration and work of the late Miss Ann White, CBE. General intensive care units were then established at Kettering (Crocket and Barr, 1966) and at Whiston (*Lancet*, 1966) and are now ubiquitous. The acute wards continue to form the back-bone of in-patient care but units for self-care have fallen out of favour. This is probably because social conditions have facilitated early discharge to home. Many large hospitals now have several intensive care units, e.g. post-cardiac intensive care, coronary care and a dialysis unit. The Royal Prince Alfred hospital has the following: general, neurosurgical and coronary care. A notable milestone in the development of intensive care was the proper organization and supervision of nurse training. This was brought about in 1970 by the setting up of an independent educational body, the Joint Board of Clinical Nursing Studies (JBCNS) which was subsequently

Table 1.2 Milestones in the development of general intensive care

*1954	Hôpital Claude Bernard (Mollaret *et al.*)
	Hôpital Necker (Hamburger *et al.*)
*1958	Hôpital Marshal Foch (Nedey *et al.*)
	Progressive Patient Care USA (US Department of Health, Education and Welfare)
1959	Mid-Ulster (Ann White, CBE)
1966	Kettering (Crocket and Barr)

* The French contributions are documented in a paperback *La Réanimation*, by Jean-Roger Le Gall (1982)

incorporated into the English National Board (ENB). The Board consists of representatives of the Medical, Nursing and Midwifery Royal Colleges and the Health Service, together with a team of full-time officers. The Board is responsible to the Secretary of State for Health and the Secretary of State for Wales. The ENB has designed outline curricula on almost every topic of post-basic, nursing, including intensive care courses. Before the teaching department of a hospital can obtain approval to run a training course, the ENB must be satisfied that the ICU will provide the nursing experience, that the nurse will be well taught and, above all, that the course will not be used as a confidence trick to provide staff. These approved courses have now ensured an adequate supply of properly trained nurses to staff ICUs.

The training structure differs somewhat in Australia. The Nurses Registration Board (equivalent to the ENB) does not control the post-basic courses. Consequently, tertiary colleges and hospitals design their own courses and may, if they desire, have these accredited by the State College of Nursing. We are sure that both countries will claim advantages.

III CODES OF PRACTICE

The heart of the matter is a new organization of patient care with clearly defined aims and objectives. This implies that there is something wrong with the preceding system, a topic now considered. This analysis is prefaced by a statement on the codes of practice. The principles guiding the practice of intensive care are also those governing the whole of medicine, and are three in number.

'Has this person (or, if he is incapable, his guardian) been given all the necessary knowledge and freedom to decide whether he accepts the course of action recommended, that is, is his consent informed, intelligent and voluntary?

Is my recommendation based on the best scientific probabilities?

Is my proposed course of action one that I would advise for someone I love, and if I were similarly circumstanced would I wish this done for me?' (Lord Cohen, *The Cost of Life*, 1967).

On rare occasions the doctor has to start resuscitation before informed consent can be obtained. There are additional codes of practice which, although not exclusive to intensive care, are integral with this type of care.

(1) Intensive care should only be considered when the patient is deemed recoverable. Thus, it is quite wrong to use artificial ventilation for a patient with advanced end-stage disease of any kind. The criteria for intensive therapy alter with advances in medicine.

(2) Intensive care, like many treatments, is started on the assumption that the patient wishes to survive the critical illness or injury. Because of the acuteness of the illness or its severity there may not be time to determine the patient's wishes and often the doctors and nurses later have to accept the fact that the patient has lost the will to survive.

(3) Intensive care should be stopped when a patient shows evidence of brain death, thus avoiding unnecessary distress to relatives and hospital staff. Brain death can easily and quickly be diagnosed by the signs to be described later. There is a further indication for stopping intensive therapy, that is, when it becomes clear that the pathological processes are irreversible, even though the patient has not suffered brain death. In such instances, treatment of symptoms is continued, but specific therapy is stopped.

(4) The interest of the patient takes precedence over those of the doctor. This code is of cardinal importance to general intensive care. Doctors are often reluctant to accept priorities in medicine, and allow their own interest in some disease or operation to take priority over the diseases which have the highest priority. The obligations of the intensive care staff must be centred on those patients most likely to benefit from intensive care. In other terms, a general intensive care unit should have clearly defined aims, stated in terms of the anticipated death rates.

(5) We do not believe that the intensive care doctor should play 'God' and base his actions on the predicted effects on society – 'what use is a newborn babe?' as the late Sir Henry Miller reminded us (*Cost of Life*, 1967), and Benjamin Franklin long before. The intensive care doctor is at a great disadvantage in comparison to the old-fashioned general

practitioner, who knew his patients and their relatives, and might then judge the best action for the individual patient. There could be no clearer statement on this aspect of the doctor–patient relationship than that made by the transplant surgeon, T.E. Starzl (1967).

'It is doubtful if many doctors who actually care for the sick and the infirm plan their actions on the basis of the predicted effect upon society. Instead, the dominant tradition is for the physician to provide the best care of which he is capable for those who either seek his services or are assigned to his responsibility; by and large this is done without regard for the conceivable broader issue of whether treatment is justifiable on social grounds. His reasons may include pride, altruism, compassion, curiosity, a spirit of competition, even avarice, or a combination of all these things. Whatever the motives, the reflexes that follow are sure and respond similarly to the needs of the productive members of the community, the insane and feebleminded, children with incurable birth defects, condemned criminals, or even soldiers who moments before were members of a hostile army.

The foregoing viewpoint is a narrow one, but there is no reason to believe that it should be abandoned in the face of advancing technocracy. It has shielded the ill from the caprices and the mural judgements of other men through centuries of evolving philosophical, religious, and legal doctrines. It has placed the concept of the sanctity of human life on a practical foundation, since the responsibility of one person for another could not be more clearly defined than through the doctor–patient relationship, irrespective of the reasons for the contract entered into between the two involved parties.'

To return to the central theme – the right patient in the right place at the right time. This aim needs correct decisions on patient management (not by the sort of people who hide in office blocks!) and the decisions must be made throughout the hospital – from casualty to obstetrics and gynaecology, from ENT to the recovery room at any time of day or night every single day of the year. To grasp what this means it is essential for the beginner to re-consider the older system of decision-making. Reflect on the variables given in Table 1.3; the place of action, the experience of the medical staff and the time course. The latter means the time during which the management decision must be made to enable the individual patient to get the right treatment. As a generalization, an out-patient will lose nothing if the right

Table 1.3 Decision-making in hospital

Place	Medical staff	Time course
Clinic	Staff specialist Registrar SHO	Days, weeks, months
Wards/A & E		
Majority	Consultant Registrar SHO HO	Days
Minority	Registrar SHO HO	Minutes, hours

diagnosis and treatment are made in days or even weeks; if the consultant gets it wrong at the first consultation, only rarely does the error cause harm. The same holds good for the majority of patients in the A & E department and wards. Two facts make the decision-making more risk for the patient. Firstly, initial assessment is often made by the most inexperienced, especially after office hours – the pre-registration house officer or SHO. The reader will be familiar with the difficulties. 'The central dilemma of learning the practice of any branch of medicine is that training requires responsibility but the patient's interest requires that responsibility should only be given those who have been trained.'(BMA, 1967). If our new system of general intensive care is to be effective – anecdote suggests that this is not always the case – then the entire medical staff of a district general hospital must be taught when to summon aid – when to 'press the button'.

'The second fact is that for only a minority of patients in the A & E department and wards is urgent action essential, even life-saving. Examples would be asthma, haemorrhage or diabetic keto-acidosis. The key to success is to teach all the doctors to recognize the right patient at the right time. The result would be the credit or benefit side of the story. Unfortunately too often the wrong patient is admitted to an ICU – the burden side of the equation. In later chapters we will learn that many patients cannot possibly benefit from intensive care. This is an appropriate place to crystallize what intensive care does not do, self-evident from Table 1.4.

Table 1.4 What intensive care does not do
(From *Essential Intensive Care*, with permission)

(1)	Save life at any cost
(2)	Substitute for the recovery room
(3)	Excuse poor standards – 'rescue operation'
(4)	Rob other services of staff or money
(5)	Create a nursing elite
(6)	Make the nurse into a frustrated doctor
(7)	Create prestige and status for doctors
(8)	Make an 'interesting' job for bored doctors

IV RESULTS

When general intensive care is introduced into a district general hospital there is a big shake-up. Clinical 'decision-making' and medical training need radical surgery! The raison d'être must produce results. The latter are two kinds – the clinically obvious labelled 'direct' in Table 1.5 and applying to patient, nurse and doctor, The more subtle, but equally important are called 'indirect' and a brief explanation is required. The indirect results for the patient means that omissions are analysed, publicized and thus not repeated, thank you! This process has to be given a posh label – educational feedback, and applies to many conditions, some shown in Table 1.6. Here are two examples. A patient with a curable disease dies because the upper airway is not protected: this, despite the fact that diagnosis and treatment are so simple; the feedback is training and more training to prevent a second disaster. Appropriate nutrition can determine morbidity and mortality – the proof is in the books in the medical library. When the consequences of malnutrition are observed in an ICU – a patient with inflammatory bowel disease, for example – then the opportunity is seized to teach, or perhaps preach is the right word. Of course the teaching must go on and on just like in the school classroom. The principles of educational feedback were summarized beautifully by the Danish pioneer Björn Ibsen as follows. 'Intensive care units are of great value not only to patients who are a admitted for treatment, but even more so to the many patients who due to the experience gained are saved from complications later. When the patient is saved by intensive therapy it has very often been said; why was he allowed to be so ill? It would have been easier to prevent this than to cure it.' (Ibsen, 1966).

Table 1.5 Results of general intensive care (From *Essential Intensive Care,* with permission)

	Direct	
PATIENT	The right patient in the right place at the right time A few lives saved High standards of care for many	
NURSE	Increased:	Knowledge Skills Responsibility Diagnosis Therapy
DOCTOR	Increased:	Knowledge Skills
	Management decisions	
	'Responsibility should only be given to those who have been trained'	
	Indirect	
PATIENT	Feedback, e.g. asthma, shock, etc.	
NURSE/DOCTOR	Educational: A teaching machine	
	– Segregation of the patients – Continuous training, programmes – Regular teaching (day and night!)	

V AUDIT

Both staff and patients know that intensive care is both extensive care and expensive care. The justification – the raison d'être – of intensive care must be subjected to audit, defined as 'the systematic regular review of medical work by doctors themselves' (Jennett, 1986). How intensive care is to be reviewed is next briefly described. The newcomer will already be familiar with some medical audit. In hospital **A** a cholecystectomy costs three times as much as in hospital **B**. But intensive care is not so straight- forward. As one of the writers said on his daily rounds 'I know that you are doing a fine job, the only problem is proving it'. The audit problem can be broken down into two parts.

Table 1.6 Educational feedback from intensive care
(From *Essential Intensive Care*, with permission)

Coma and impaired consciousness

Cardiac arrest

Respiratory arrest

Major injury

Shock

Starvation

Acute asthma

Thromboembolism

Renal failure

Acute inflammatory bowel disease

---

1. The patient

A miraculous recovery in your unit impresses the local media, but how severe was severe? What is needed is an international scale of severity, as there is for body temperature. Some progress has been made in grading disease or failure of a body system. These will be detailed in this book, but examples are given at this early stage. The severity of trauma or asthma can be graded by widely used methods. The beginner will be familiar with an internationally used scale for impaired consciousness – The Glasgow Coma Scale. In intensive care we can now compare groups of patients with similar diseases. The system needs the physiological information which is invariably available and this is labelled the acute physiological assessment (APA). To this is added the severity of pre-existing disease, chronic bronchitis for example; this facet is called the chronic health evaluation (CHE). The total assessment becomes the APACHE score. The real strength of the APACHE system is that it has been tested on thousands of patients and not only grades the severity but can be used to predict risk of death. Having gained some insight into the patient on admission, what about audit of the end result? Consider a patient who, during three weeks of intensive care, had the full works but died. The result is a sad one and the cost effectiveness is zero; the unit budget is significantly spent. The audit is: did admission fulfill agreed criteria; were mistakes made during intensive care; should therapy have been stopped after the first few days when predictors indicated a near-hopeless outcome? Patients who survive are also subject to audit. What

Table 1.7   Audit of hospital care: some definitions (After Jennett, 1986)

Label	Definition
Cost effective treatment	The cheapest means of achieving a specified beneficial end, e.g. dialysis versus transplantation
Cost-benefit analysis	Use of resources to relieve different conditions: the end-result, not the means.
Quality of life after intensive care	Physical and mental states financial position loss of earnings cost of dependency
Quality adjusted life years (QUALY)	A single measure to combine mortality and morbidity

is life like for the individual five years later? Recovery from a head injury cannot be 'remarkable' when you find that the patient is totally dependent upon others for daily living; the burdens may exceed the benefits. This kind of audit must continually influence the practice of intensive care.

2. The methods

Those for diagnosis and treatment are regularly subject to audit. The learner should not assume that the methods are necessary because they are impressive ('state of the art') or involve high-tech. Consider a few examples in the field of diagnosis and monitoring. To sort out the head- injured we often need computerized tomography (CT) of the brain; this is expensive. Audit will decide which patients need a CT scan and how often. Audit of the clinical chemistry of intensive care may reveal that the unit consumes a large portion of the entire hospital budget; the remedy is straightforward. Some investigations are invasive and can cause death or disability. These 'complications' must be reduced by a study of the indications and competence of the staff. Finally, therapy, the heart of the matter. In this field it is so easy to conclude that the team is 'doing good', but so difficult to prove that a particular treatment is effective and cost-effective. Reflect on routine treatments for acute self-poisoning. Gastric lavage and forced diuresis cost time and effort; both caused serious morbidity and neither could be shown to be effective. Moving into the high-tech arena. Blood was circulated outside the body and perfused over charcoal to remove poisons or toxins – very expensive and rarely effective. Antibiotics are necessary but their misuse causes harm and wastes money. Audit makes antibiotic policies mandatory. This makes treatment more effective, safer, more rational and saves money.*

This account is just a glimpse into a wide ranging but essential practice. Newcomers should study the matter further and themselves participate in audit.

---

* At the Whiston Hospital such policies were enforced from 1978 and saved £36,000 in the first 6 months

2
The five essentials

I   THE NURSING TEAM
II   THE MEDICAL TEAM
III   STANDARDIZED METHODS
IV   THE UNIT
V   PHILOSOPHY OF PATIENT CARE
       APPENDIX: PLANNING AND DESIGNING
       A GENERAL ICU

In 1966 we developed a formula for successful general intensive care. This was based on the first few years of personal experience and on discussions with surgeons and anaesthetists involved in specialized intensive therapy. The recipe for success consists of five components listed in Table 2.1 in order of importance, and these are now considered.

Table 2.1 Essentials of intensive care in order of their significance (From *Essential Intensive Care*, with permission)

1. Permanent nursing team, specifically trained and giving continuous service.

2. Readily available medical (service) team.

3. Standardized techniques of investigation and treatment.

4. An 'area', 'facility' or unit.

5. Revised philosophy of patient care.

I THE NURSING TEAM

This is the key to success, a fact recognized many years ago (Table 2.2). The first role of the unit is that the nurses are permanently allocated to the unit and are never seconded elsewhere, even when there are no intensive care patients. After training (Chapter 3) the nurses assume responsibility for most of the caring, most of the observations and the specialized therapy. The duties and responsibilities of the nurses are three-fold: firstly, intensive

Table 2.2 The first essential of intensive care, the nursing team: Quotations from the literature (From *Essential Intensive Care*, with permission)

'... the essentials for such a unit. The first unquestionably is provision of specifically trained nursing staff. These nurses must be confident and competent...' Bates, 1964

'... a nursing staff with an 'esprit de corps' working permanently in the unit is essential ...' A group of nurses should be trained specifically for working in an intensive care unit. Safar, 1965

'... A dictum of non-rotation of personnel has been followed. We consider this to be the most important feature of the programme... It has resulted in an almost unparalleled esprit de corps.' Beardsley, Bowen and Capalbo, 1956.

Table 2.3 Allocation of nurses according to the needs; figures are nurse-to-patient ratios used at Whiston Hospital

Class A	Mechanical ventilation, daily or continuous dialysis/filtration	Ratio 1.2 to 1.0
Class B	Infections, dysrythmias, impaired conciousness	Ratio 1.0 to 4.0

nursing care, which means a detailed and enlightened care of the whole patient, that is appropriate rest and movement, feeding, care of the skin, and hygiene of excreta; clinical observation of the mental state, circulation and so on, and specialized observations needed for a particular treatment, for example interpretation of the electrocardiogram, or readings taken on a ventilator; specialized therapy given to some of the patients, for example intravenous injections, defibrillation of the heart, ventilator treatment. The second and third responsibilities were not accepted by the nursing profession until some 30 years ago. It should be explained that these and other responsibilities, formerly rightly regarded as medical, are only accepted by those who have been specifically trained; the nurse then expects and appreciates increased responsibility and enhanced status. From this it is clear that the creation of intensive care nursing teams meant a big change in the philosophy of patient care especially that relating to responsibility. High standards can be maintained only by large nursing teams working in two or three shifts. Most members of the team are full-time and a minority are part-time. But how many? Rather than snatch a figure out of the air, we can use that proved at St. Bartholomew's hospital, where the ratio is 5.5

Table 2.4 A formula for staffing levels at the Royal Prince Alfred Hospital

1. For 1 to 1 nursing 26 h is required to allow for shift changes. For a week the figure then becomes 182 h.

2. The nurses work a 38 h week so that the number of nurses per week is 4.79.

3. Annual leave is 6 weeks and 1.9 weeks sick leave is allowed; this adds up to 0.73 extra full time equivalents.

4. The final ratio then becomes 5.52 full-timers for each bed nursed 1 to 1.

5. The nursing complement is altered according to the needs which vary as shown in Table 2.3

whole time equivalents per bed. This complement will provide 1 : 1 nursing. The workload of a patient on a particular day can be quantified by means of scoring systems. The simple systems used at Whiston and the Royal Prince Alfred hospitals are shown in Tables 2.3 and 2.4 The salaries of the nurses constitutes the largest part of the running costs. The team is maintained by replacing the leavers by nurses trained on the post-basic course. An intensive care unit is an additional department of a hospital and requires a nursing manager. The duties amount to 20 h work a week so that the administrative requirements of a unit can be shared with a second department. The responsibilities of the nursing manager are set out in Table 2.5. It is important that the nursing officer was, at some previous time, a member of the nursing team of an ICU and is therefore fully conversant with the knowledge, skills and attitudes. The nurse–patient relationship is almost exclusive to intensive care. The only earlier practice resembling the intensive care situation is the patients 'specialed' in a single room. Two general factors influence the relationship. Firstly, whether communication is possible or impossible and secondly the length of stay. Since the nurse has an adequate knowledge of the disease and its treatment, she is able to talk intelligently with assurance to the conscious patient. The patient (and the relatives) soon come to appreciate that the nursing team know their job and thus establish confidence. When the stay in the unit is short-lived (acute myocardial infarction, poisoning) the nurse–patient relationship is incompletely developed and the corresponding dehumanization leads to a feeling of production-line care. Patient–nurse communication was deliberately placed first because of its key role. The student has to learn new techniques of

Table 2.5 Responsibilities of the Nurse Manager (From *Essential Intensive Care*, with permission)

---

1.   Maintaining the nursing team; its numbers, quality, standards of work and morale.

2.   Planning the nursing duty rota.

3.   Planning, supervising and participating in the course in intensive care nursing.

4.   Maintaining a liaison with the teaching department, accident and emergency and operating theatres.

5.   Supervising the maintenance of equipment and supplies and the work of the unit technician and ward clerk.

6.   Maintaining unit records.

---

communication; how to communicate with the patient who is conscious, pain-free, and adequately sedated but receiving muscle relaxants. At some stage of the illness the patient is, usually also dependent on the nurse for intensive nursing care (heavy nursing) which can be defined as follows: 'the detailed and enlightened care of the whole patient; the appropriate rest and movement; the feeding, the care of the skin and hygiene of excreta' (Jones, 1967a). To this is added the specialized observations, and of course the intensive therapy! This patient–nurse relationship is both demanding and challenging. The nurse soon comes to appreciate that nursing care alone will not guarantee recovery and that she must advance her knowledge and accept greater responsibilities (Jones, 1976b). Provided that the following conditions are satisfied, then intensive care nursing is rewarding and intellectually satisfying: logical patient selection; a work-load to match the staffing; a medical team as good as the nursing team! A few points on the nurse–doctor relationship requires emphasis. Of the many factors which much influence the nurse–doctor relationship, three stand out. Firstly the professional competence of the medical service team; secondly the doctors' attitudes to nursing and particularly to the role of the nurse in intensive care; lastly the system of communication. The first two problems will be dealt with when the training of the service doctor is described. The efficient working of the therapeutic team depends on free communication. The factors influencing this communication were studied in 1966 with the help of

R.R. Hetherington. It goes without saying that there is an efficient telephone service and system of 'bleeps'. The first communication system is to organize the medical instructions relating to the patient. Unless this is organized, the nurses will be bombarded with confusing and conflicting instructions from various doctors who 'pop in' to see the patient. Such chopping and changing of treatment is disastrous for the patient and demoralizes the nursing team. The problem is resolved by designing a rigid policy which is included in the *Rules and Regulations*. Excluding unexpected changes, the treatment is planned at the regular daily rounds and nothing is altered without discussion with the unit's service doctor, who is immediately available at all times. This plan of communication is greatly facilitated by the use of standardized methods, the fourth essential of intensive care. The important barriers to communication are not electronic however, but are decidedly physiological and they are two in number. The status (or hierarchical) barrier operates in one or both groups of the team and between each group. 'In a team all should be equal' wrote Lord Cohen in 1946. This obstruction to free communication can endanger the care of the patient and impede learning by the nurse. To take an example: a nurse observes a change or some sign in her patient; unless she reports this sign to the service doctor or directly to a consultant then harm could come to that patient; a communication barrier can easily stop her reporting the observation. The appropriate doctor–nurse relationship is such that the doctor welcomes the information even when received at unsocial hours. The second barrier is one of language. A newcomer to intensive care is at first bewildered by the names of the measurements or treatment; the terminology (and the jargon) can impede communication. To facilitate this aspect of nurse–doctor communication, the medical staff should design teaching methods and visual aids to make things simple. This book was written with this principle in mind.

II THE MEDICAL TEAM

Before summarizing the essentials, it should be made clear that the formula refers only to general intensive care and not to the specialized (tertiary) class, for example organ transplant or neonatal.

The patients in a general ICU are investigated and treated, and when appropriate not treated, by two groups of doctors, who must clearly collaborate closely. These are the staff specialist and their junior staff who both refer patients and decide some of the treatments, e.g. accident surgeon, general surgeon, obstetrician, physician. If these specialists are to use the ICU. they must appreciate which of their patients are likely to benefit from intensive care and at what stage of a disease will the best results be obtained – intensive care too late often fails.

Junior medical staff are expected to visit their patients referred to the unit and learn some of the principles of intensive care. When a patient is transferred back to the referring 'firm' then the ward doctor is briefed on the further management. On the other hand, when a patient dies in the unit the referring staff specialist is informed by telephone of this event and of the natural history of the terminal illness. An additional class of doctor is concerned with the care of the patient during his stay in the unit; this is the group or team running the service. In Australia the majority of staff specialists* are full time – the intensivists. In the UK the majority are part-time and their other duties are in anaesthesia or internal medicine. During the evolution of intensive care the function of the service doctor was neither defined nor understood; put in other terms, there was no job description. The confusion was made worse because hospital staff confused general intensive care with the specialized variety, and because, believe it or not, nobody sat down to consider which diseases should be treated. These problems are now easily resolved. Current practice, based on experience or trials, has shown which medical and surgical emergencies need intensive care to get the best results (Chapter 3). From this information it is then possible to formulate a job description of the service doctor, and a training scheme.

The patients will then have the right doctor at the right time in the right place. One set of facts will be obvious. The staff specialist and junior service doctors will possess more knowledge of the natural history of the diseases than the remaining members of the junior hospital staff; they will have greater skills (a skill can be defined as a practical ability, facility in doing something) in performing some investigations or treatments – excluding surgical operations. Lastly, they will posses the right attitudes to emergency care. (a) Essential knowledge. This has been summarized in Table 2.6. The service doctor will have detailed knowledge and long experience of the emergencies of internal medicine; the natural histories of these diseases can only be mastered and taught by continuing experience. This old-fashioned truth was aptly stated in 1967. 'It is ridiculous to suppose that intensive therapy of all acute medical and surgical emergencies can be learned in isolation from the relevant branches of medicine' (British Medical Association, 1967). The knowledge extends well beyond the boundaries of internal medicine, and includes the care of the injured, head injuries, chest injuries

---

*   Staff specialist. This label is used to embrace the UK one of consultant, a
name now outmoded.

Table 2.6 Essential knowledge for the doctor in general intensive care
(From *Essential Intensive Care*, with permission)

• Natural history; all emergencies of internal medicine, multiple injuries, some surgical emergencies, occupational toxicology of the area.

• How and when the intensive care can modify the natural history of disease, e.g. diabetic keto-acidosis, head injury, asthma.

• How at times, treatment in the form of resuscitation, must precede diagnosis.

• When not to advise intensive care – life threatening acute illness in the chronically disabled or infirm.

• Programmed investigation, e.g. head injury, uraemic emergency.

• Learning processes and modern methods of teaching and assessment.

• The feed-back from intensive care to wards, casualty and outpatient.

• Organization and administration of hospital departments.

---

or closed injuries to the abdomen for example. The intensive care doctor must know the indications for operative intervention in such cases. Much of the therapy is based on restoring or preserving the composition of the body fluids – the internal medium – until the pathological process has resolved. The same doctors will need to understand the basis of fluid therapy, nutrition, oxygen therapy and so on. Many, but not all patients in a general ICU require prolonged intermittent positive pressure ventilation (IPPV). It follows that all the staff specialists will have learnt the basics of anaesthesia and then learnt the methods of IPPV relevant to general intensive care.

From his knowledge of the natural history, the service doctor will advise when or not to employ intensive care. This entails an enquiry into the patient's disabilities, his attitudes to these, the support of his family and the predicted quality of life, should the patient survive. In intensive care, enthusiasm should be tempered by wisdom. Knowledge on programmed investigation is essential for general intensive care. This is because time for a diagnosis is often short, and omissions are readily made. The staff specialist responsible for the service requires an elementary knowledge of current concepts of learning, and of modern methods of teaching and of the assessment of the course. The therapeutic team must know how

Table 2.7 Particular skills required by a service doctor in general intensive care (From *Essential Intensive Care*, with permission)

(A)	INVESTIGATORY	Percutaneous cannulation of blood vessels.
		Needle biopsy
		Endoscopy
(B)	THERAPEUTIC	Resuscitation
		Ventilatory support
		Endocardial pacing
		Dialysis
		Nutrition
		Clinical pharmacology
(C)	COMMUNICATION	Basic skills
		Counselling techniques including
		those related to the dying and the bereaved

intensive care can benefit patients who never enter the unit; this is by a process labelled educational feedback. Asthma and diabetes are classical examples of this principle. Education of the patient, early admission to hospital and the correct therapy will entirely avoid the need to resuscitate the patient. (b) Essential skills. ThOse required by the medical team are, with two exceptions, of a low order and basic to hospital practice (Table 2.7) After all, nine-tenths of the skilled observation and therapy is carried out by the nursing team!

For investigation the junior staff can readily learn the percutaneous method of cannulating blood vessels, and needle biopsy. Resuscitation is taught to all hospital staff and selected ambulance personnel. We are left with the skills necessary for prolonged ventilator treatment and for dialysis. As already stated the staff specialists to the unit will possess both knowledge and skills relevant to these treatments and he can teach the junior members of the medical team. Learning these skills is greatly facilitated by the use of standardized methods and programmes of IPPV or dialysis, tailored to the particular disease. From this account the job description of a staff specialist can be drawn up. How did the doctor acquire the necessary knowledge, skills and appropriate attitudes? During the years 1960–80 many of the staff specialists were ill-prepared for the job 'learn as you go'. By 1980 two national schemes were running in Australia. British doctors got around to considering formal training some 17 years after the UK nurses! There is now a choice between appointing full-time or part-time (but readily available) staff specialists. The number of such doctors needed to provide a well-organized rota will depend on the number of admissions and the man-hours for each patient; we do not yet have a formula as applied in nursing. This section closes with a short comment on administration. We can leave out the administrative aspects of the domestic services, pharmacy, laundry and lots more to concentrate on the two facets of the medical administration. In contrast to the clearly defined position in nursing, medical administration is a shambles! Let us start with the easy aspect of medical administration. This is a medical contribution to the general running of the unit – medical staffing, teaching, and equipment. The difficult administration is clinical and, alas, in many units is untouched upon, with disastrous consequences. The staff specialist in intensive care must exercise considerable power over the hospital divisions which have patients who can benefit from intensive care. We are back to the fundamental of 'the right patient in the right place at the right time'. Let us assume that the initial assessment of the potential customers are made by a SHO or registrar in medicine, A & E, surgery, orthopaedics, or obstetrics. The criteria for intensive care (Chapter 4) may be published and taught but young doctors may not want to follow the rules amd may prefer to go it alone, or resent the interference from intensive care. It follows that the staff specialist in intensive care must wield power to get the right patient transferred at the right time. This applies both to the patient who should survive and to the potential organ donor. The worst administrative practice of intensive care exists when the staff specialists have not been trained to do the job or have personality problems which wreck the system.

III STANDARDIZED METHODS

At some time or another it should occur to all hospital doctors that if the day-to-day investigations or treatments are to succeed then they must be standardized; such standardization avoids omissions and the errors and omissions which occur because staff change and communication fails. In the pursuit of standardized methods the authors found encouragement in the literature (Table 2.8) – the newer aids to problem solving, the logical tree and the algorithm. Later in this book there are accounts of standardized methods, and at this stage a few general remarks are necessary. There are three principle reasons for adopting standardized procedures; to prevent omissions when time is short because the chips are down; to preserve continuity of care when nurses change shifts and to obtain results from methods which take the form of an uncontrolled trial. From 1960 we applied this principle to wards and intensive care and more recently added the newer aids to problem solving, the flow diagram (logical tree) and algorithm. Standardized methods are based on current world practice and are enforced by consensus management. They seem logical and make life easier, but are they effective? Rigorous and critical review (monitoring) of these variables

Table 2.8 The third essential of intensive care, standardized methods; quotations from the literature (From *Essential Intensive Care*, with permission)

'It was found advisable to establish simple and precise routines for the nursing staff and house staff concerning procedures in general unconscious patient care, continuous intravenous administration of potent drugs, asepsis, emergency cardiopulmonary resuscitation, tracheostomy care and prolonged hypothermia'. (Safar, 1965)

'...techniques of treating seriously ill patients can be standardized'. (Crockett and Barr 1965)

is just as necessary as is the costing of diagnosis or treatment. The auditing of intensive care was outlined in Chapter 1.

IV THE UNIT

To state the obvious: an ICU is an area within which patients receive intensive therapy; it never closes. A little thought on the requirements of a specialized, regional, divisional, referral unit will inevitably lead to the conclusion that it is not possible to generalize on the design of such a unit, because of the varied types of therapy carried out in these units. Thus, a unit for organ transplant will be unsuited to the thoracic surgical patient. Another fundamental principle is that the design of the unit and the amount of equipment are of little importance in comparison with the quality of members of staff. It is unfortunate that when a hospital sets up a new unit, far too much time and money is devoted to the design and equipment and so little to its staffing. As usual in medicine, much can be learnt from history; in this instance recent history. Two of the best respiratory units in Europe, those at the Churchill Hospital in Oxford and the Blegdam Hospital in Copenhagen were established in a 'brick-built' bungalow and in an old infectious diseases ward respectively! The world-famous regional poisoning centre in Edinburgh was established in 1930 and still occupies the same building! The important features of the design of a general ICU can be laid down, because there is now adequate knowledge based on experiment and experience. The essentials are given in the Appendix to this chapter).

V PHILOSOPHY OF PATIENT CARE

This, the last component of general intensive care, is by no means the least important. The philosophy of patient care in the unit is an important factor in determining the results for the patient and the job satisfaction and happiness of the therapeutic team. Inappropriate attitudes are a frequent cause of stress and even conflict in the intensive care unit. The newcomer to intensive care should appreciate that the philosophy of patient care differs considerably between this unit and a ward or operating theatre. The correct attitudes will now be highlighted as they relate to the patient, the doctor and the nurse.

The staff specialist's obligations to the patient require many more hours of doctoring than in the wards and, except when the patient is unconscious, a much closer relationship. A similar relationship is developed between the doctor and the patient's relatives. The patient is less likely to be dehumanized by the doctor than in other parts of the hospital. Each doctor working in the unit must also possess the appropriate attitudes to the care of the dying, noticeably absent or inadequate in ward practice.

Medical attitudes to the diseases treated in a general intensive care unit are of two contrasting patterns. Consider the appropriate attitudes to asthma, acute poisoning or diabetic acidosis. Should the doctor regard these diseases as 'well recognized causes of death' then the highest standards of care will never be attained. For some diseases an attitude of survival at all costs is appropriate. But for other diseases this attitude is totally incorrect. When a patient with chronic lung disease is severely disabled by dyspnoea and is then admitted to hospital with acute respiratory failure then the doctor should not advise or offer treatment by means of artificial ventilation, since this is equivalent to prolonging death rather than the slender chance of saving life. We are reminded of Lord Cohen's comment 'the feasibility of an operation is not the best indication for its performance'. Should a patient undergoing intensive care develop new signs which indicate irreversible organ failure, then the doctor should accept this situation rather than continue a battle that cannot be won; failure to do so causes unnecessary suffering and distress both to the patient and his relatives.

Correct attitudes should exist between the various members of the medical team, which includes doctors of different specialities. A closed-shop attitude will invariably lead to friction. Each doctor working in that unit must appreciate that it does not matter who does what but that the task is well done at the right time. There is no place in intensive care for the doctor who resents the achievements of his colleagues, either junior or senior.

The doctor–nurse relationship requires attitudes which are quite different from those in most wards. We all recognize the key role of a ward sister; the ICU is a ward with 20 sisters! The newcomer must acknowledge that the nurse is indispensable; the chief observer and the chief therapist. Because the nurse takes on greatly increased responsibilities the doctor should recognize her increased status. A consequence is that the status barriers, so noticeable in hospitals, must not exist in the ICU.

APPENDIX

Planning and designing a general intensive care unit

The following recommendations are based on the experiences described at a seminar organized and published from the WHO regional office for Europe (1971):

(a) A procedure for setting up a general ICU. A working party is formed to make recommendations to the medical and nursing staff and to the hospital managers. The working party is composed of the following; a hospital manager; representatives of internal medicine, surgery (including accident surgery) and anaesthesia; nursing administrator and, when possible, the nurse who will have charge of the unit; an architect and possibly an engineer. Members of this working party carry out a survey of the acute hospital beds in order to list the diseases which may be treated in the proposed unit; for example, multiple injuries and acute poisoning. At the same time the working party studies the literature on the design of an ICU and the organization, administration and results of general intensive care. Visits are made to established units.

(b) Design of a general unit. Extensive experience suggests that a general unit of 6–8 beds is the optimum size. If a unit of this size is too small, a second unit of similar size is probably better than a single unit of 16 beds. This practice resembles the establishment of ICU within the specialist divisions of a large teaching hospital; for example, the RPA hospital has the following; general (which includes organ transplantation), coronary care and neurosurgical.

Hand basins are fitted, one for each single room and one for our open-plan beds. The following services are necessary (i) eight electrical socket-outlets per bed (ii) piped gases and suction. Compressed gas is essential if respirators are used which are driven by compressed gas. A clear distinction should be made between ventilation and air-conditioning. Natural ventilation by conventional windows and by the movement of air caused by central heating fulfils most of the requirements of a general ICU. Air-conditioning must be of a type specifically designed for bacterial filtration, in addition to controlling the temperature and humidity of the air; it then becomes very expensive. This type of air-conditioning reduces the bacterial content of the air and provides pleasant working conditions for the staff. Individual temperature control of a single room makes it an easy matter to cool or warm the body. Air-conditioning cannot prevent hospital infection caused by bacteria transmitted by the staff or equipment. The control of infection in an ICU depends largely on good techniques performed to a high standard. The lavatories and sluice have extractor fans fitted to the windows and springs fitted to the doors. A small laboratory is necessary, preferably adjoining the patient treatment area. In this laboratory the staff make emergency measurements on blood and urine. The unit workshop is fitted with a bench and hand tools for servicing equipment and emergency repairs. Sterilization of equipment or bedding can be carried out in the workshop or elsewhere.

The patient accommodation can be one of two types: (i) open-plan, with the bed centres at about 2.5 m or with the beds grouped around a nurse station. Each bed requires 18.5 m^2 of floor area (ii) individual rooms for each patient, each having a floor area of 20 m^2. Many units have a combination of single rooms and open beds, often in the ratio of one to three. The chief advantage of the single room over an open-plan bed is that noise and high intensity lighting do not interfere with the other patients. The single rooms are often used for patients with severe infection or in an attempt to exclude infection to which purpose the cumbersome label of 'reversed barrier-nursing' is applied. There is no evidence which would withstand scientific scrutiny to show that the single rooms reduce cross-infection. The chief disadvantage of single rooms is that more nurses per patient are required. When glass is used in the construction of the walls of single rooms, several patients can be observed from the nurses' station. The total floor area of an eight-bedded unit ICU should be 400 m^2, of which 200 m^2 is for patient treatment. The walls, floors and ceilings of a unit have a smooth finish for easy cleaning. The lighting intensity in the patient area should be 300 lux with a facility for dimming the lights; in the remaining area 150 lux is adequate. The unit laboratory needs lighting of 200 lux. Blinds are required to reduce sunlight. Fixed storage cupboards or mobile storage shelves are essential for rapid and easy supply, and to reduce traffic by the staff. In addition to the area for patient care, the following facilities are needed: (a) lavatories and washrooms (b) a room or rooms for relatives (c) staff changing rooms with lavatory, hand basin, shower and lockers (d) staff lounge (e) small kitchen (f) unit office (g) study-library (h) storage areas or rooms for clean equipment and disposables (i) workshop for the maintenance of equipment (j) room or area for the sterilization of machines, anaesthetic equipment etc. The total area of these facilities is roughly equal to that necessary for the patient care. A doctor's bedroom is included in some units, but other units disapprove of this idea, and prefer a doctor to be readily available.

3
Criteria for admission

There is abundant evidence that disproportionate amounts of
resources in many ICUs are expended on patients whose lives are not
saved. Bryan Jennett, 1986

...Clinical freedom is dead and should have been buried years ago.
John Hampton, 1983

I INTRODUCTION
II CRITERIA FOR ADMISSION

I INTRODUCTION

When properly organized, general intensive care is part of progressive
patient care. This fundamental can be stated alternatively: intensive care
must be fully integrated with other types of care: intermediate stay ward,
the A & E department, obstetrics, and with regional units for neurosurgery
and spinal injuries to list only two. Hearsay points to the disappointing fact
that this goal is rarely achieved. The central theme is to get the right patient
in the right bed at the right time. The alternative is the highly ineffective use
– rather misuse – of intensive care. What happens then is that the wrong
patient is admitted, or the right patient at the wrong time – too late. The
results are then very poor and the service cannot be justified (Table 3.1).
Too often the unit is used to rescue a patient who had suffered the
consequences of neglect; examples are hypovolaemic shock, malnutrition,
aspiration into the lungs. Another serious misuse of intensive care is to use
the unit as a substitute for proper standards in intermediate care wards or
to avoid the effort and expense of a recovery room service. Our joint
experiences in the UK and Australia add up to a hundred years – plenty of
time to organise admissions! Although the objective is common, the methods are very different and are therefore described separately. Neither system
is perfect in that patients who need intensive care are still hidden away in
various corners of our hospitals – you can't win 'em all.

II CRITERIA FOR ADMISSION

(a) Royal Prince Alfred and St. Bartholomew's hospitals. The indications
fall into two categories, based on the failure of one or more body
systems or the probability that this will occur. (i) Those by reason of

Table 3.1 Inappropriate intensive therapy (After Jennett, 1976)

1	UNNECESSARY: because the desired objective can be achieved by simpler means
2	UNSUCCESSFUL: because the patient has a condition too advanced to respond to treatment
3	UNSAFE: because the complications outweigh the probable benefit
4	UNKIND: because the quality of life after rescue is not good enough (or for long enough) to have justified the intervention
5	UNWISE: because it diverts resources from activities that would yield greater benefits

surgery, trauma or other acute disease require intensive monitoring and are very likely to need intensive therapy. (ii) Those patients with life-threatening but potentially curable diseases which need intensive therapy.

(b)   At Whiston Hospital the criteria given below were disseminated by repetitive teaching and were published in a booklet. This example of consensus practice might be seen as an infringement of clinical freedom; hence the quote from Professor Hampton at the start of the chapter.

1. Acute myocardial infarction

(a)   Patients presenting within 4 hours of the onset of pain.
(b)   Patients with significant ventricular dysrhythmia (frequent ectopic beats, ventricular tachycardia).
(c)   Patients with hypotension on admission (systolic blood pressure less than 100 mmHg).
(d)   Resuscitated cardiac arrest.
(e)   Patients with heart block.

2. Asthma

(a)   Patients presenting to hospital in Grade III or Grade IV asthma, using the Whiston method of grading.

(b)   Patients with less severe symptoms but in whom two of the following signs are found on examination:
  (i)   pulse rate 120/min
  (ii)   pulsus paradoxus
  (iii) hypotension
  (iv)   impaired mental state
  (v)   inappropriate sedation
  (vi)   exhaustion

3. Poisoning

(a)   Patients presenting with coma sufficiently deep to tolerate an endotracheal tube.
(b)   Patients presenting with impaired consciousness not deep enough to tolerate endotracheal intubation but where the predicted trend is downward.
(c)   All patients with hypotension (systolic blood pressure less than 90 mmHg.
(d)   Acute salicylate poisoning when the plasma level is 60 mg/100 ml or above, within 6 hours of ingestion.
(e)   Tricyclic antidepressant overdoses when a large dose has been swallowed, the heart rate exceeds 120 beats per minute, or the ECG shows a dysrhythmia or conduction defect.
(f)   All cases of poisoning with paraquat or diquat.
(g)   All cases with symptoms due to the inhalation of acid fumes or irritant gases, such as chlorine.
(h)   When the inhalation of vomit is either overt or suspected on circumstantial evidence – vomit on the clothing or in the mouth. Remember that an early radiograph can be normal.

4. Diabetes

(a)   Impaired consciousness unless this is due to hypoglycaemia and responds rapidly to intravenous dextrose.
(b)   Patients with two of the following signs:
  (i)   pH less than 7.2
  (ii)   blood sugar greater than 35 mmol/l
  (iii) hypotension (systolic BP less than 100 mmHg
  (iv)   suspected myocardial infarction
  (v)   suspected bacteraemia
  (vi)   impaired renal function

5. Gastrointestinal haemorrhage

(a)   Patients demonstrating three or more of the following features:
 (i)   age over 60 years
 (ii) past medical history of respiratory, cardiac or renal disease
 (iii) teetotal
 (iv) no drugs for one month prior to admission
 (v)   congestive cardiac failure on admission
 (vi) an ulcer found on endoscopy
(b)   Patients with profound hypotension complicating a massive haematemesis; arterial BP less than 90 mmHg
(c)   Recurrent bleeding in a previously stabilized patient

6. Inflammatory bowel disease

(a)   Severe exacerbations with systemic manifestations of fever (temperature above 38°C), raised ESR, hypoalbuminaemia (less than 30 g/l) and profuse bloody diarrhoea (more than 10 stools/day)
(b)   Pre-operatively, in debilitated patients requiring metabolic balance and intravenous nutrition
(c)   Patients with complications of their disease
 (i)   acute toxic dilatation
 (ii) perforation
 (iii) haemorrhage

7. Severe injury

Any of the following require expert assessment and probable admission to ICU:

(a)   Respiratory:
 (i)   chest pain
 (ii) dyspnoea
 (iii) altered breathing pattern
 (iv) external injury
 (v)   rib fractures
(b)   Circulation – hypotension systolic BP less than 100 mmHg
(c)   Head – decreased level of consciousness
(d)   Abdomen:
 (i)   pain and tenderness with rebound, absent bowel sounds or haematuria
 (ii) abdominal distension
(e)   Spinal injuries

8. Neurological

(a) All undiagnosed cases of coma not thought to be due to a cerebrovascular accident.

(b) All cases of spontaneous subarachnoid haemorrhage who may fulfil criteria for organ donation.

(c) Patients with progressive ascending polyneuritis (Guillain-Barré syndrome) where paralytic respiratory failure is likely (vital capacity less than 30% of the predicted; impaired deglutition. Blood gases are misleading and patients require mechanical ventilation before the gases become abnormal.

(d) Myasthenia gravis, where there is dyspnoea, dysphagia or laryngeal incompetence.

9. Renal failure (We use the definition of a raised blood urea or creatinine)

(a) All patients with symptomatic uraemia where the diagnosis is not yet established.

(b) Patients with acute exacerbations of previously diagnosed chronic renal failure where uraemia is normally controlled by conservative management or the patient can be treated by means of dialysis and transplantation.

(c) Acute renal failure. All cases should be considered as soon as the diagnosis is made.

10. Addison's disease

Patients with any of the following features:

(a) vomiting

(b) diarrhoea

(c) abdominal pain

(d) trauma, including minor injuries

(e) hypotension

(f) impaired consciousness

(g) syncope

(h) surgery

11. From the recovery room

(a) Patients with severe pre-existing disease (e.g. chronic lung disease)

(b) Inadequate spontaneous ventilation

(c) Serious dysrhythmia and cardiac arrest

(d)   Prolonged hypotension

12. Thyrotoxicosis

(a)   Delirium
(b)   Tachycardia greater than 140/min
(c)   Hyperpyrexia
(d)   Heart failure

13. Myxoedema

(a)   Hypothermia
(b)   Impaired consciousness
(c)   Cardiomyopathy (myxoedema heart) or pleural effusions

14. Obstetric indications

(a)   Excessive bleeding associated with hypotension
(b)   Coagulopathy
(c)   Resistant dysrhythmia
(d)   Acute heart failure
(e)   Convulsions due to toxaemia

15. Obstructive bronchitis and emphysema

(a)   Before and after elective surgery to abdomen or thorax
(b)   Where there is a reversible second pathology (e.g. pneumonia, diabetic ketosis)
(c)   Therapeutic errors: oxygen toxicity, sedation

SECTION TWO
SYSTEM FAILURES

4
Disorders of the body fluids

I   THE COMPARTMENTS
II   THE EXTRACELLULAR FLUID
III   INTAKE AND OUTPUT IN HEALTH
IV   ABNORMAL METABOLIC BALANCE
V   ASSESSMENT OF FLUID BALANCE AND NUTRITION

In a general hospital, most of the patients have disorders of the body fluids. In the intensive care patient the assessment of these disorders starts on admission and goes on round the clock. The newcomer must appreciate that restoring and then maintaining the body fluid is part of the very fabric of intensive care. The subject is therefore considered in this early chapter in which the information is broken down into five sections.

But the exchanges between the compartments show differences important to fluid therapy, and a little revision is essential. The gradients between the ICF and interstitial fluid is called active transport and is governed by cell metabolism; that between the interstitial fluid and the blood volume – the capillary membrane – is governed by osmotic force. This physiology is very pertinent to the applied physiology of i.v. fluid therapy and is, therefore, mentioned here. Intravenous water causes haemolysis, but isotonic glucose is the safe equivalent since the glucose is quickly metabolized. This i.v. fluid will be rapidly distributed across the capillary and cell barriers. An infusion of normal saline will remain in the vascular compartment for minutes or hours, thus expanding the blood volume, but a proportion will pass through the capillary membrane and expand the interstitial spaces. But this infusion will be repelled by the ICF. Lastly, i.v. albumin or gelatine will remain in the blood until the protein is catabolized. This essential knowledge will make i.v. fluid therapy logical and avoid spurious debate on the choice of infusion.

The ECF now needs to be singled out for attention because its preservation is vital in health and in our patients.

I THE COMPARTMENTS

To understand the disorders of the body fluids it is necessary to know a little about the intracellular and extracellular compartments and the functioning of the extracellular fluid.

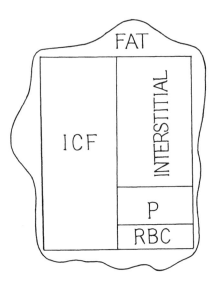

Figure 4.1 The body fluid compartments in health. The volume of each compartment approximates the area shown. ICF, intracellular fluid; P, plasma; RBC, red cell mass

About half the weight of a healthy adult consists of water. The intracellular fluid (ICF) consists of about 75% water and the extracellular fluid (ECF) is 90% water. The latter consist of the blood plasma and the interstitial fluid, which lies outside the circulation but in intimate contact with the cells.

Using isotopes it is possible to dissect the body into major compartments as shown in Figure 4.1. The blood volume occupies about 5 litres and the other compartments larger volumes; body fat is shown as a separate compartment which is very variable between individuals! A few more facts require to be recalled. It is essential to understand the relationships between volume and concentration. For example, the plasma volume is 3.0 litres and the concentration of sodium (Nap) is 140 mmol/l. Such a result for Nap does not tell one either the volume of the plasma nor the total sodium in the plasma. The concentration of potassium in the ICF is about twenty times that in the plasma (Kp) or interstitial fluid, but the Kp result on a patient will not give information on the concentration of potassium in the ICF. Turning next to protein, the ICF is rich in protein, the plasma contains much less (70 g/l) and the interstitial fluid contains negligible amounts. The last fact on this topic is to remember that there is a continuous exchange of ions between the three compartments; thus sodium moves in and out of the individual cell, but in health the rates of exchange ensure that the concentrations remain within close limits.

II THE EXTRACELLULAR FLUID

To understand the role of the ECF in health and disease it is helpful to learn a few facts about the evolution of the body fluids. The idea of viewing the ECF in this way was conceived by the French physiologist Claude Bernard in 1878. On the planet Earth, life began in the oceans and sea water has a striking similarity to interstitial fluid except that it is more concentrated. Life in the oceans was dependent on the constancy of the sea water; the concentrations of electrolytes, the osmolarity, temperature and so on. When organisms became terrestrial, their bodies had evolved to include the body fluid compartments. The ECF became the internal environment or *milieu intérieur* of Claude Bernard. Put crudely, the cells of the body were bathed in an internal sea. In man the *milieu intérieur* consists of the interstitial fluid and the blood plasma. These fluids possess properties – such as volume and temperature and are composed of electrolytes), not forgetting oxygen and carbon dioxide. Table 4.1 is an impressive list, but still incomplete. The newcomer to intensive care should apply the concept of the internal medium to all the patients as early as possible. A start can be made by analysing an emergency which is already familiar, likely diabetic keto-acidosis. In this condition the ECF is severe, deranged and the organs and cells of the body therefore cannot function properly; the ECF then becomes a hostile environment of the cell. The ECF becomes extremely acid from the acetoacetic acid; the concentrations of sugar and urea are raised exerting an increased osmotic force on the cells; the volume of the ECF Is greatly reduced. The coma or shock of diabetic acidosis should be analysed in terms of the disturbed ECF. An important general principle is that the more severe these and other changes, and the longer they persist, the greater the damage to cell function and the higher the morbidity and mortality.

III INTAKE AND OUTPUT IN HEALTH

1. Intake

In order to maintain a state of metabolic balance, an adult kept at rest needs the fluid and food shown in Table 4.2; for the sake of simplicity vitamins and trace elements are omitted. The majority of the patients treated in an ICU require more than these basic needs and the minority require less. The essential needs of our resting physiological man can be met by conventional hospital beverages and food. However, the slightest experience of hospital

Table 4.1 Properties and composition of the extra-cellular fluid. Units are mmol/l unless shown otherwise

	Properties
Volume (litres)	
plasma	3
interstitial	14
Temperature	37°C
Osmolarity	290
Hydrostatic pressure	
Viscosity	
It moves!	
	Composition

Oxygen, carbon dioxide, amino acids, trace elements, enzymes, hormones

Protein	
plasma	70 g/l
interstitial	14 g/l
Na	140
K	4
Ca	2.5
Mg	0.9,
Hydrion	40 nmol/l
Cl	103
HCO_3	23
PO_4	1.0
SO_4	0.5
Organic acids	6
Urea	6
Creatinine	80 μmol/l
Glucose	5

practice will have taught the reader that ill patients cannot cat enough hospital food to fulfil the basic needs and semi-starvation must result. Similarly, when disease prevents the proper digestion and absorption by the gastrointestinal tract, dehydration and starvation must follow. Our physiological man takes in, as beverages and food, about 2.5 litres of water and the electrolytes shown in Table 4.2. A conventional western diet provides carbohydrates, fat and protein in balanced proportions. For optimum nutrition 50% of the total energy should be obtained from carbohydrate, 40% from fat and 10% from protein. Again, for the optimum utilization of protein, the ratio, energy from carbohydrate divided by protein should be about 20. Quality of protein is important and the standard of reference for this is the hen's egg, which contains essential and non-essential amino acids in the 'ideal' proportions The casein of cow's milk is a good second best. This

Table 4.2 Dietary requirements of an adult per day
(From *Essential Intensive Care*, with permission)

Water	2.5 litres
Energy	2500 kcal (10.5 MJ)
Sodium	100 mmol
Potassium	80 mmol
Calcium	500 mg (125 mol)
Iron	10 mg (1.8 mol)

information is needed when preparing diets for the IC patients either in the form of conventional food, tube feeds or intravenous diets.

The intake of water and salt even in resting subjects varies greatly; according to habit and custom, as well as the physiological stimuli of thirst or hunger. However, the figures in Table 4.2 are useful hat-pegs for the practice of metabolic care.

2. Output of water, electrolyte and nitrogen

In health, each of these components enters the body pool, the nitrogen in the form of amino acids, and are excreted via the urine, skin and expired air. The approximate amounts lost in this way are shown in Table 4.3. From this information it is apparent that a rough but clinically useful balance can be obtained by analysis of the urine alone. When the weight of a healthy adult is steady over a week or more and the diet is a reasonably balanced one, then the urinary output will be approximately 0.8 litre less than the intake. The sodium and potassium in the urine will be about 11.0 and 18.0 mmol respectively, less than the intake in fluid or food. If the diet of our physiological subject contains 14.4 g of nitrogen (75 g protein) then the 24 h urine will contain 13.3 g of nitrogen, that is about 57 g of urea.

IV ABNORMAL METABOLIC BALANCE

1. Terminology and causes

A state of imbalance occurs when the intake and output (losses) do not match the metabolic state of the patient. In a general ICU deficits are more common than excesses, but in an individual patient both can exist at the same time; for example an excess of salt and water and a deficit of potassium. The nutritional needs of the IC patient are equal to or greater than those of the same subject when healthy but at rest. During acute illnesses, nutrition is described in terms of energy (calories or Joules) and

Table 4.3 Balance data on healthy adults fed on Complan-glucose (From *Essential Intensive Care*, with permission)

	Water (litres)	Sodium (mmol)	Potassium (mmol)	Nitrogen (g)
Intake per day	2.56	116	84	14.4
Output in urine	1.77	105	66	13.3
Balance	0.79	11	18	1.07

protein (or nitrogen), and the deficits of either or both (protein-calorie deprivation) are equivalent to the familiar terms of semi-starvation or malnutrition. A useful rule is that when there are deficits of fluid and electrolyte, there is semi-starvation.

The causes of imbalance are legion and can be grouped under symptoms or equated to failure of a particular organ. From Table 4.4 it is evident that in many intensive care patients the losses of fluid and electrolyte exceed those in health. For example fever, sweating or increased breathing can readily cause deficits. In a similar manner fever, surgery, injury, infection, shivering or increased work of breathing, all increase the energy requirements above the physiological. A proportion of the patients with one or more of these conditions develop a pathological acceleration of metabolism, referred to as the hypercatabolic state. In addition to varied pathological processes leading to metabolic imbalance, many of the treatments commonly used during intensive care affect metabolism. Fluid therapy and nutrition (Chapters 16, 17) have the obvious aims of both restoring and maintaining metabolic balance.

Other non-specific treatments such as dialysis or diuretics can help to restore balance. Some therapies are, unfortunately, double-edged, improving some facets of the metabolic balance and at the same time producing a new imbalance; examples are diuretics, artificial respiration or steroids. In addition to the natural history of each disease and its treatment, three non-specific factors can, alone or in combination, influence the consequences of a metabolic imbalance. These are the duration of the illness, the previous nutritional state of the patient and the rate of metabolism. An almost infinite number of permutations and combinations of imbalance are seen in disease, but there is only a handful of common patterns and these are now prescribed.

Table 4.4 Some causes of metabolic disturbances (From *Essential Intensive Care*, with permission)

Non-specific	Anorexia, nausea, dysphagia, apathy, confusion, coma, fever, sweating, increased breathing
Specific diseases or syndromes	Diabetes mellitus, diabetes insipidus Pyloric obstruction intestinal obstruction Paralytic ileus Ulcerative colitis, Crohn's colitis Malabsorption syndrome Extensive burns Multiple injuries
Organ or system failure	Cardiac failure Renal failure Hepatic failure
Treatments	Diuretics Steroids

2. Saline depletion (dehydration)

This means combined deficits of water and sodium. In adult hospital practice the deficits involve water and salt in the proportions normally found in the ECF, and the patient's plasma sodium therefore remains normal or nearly so. On occasions, there is a significant disproportion, resulting in severe hypo- or hypernatraemia. Dehydration can be caused by an inadequate intake due to nausea or coma; or increased losses due to vomiting, gastric suction, diarrhoea, burns, diabetes or renal failure. Total deficits of sodium can vary from 250–500 mmol (moderate) to 500–1000 mmol (severe) and these values correspond to water deficits of 2.0–7.0 l. The clinical manifestations depend both on the size of the deficit and the rate at which it was incurred. Irrespective of the route by which the fluid is lost, rapid adjustments take place between the extracellular and intracellular compartments (Figure 4.2). The volume of the interstitial fluid falls, so that the mucous membranes become dry and the skin and muscles show reduced elasticity. The blood volume falls and the haematocrit and viscosity increase. The deficiencies have important effects on the mental state and can result in apathy, depression, confusion or restlessness. The body responds to dehydration by increasing the peripheral vascular resistance so the veins are narrowed and the skin temperature falls in the legs and arms. In the surgical patient, thirst is the exception rather than the rule. In the absence of renal

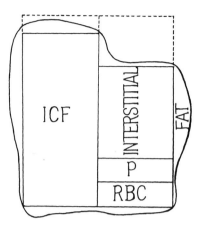

Figure 4.2 The body fluid compartments in saline depletion; compare with Figure 4.1. The broken lines represent the compartments in health

disease, there is oliguria and the urine shows a high specific gravity. Increased osmolality, low sodium concentration and high urea. As previously explained, the Nap is usually normal, or there is moderate hyponatraemia. The blood urea rises due to a fall in glomerular filtration rate although the kidney is capable of normal function. This state can either be termed pre-renal failure, or renal failure, depending on one's definition (Chapter 9). Very large deficits of salt and water result in shock. There is tachycardia, hypotension and cold extremities; the CVP and cardiac output are low. An ensuing metabolic acidosis further aggravates the circulatory collapse. At this stage unless treatment is prompt and adequate then acute renal failure and brain damage will surely follow. The external balance during saline depletion will be described later.

3. Saline excess

Saline excess (overhydration) is the converse state of saline depletion. This harmful disturbance of balance occurs when the intake of saline exceeds the output and the body is already in saline balance. Saline excess can occur either because the intake is inappropriate or the kidney Is unable to excrete the excess; the end result is a positive balance of sodium and water. The excess of saline is distributed throughout the ICF and ECF and it should be understood that the intravascular volume (the blood volume) may be normal or increased (Figure 4.3). It follows that in saline excess the central venous pressure and blood pressure can be normal. Saline excess must be carefully

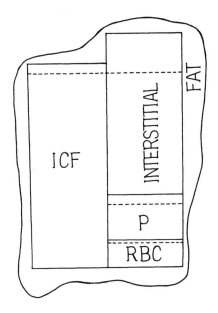

Figure 4.3 The body fluid compartments in saline excess with hypervolaemia; compare with Figure 4.1. The broken lines represent the compartments in health

distinguished from acute circulatory overload (over-transfusion), although the two can co-exist. In the former the blood volume is increased, the central venous pressure raised, and the blood pressure may be elevated. Saline excess will cause an increase in body weight and generalized oedema – the latter may be seen in the skin, subcutaneous tissue, conjunctivae or lungs, where it is especially dangerous. The pulmonary oedema starts in the interstitial tissue of the lung and can progress to become alveolar. Saline excess is an important – but largely avoidable – cause of acute respiratory failure in the intensive care patient. Early recognition depends on the external balance of sodium and water because the clinical signs and the changes in the chest radiograph are late. The diagnosis, and better still prevention, of saline excess depends on knowing when it is likely to occur. Which patients are at risk? Recognition requires an elementary knowledge of the responsible mechanisms. Saline excess can only occur when one of the following processes operates – (a) saline is given at a rate which exceeds the capacity of the normal kidney, (b) during acute or chronic renal failure, or (c) when the kidney is stimulated to retain saline by an excess of aldosterone or antidiuretic hormone. These are now briefly considered in turn. (a) The kidney has a huge capacity to excrete water (up to 1.0 l/h) but that for sodium is much less. Data on the capacity of the healthy subject to excrete intravenous saline are inadequate. For intensive care some generalizations are necessary. Firstly, saline excess is much more likely to occur when the sodium and water are given intravenously rather than intragastrically. Secondly, the maximum excretory capacity for saline is far less than for water alone, e.g. isotonic dextrose. (b) Renal disease can cause retention of sodium and water leading to saline excess. The disease may be acute or chronic and the lesion may be predominantly glomerular or tubular. In these patients the risk of saline excess developing is readily understood. (c) A more subtle pathological process which can cause saline excess is seen following severe injury or in the patient who has undergone major surgery or who has been resuscitated for shock. The kidney is normal but retains saline inappropriately. The mechanism is hormonal and part of the metabolic response to stress. The stimulus can persist for hours, days or even weeks, during which time there is a continuing risk of the patient developing saline excess. Since the stimulus to retain saline varies greatly from patient to patient the only safe management is by means of the balance technique. In addition to trauma. surgery and shock the inappropriate retention of saline may be caused directly by prolonged intermittent positive pressure ventilation.

4. Water intoxication

Water intoxication is a variation of saline excess in which an excess of water predominates over sodium. Clearly this can only occur when the kidney is unable to make the necessary adjustments or when an excess of hypotonic fluid is given by mouth or by vein. In most cases of water intoxication two or three factors operate simultaneously. The condition is often preventable. A source of water which can easily escape attention is that produced in the body from the catabolism of fat and muscle. A renal inability to excrete an average water load is seen in two conditions requiring intensive care. An excess of antidiuretic hormone occurs as part of the metabolic response to trauma and can also occur during prolonged ventilator treatment. A few cases of acute renal failure develop water intoxication because the kidney cannot excrete an excess of water given as beverages or hypotonic infusions. Rare causes of water intoxication are acute adrenal insufficiency or freshwater drowning. Water intoxication manifests itself as psychological or neurological disturbances which can readily escape attention, or be attributed to the primary illness. The possible symptoms are headache, confusion, restlessness, apathy, drowsiness, fits or coma. Other symptoms are nausea, vomiting and hypertension. The patient is normally hydrated or shows oedema. Hyponatraemia is invariable, with Nap values in the range 110–120 mmol/l.

5. Hyperosmolar syndromes

A severe increase in the osmolarity of ECF causes cellular damage and the brain is the most sensitive organ. The substances in the ECF responsible are glucose and sodium (Table 4.5), but a rapid rise in the urea can also exert an osmotic force on the brain because of the lag in equilibration across the blood–brain barrier. Hence, hyperglycaemia, hypernatraemia and urae-mia, alone or in combination are found. Hyperglycaemia causing hyperos-molar brain damage can occur in diabetes mellitus or stress diabetes; hypernatraemia follows the misuse of saline or sodium bicarbonate usually in the 'surgical' patient with intestinal obstruction. paralytic ileus or acute pancreatitis and more rarely following head injury. The remaining patho-logical process, i.e. uraemia can be pre-renal due to saline depletion or due to intrinsic renal disease. The symptoms of the hyperosmolar syndrome are neurological – drowsiness. apathy, confusion, fits and coma. Prevention is of the utmost importance and this depends on routine measurement of the blood sugar, urea and Nap on all acutely ill patients; on the correct use of intravenous saline and alkali and on the early recognition of uncontrolled diabetes mellitus.

6. Starvation

Starvation produces its own pattern of metabolic imbalance although this is modified by age, sex, the previous nutritional state, physical activity, the environment of the subject and the duration of the starvation. An elementary knowledge of the natural history of starvation is necessary because it frequently complicates serious illnesses or injury. The effects of starvation can be illustrated by referring to a 50-year-old man weighing 70 kg, kept largely at rest and given fluid and electrolyte but no nutrient. Hunger is soon felt and there is progressive loss of weight, with wasting of both fat and muscle. Striking psychological changes follow starvation: low morale, apa-thy and depression and the loss of willpower. Physical weakness is a late sign. The metabolic events are due to the continuing expenditure of energy which must be met by a relentless consumption of the body's energy stores. The carbohydrate stores provide only 1500 kcal (6.3 MJ) – barely enough for the first day! If our subject has about 7000 g of body fat, about 90% of this can be used as fuel. He will use 150 g per day and the fat store will be thus exhausted in 40 days. When more than 25% of the body protein has been

Table 4.5 Causes of hyperosmolarity of the ECF (From *Essential Intensive Care*, with permission)

Hyperglycaemia	Diabetes mellitus Stress diabetes Strong dextrose infusions without insulin*
Hypernatraemia	1. Disproportionate loss of water in sweat; urine – K depletion diuretics 2. Infusion of hyperosmolar solutions, saline† or sodium bicarbonate
Uraemia (raised blood urea)	Renal failure

*In health huge quantities of dextrose can be infused without causing hyperglycaemia
†Normal saline is somewhat hyperosmolar (300 mmol/l), plasma 280–295 mmol/l)

metabolized, then death follows. Our subject will use up 60 g per day and he will therefore die after 40 days of starvation. The catabolism of body protein is shown as a negative nitrogen balance throughout the illness. By the 20th day, the urinary nitrogen has fallen from the basal value of 18 g to 8 g and a slow fall continues. Trauma, surgery or infection produce a metabolic imbalance known as 'the metabolic response to injury'. It might be emphasized that this is quite different from starvation of the healthy subject. Some of the changes are illustrated in Section V (p. 52) and more information is given in Chapter 12.

7. Potassium depletion and hyperkalaemia

Potassium depletion is a common imbalance with many life-threatening consequences. It is often missed, and is largely preventable. Potassium depletion arises when the intake is deficient and/or the losses are excessive. In comparison to sodium, the renal conservation of potassium is much less efficient, and a daily intake of less than 50 mmol leads to depletion even in the absence of an increased loss. The patient with a moderate potassium deficit is short of about 500 mmol and a severe deficit amounts to 1000 mmol. Potassium is lost in excess either from the gastrointestinal tract or in the urine. Gastric suction for intestinal obstruction or ileus, diarrhoea, a recent ileostomy, or intestinal fistula soon lead to moderate or severe deficits. Large amounts of potassium are lost in the urine in diabetic acidosis; during a diuresis, whether caused by an osmotic load (glucose, urea or mannitol) or a diuretic drug; during starvation or hypercatabolism. A few patients with chronic pyelonephritis waste potassium inappropriately and develop severe depletion despite a normal intake. Table 4.6 shows that potassium depletion can affect the functioning of most systems of the body. In some conditions potassium depletion is self-perpetuating. For example, paralytic ileus leads to potassium depletion which can itself cause ileus.

The concentration of potassium in the ECF bears no relationship to the total body potassium. Moderate potassium depletion can exist, yet the Kp is normal or even high, as in diabetic acidosis. Hypokalaemia invariably means potassium depletion but gives no guide to the size of the deficit. The development of potassium depletion is readily seen from an external balance. An example will be described in a later section.

Hyperkalaemia occurs when the kidney is unable to excrete potassium in a normal manner although the total body potassium is normal. The renal failure can be either acute or chronic. An excess of potassium will enter the ECF when the cells are losing potassium at a pathological rate. This occurs in acidosis, both metabolic and respiratory, during starvation and in the hypercatabolic state. The abnormal egress of potassium is reduced by glucose and insulin and when alkali is given to correct a metabolic acidosis. Unlike potassium depletion, the effects of hyperkalaemia are limited to the heart and skeletal muscle. Cardiac arrest occurs when the Kp rises above 7.0 mmol/l. The likelihood is increased by hypoxia or acidosis. A clearly defined sequence of ECG changes precedes the arrest; these include tall and peaked T waves, then widening of the QRS complex.

Table 4.6 Effects of potassium depletion (From *Essential Intensive Care*, with permission)

1. Respiratory	Weakness of the respiratory muscles; apnoea
2. Cardiovascular	hypotension; dysrhythmia; ECG – ST depression, negative T wave, prolonged Q–T, prominent U wave
3. Gastrointestinal	Anorexia, thirst, reduced gastric acid secretion, abdominal distension, ileus, defective absorption of electrolytes
4. Neurological	Confusion, apathy, irritability, tetany, muscle weakness and paralysis
5. Renal	Inability to concentrate, uraemia, 'wasting' of acid and water
6. Metabolic	Hypokalaemia, metabolic alkalosis, defective glucose utilization, defective protein synthesis

8. Phosphate depletion

You will recall from elementary human biology that most of the body's phosphate lies in the cell, but that cell function is dependent on a constant amount of inorganic phosphate in extracellular fluid. In healthy subjects, the plasma inorganic phosphate is 0.7–1.4 mmol/l. Phosphate depletion was recognized many years ago in diabetic keto-acidosis and starvation, but only during the past 20 years have we recognized that many intensive care patients are likely to become depleted, and equally important, prevention is better than cure. The group of patients most at risk are those dependent on intravenous fluid therapy and nutrition. In such patients phosphate depletion and hypophosphataemia are likely to develop in a few days. The depleted patient can show confusion and disorientation. Since there are so many causes of this mental state in the intensive care patient, then daily measurements of plasma inorganic phosphate are the rule; a result of less than 0.4 mmol/l indicates severe depletion. Depletion also impairs two other body functions, namely, the delivery of oxygen and the immune system.

9. Zinc deficiency

Zinc deficiency was recently added to the list of deficiencies likely to occur in the intensive care patient. This deficiency is most likely to be seen in the patient with inflammatory bowel disease. The clinical signs are two in number: eczema of the face and hands which is photosensitive, and diarrhoea. To the clinical signs must be added two physiological effects: deficient protein synthesis, for example, hypoalbuminaemia, and immune incompetence. In day to day intensive care the diagnosis is confirmed by giving zinc salts, when the manifestations are reversed.

V ASSESSMENT OF FLUID BALANCE AND NUTRITION

1. History

The history may or may not be relevant to the assessment. Following recent trauma or acute myocardial infarction and in acute poisoning,it can be assumed that the metabolic balance was normal prior to the illness. This contrasts with a disturbed balance in the 'complicated' surgical patient, in diabetic acidosis or a case of renal failure, either acute or chronic. A history is then required to try and ascertain the deficits or excesses and the preceding nutrition. The intake of fluid and food, intravenous infusions (not forgetting drugs) during the illness is attempted. This information is obtained from the patient, his relatives or the ward staff. Although the results are crude when compared with the quality of the information obtained in the ICU, general conclusions can always be reached. For example, large deficits of saline due to gastric suction; inadequate intake of potassium; excessive intake of saline in a case of chronic glomerulonephritis are common findings. When a patient has been in hospital for some days, and especially when intravenous fluid therapy has been used, then the fluid balance charts are examined with the aim of determining the state of balance. Similarly the preceding intake of energy and nitrogen is assessed and the nutrition classified as starvation, semi-starvation or adequate – a rare event!

2. Symptoms and signs

Disturbances of metabolic balance may or may not lead to symptoms or signs, although in the intensive care patient symptoms and signs are usual. Some correlation between signs and metabolic balance are given in Table 4.7, but it should be emphasized that each and every symptom can be caused by an alternative pathological process. For instance, increased breathing could be due to metabolic imbalance – saline excess causing pulmonary oedema or the respiratory compensation of a metabolic acidosis; alternatively the increased breathing could be due to pulmonary oedema without saline excess – left ventricular failure for example. Likewise paralytic ileus could be caused by potassium depletion or peritonitis. Despite these limitations a metabolic imbalance should always be considered in the differential diagnosis of any of the following: muscle weakness, mental disturbance, ileus, abnormal pattern of breathing and shock. The search for clinical signs is straightforward. The interrogation to assess the mental state; testing for muscle weakness; auscultation of the abdomen, etc. The beginner should not minimize the difficulty of assessing the state of hydration of the skin or subcutaneous tissue. It is an easy matter to mistake oedema for dehydration; in both conditions the elasticity is decreased and pressure causes pitting. A shiny skin means oedema. This distinction is facilitated by attempting to lift a fold of skin, a test which should be carried out at several sites on the body. In saline depletion a fold of skin can readily be lifted up and the normal elastic recoil is lost; in saline excess it is difficult or impossible for the fingers to raise a fold of skin.

3. Blood analysis

(i) Before describing the measurements on the blood necessary for the recognition and treatment of metabolic disturbances, it is essential to recall

Table 4.7 Signs of a disturbed metabolic balance (From *Essential Intensive Care*, with permission)

Delirium	Saline depletion
	Potassium depletion
	Hypo- or hypercalcaemia
	Hyperosmolarity
	Water intoxication
Weakness of voice	Saline depletion
Tetany	Hypocalcaemia, alkalosis
Increased breathing	Saline excess
	Metabolic acidosis
Dry tongue; inelastic skin and muscles	Saline depletion
Oedema of skin and subcutaneous tissues	Saline excess
Muscle weakness	Potassium depletion
Muscle wasting	Starvation
Hypotension	Saline depletion, potassium depletion
Cold pale skin of hands and feet	Saline depletion, metabolic acidosis
Hypertension	Saline excess
Paralytic ileus	Potassium depletion

their limitations. Biochemical analysis of the blood can only tell us the concentrations of various components of the extracellular fluid. The volume of ECF, interstitial fluid and ICF cannot be deduced from analysis of the plasma; this was explained on page 45 in relation to saline depletion (dehydration). Despite this irrefutable fact, many hospital doctors still try to recognize and treat fluid imbalance by means of the plasma electrolytes. If changes in the plasma sodium (Nap) or potassium (Kp) cannot be used to diagnose or treat an excess or deficiency of these ions, why measure them? The answer is both important and straightforward. A significant change in the concentration of one or more components of the ECF can itself disturb cell metabolism and organ function. The same events occur when there is a precipitous drop in arterial oxygen or pH, or an extreme rise in temperature. Restated in the words of the pioneer Claude Bernard (1878) the constancy of the internal medium (ECF) is essential for life. The second principle is that the more rapidly a pathological process causes a change, the less time the body systems have for adaptation (compensation). It is with these principles in mind that the 'urea and elecs' should be measured throughout hospital practice. An abnormality may be the reason for referring a patient to the ICU. During intensive care blood analysis is made according to the priority list of treatment and is also varied according to the specific disease. Thus one or two blood analyses will suffice for coronary care, asthma and acute sedative poisoning. In contrast multiple injuries, renal failure and prolonged ventilator treatment will require measurements each day or on alternate days.

In such cases it makes for efficiency to organize the procedure. It is our practice to plan the biochemical, haematological and bacteriological investigations on each patient following the first unit round of the day (09.00 hours). An appropriate blood sample is then taken. The results are later entered in a table. Broadly speaking the tests on blood fall into two classes. The primary analyses (Table 4.8) are necessary on all acutely ill patients whether their illness is medical, surgical, obstetric or traumatic. During intensive care they may be repeated daily or in some diseases at intervals of a few hours. A more selective approach is used for the secondary tests shown in Table 4.8. Interpretation of the primary blood tests is considered next. As with all laboratory investigations the interpretation requires information on the history, signs and previous treatment.

(ii) Blood urea. The normal range is 3.5–8 mmol/l (20–50 mg/100 ml). The plasma urea is a balance between the production and excretion of urea (cf. $PaCO_2$). More urea is produced in the body during fever and as part of the metabolic response to injury but such an increase does not of itself cause a rise in blood urea; the increased excretion is part of a negative nitrogen balance. It follows that a raised blood urea means renal failure which can be due to saline depletion (dehydration), potassium depletion or obstruction nephropathy and there are hundreds more causes. The urinary volume can be normal, reduced or increased. In acute renal failure the rate at which the blood urea rises depends on the severity of the failure and also on the rate of urea production. Consequently, when injury of sepsis causes a state of hypercatabolism, the blood urea rises by daily increments of 8–16 mmol/l (50–100 mg/100 ml).

(iii) Plasma sodium. The normal range is 135–146 mmol/l. A decrease or increase in the Nap can be graded as moderate or severe (Table 4.9). It is our experience that during a critical illness the kidneys manage to adjust Nap to within the limits of moderate hypo- or hyper-natraemia and that severe disturbances are the fruits of error or omission! When interpreting

Table 4.8 Biochemical tests on blood and urine (From *Essential Intensive Care*, with permission)

	Primary	*Secondary*
Plasma/serum	Urea	Osmolarity
	Sodium	Albumin
	Potassium	Creatinine
	Sugar	Calcium
		Magnesium
		Phosphate
Urine	Protein reagent strip	Protein
	Sugar reagent strip	Sugar
	Blood reagent strip	Osmolarity
	Specific gravity	Sodium
		Potassium
		Urea
		(or total nitrogen)
		Creatinine

hypo- or hypernatraemia the following questions should be asked: is there renal failure? Has the fluid therapy been inappropriate – hyperosmolar or hypo-osmolar solutions? It is important to again stress that the Nap cannot be used to diagnose deficiency or excess of sodium, that is the state of balance. The Nap can be used to guide the type of fluid to be used in the treatment of dehydration but cannot help to determine the total amounts of sodium and water required. Severe hypo- or hyper-natraemia require immediate therapy to restore the Nap to near normal. Moderate changes in Nap call for a revision of the fluid therapy in order to prevent the occurrence of more severe changes.

(iv) Plasma potassium (Kp). Normally lies between 3.5 and 5.2 mmol/l and it is useful to grade changes as moderate or severe (Table 4.9). In the interpretation of hypo- and hyperkalaemia we are on easier and surer ground than for sodium. The rules of the game are: hypokalaemia = potassium depletion; potassium depletion can exist with a normal Kp; hyperkalaemia = failure to excrete due to renal failure. During hyperkalaemia the body potassium is usually normal with a notable exception of diabetic keto-acidosis. when there is potassium depletion. In this disorder the cellular potassium is rapidly lost to the ECF and the kidney cannot excrete potassium quickly enough, so that the Kp rises.

Table 4.9 Some abnormalities of blood chemistry (From *Essential Intensive Care*, with permission)

	Normal* (plasma)	Disturbance	Moderate	Severe
Urea	3.5–8.0 mmol/l	Uraemia	8.0–30.0	30–100
Sugar	3.0–7.0 mmol/l	Hyperglycaemia	10–16	16–50
		Hypoglycaemia	1.7–2.8	0.85–1.7
Sodium	135–146 mmol/l	Hypernatraemia	150–160	160–170
		Hyponatraemia	120–130	110–120
Potassium	3.5–5.2 mmol/l	Hyperkalaemia	5.5–6.5	>7.0
		Hypokalaemia	2.5–3.2	1–5–2.5
$PaCO_2$	4.7–6.0 kPa (35–45 mmHg)	Hypercapnia	6–7–8.0 (50–60)	8.0–12.0 (60–90)
		Hypocapnia	3.3–4.0 (25–30)	2.0–3.3 (15–25)
pH	7.35–7.45	Acidosis	7.1–7.3	6–8–7.1
		Alkalosis	7.5–7.6	7.6–7.8
Osmolarity	280–295 mmol/l	Hyperosmolarity	320–350	350–370
Calcium	2.3–2.7 mmol/l	Hypercalcaemia	3.0–3.5	3–5–5.0
		Hypocalcaemia	1–5–1.8	1.0–1.5

*Based on adult normal reference values quoted by Bold and Wilding 1975
[†]Blood taken at random: fasting range 3.0–5.3 mmol/l

(v) *Blood sugar*. Interpreting the blood sugar during intensive care follows the same practice as that in the wards, with which the reader will be familiar. Frequent measurements are required to treat diabetic acidosis and when concentrated dextrose solutions are used for intravenous nutrition (Chapter 17). Some of these blood sugar measurements can be conveniently made in the unit by means of Dextrostix. Three of the variables referred to above – Nap, urea and sugar are the important variables responsible for the osmotic pressure of the ECF. It follows that the plasma osmolarity can be calculated from the concentrations of these three substances measured in mmol/l.

Osmolarity (mmol/l) = Nap × 2.0 + urea + sugar
The normal range is 280–295 mmol/l

A more accurate result is obtained by measuring the osmolarity in the laboratory.

4. Urine

For assessing metabolic balance, urine analysis can follow a similar approach to that used for the blood. The primary tests (Table 4.8) are routine practice. Other essentials on urine – colour, blood, microscopy of the deposit – should not be omitted. In the ICU the daily urine volume is a measurement of guaranteed quality. The normal state of water balance was described on page 41 and the interpretation of a disturbed balance will follow. Two terms require definition and interpretation. Anuria is variously interpreted but there is no mistaking the term total anuria – 'the absence of any measurable urine volume' (D.N.S. Kerr).

Oliguria means a daily urine output of about 500 ml or an hourly output of 25 ml. During resuscitation and intensive care, oliguria should prompt a systematic enquiry (Figure 4.4). For example, measurements of the circulation are re-checked; in shock the therapy is quickly revised; the acid–base balance of the blood is measured to exclude an unforeseen metabolic acidosis. The question is now asked, is the patient developing renal failure?

Additional tests are made on the blood and urine and a diuretic test is included in the plan. The pH of the urine is of little help in the assessment of metabolic balance. An acid urine in a patient with a high blood urea and a metabolic alkalosis points to potassium depletion causing acute renal failure. The secondary measurements of titratable acidity and ammonia are used to unravel chronic disturbances of acid–base balance seen in the ward or clinic. There are limitations to the interpretation of urinary sodium and potassium comparable with those for plasma. Saline depletion and the metabolic response to injury lead to low values of sodium (approximately 25 mmol/l) and high values of potassium (100 mmol/l). On the other hand the urinary potassium is no guide to potassium balance because the concentration may be low (50 mmol/l), normal or high. The daily output of sodium and potassium are necessary for an external balance and this information is of the greatest value to the intensive care patient. In this way the balance of sodium and potassium can be used both for assessment and fluid therapy.

5. Vomit, gastric aspirate, diarrhoea, and ileostomy fluid

It is important to obtain some idea, albeit a rough estimate, of the loss of water and electrolyte when there is diarrhoea and vomiting, gastric suction

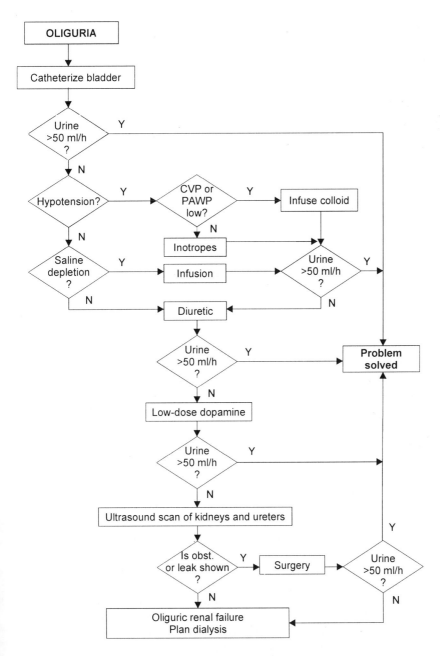

Figure 4.4 Algorithm to facilitate the management of oliguria

Table 4.10 Approximate composition of fluids lost from the gastrointestinal tract (From *Essential Intensive Care*, with permission)

	mmol/l			
	Na	K	HCl	HCO₃
Vomit or gastric aspirate				
pyloric stenosis	50	15	70	
intestinal obstruction	120	20		30
Watery diarrhoea	100	30		
Ileostomy fluid				
(recent stoma)	110	15		
Pancreatic fistula	150	10		80
High intestinal fistula	120	15		
Biliary fistula	140	15		40

or from a recent ileostomy. In our units we are unable to analyse liquid faeces or the blood-stained stools of colitis, so that in these conditions the faecal losses are just guesses – 'six loose bowel actions today'. Fluid from a recent ileostomy is measured each day and the losses calculated from Table 4.10. Gastric aspirate is collected and analysed in the laboratory. The composition of fluid differs greatly in pyloric obstruction and intestinal obstruction as seen in Table 4.10. For each 24-h period the output of water, sodium and potassium is entered on the balance chart and added to the urinary losses.

6. Metabolic balance

Metabolic balance measurements on hospital patients are used to solve quite different clinical problems. In the first instance, relatively well patients with chronic disorders of calcium or purine metabolism are admitted to a metabolic unit, are then given a controlled diet and the output measured. The other group of patients are acutely ill, often critically ill or injured. An approximate day-to-day balance is required for research on a particular disease and is also vital to the metabolic care of the individual patient. The following are examples of this application of the balance technique. In 1831 a Doctor O'Shaunessy demonstrated a large loss of base in the stools during cholera and he also showed that base was lost from the blood. In the early 1930s Sir. David Cuthbertson used the balance technique to show the negative nitrogen balance which follows trauma. Darrow used the balance technique to demonstrate a potentially lethal potassium depletion in children with gastroenteritis. In 1963 Jones and Sechiari introduced a simple technique for providing metabolic balance data to the intensive care unit.

An external balance for water, sodium and potassium, and sometimes nitrogen as well, is an essential requirement of general intensive care. Only a small proportion of the total admissions require this facility and the chief indications are shown in Table 4.11. It is nearly always possible to decide which patients will need a balance soon after resuscitation is complete and this is then noted in the clinical notes, the unit diary and lastly the name of the patient is entered on a blackboard in the sluice. The balance is continued until the nutritional needs of the patient can be taken as conventional food or in the case of chronic renal failure as a special diet. The balance of water and electrolyte is obtained by giving a known intake by mouth, a nasogastric tube or intravenously. Examples of the standardized intragastric or intra-venous diets used are given in Chapter 17. If the patient is able to take beverages or soft foods, then these are measured and charted and their composition determined from food tables.

This procedure will involve considerable work in comparison to the use of tube feeds or intravenous nutrients. The intake during 24 h periods – our 'day' starts at 08.00 hours – is drawn on a chart. The output of water and electrolyte naturally requires the careful collection of urine, gastric aspirate and more rarely liquid faeces. When the stools are formed they are discarded because their content of water, sodium and potassium will not invalidate an approximate balance; liquid stools should be collected and analysed. The critically ill patient with diarrhoea usually has faecal incontinence and the stools cannot be measured. If this situation persists for more than a day, then a rectal tube is used to collect the liquid stools directly into a plastic container. Gastric aspirate. ileostomy fluid, etc. are stored in separate polythene bottles to which is added 5.0 ml of an antiseptic. At the end of each collecting period the volumes are measured and an aliquot is analysed in the laboratory. The outputs of water, sodium and potassium can now be entered on the balance chart and the state of their balance interpreted. The clinician should decide in the first place whether the balance data are to be interpreted as they stand, or after correction for fever, sweating and so on. When time allows, the corrected data give more precise information, but the former is adequate for day-to-day management. The second procedure is to examine the state of balance for each variable, both for each day, and for the trend over 2 or 3 days. The data are interpreted as follows: A positive or negative balance for water is recorded when there is a difference of 1.5 or more litres between the intake and output. A positive balance for sodium is recorded when the measured intake exceeds the output by 30 mmol or more. Natriuresis is recorded when there is either a negative balance of

Table 4.11 Indications for metabolic balance (From *Essential Intensive Care*, with permission)

Prolonged coma
Prolonged ventilator treatment
Renal failure
Multiple injuries
Pyloric stenosis
Intestinal obstruction
Paralytic ileus
Recent ileostomy, intestinal fistula, pancreatic fistula
Forced diuresis
Acute hepatic failure

30 mmol or more or a threefold increase in urinary sodium over that of the preceding day. A positive or negative balance for potassium is recorded when there is a difference of 30 mmol or more between the intake and the output. These criteria for positive or negative balance for water or electrolyte are approximately twice those obtained on control subjects and are therefore highly significant (Table 4.3).

A nitrogen balance is only necessary on a proportion of those patients on whom a fluid balance is essential. By far the most important use is to show whether the methods of nutrition of the surgical or trauma patient are adequate to maintain nitrogen balance. When this has been established, future patients with such increased metabolic demands can be assured adequate nutrition without an individual nitrogen balance. In renal failure when nitrogen balance is disturbed it might be thought vital to carry out a balance. Unfortunately a nitrogen balance is impossible when the patient is treated by dialysis. This is because we cannot measure the amount of urea and amino acids removed during dialysis. Indications for nitrogen balance in renal failure are, firstly during the recovery phase from acute oliguric failure when dialysis is no longer required but the blood urea remains in the range of 8.0–13.0 mmol/l (50–80 mg/100 ml). The results of the balance are used to adjust the protein intake. Secondly a balance is required during the course of acute renal failure treated without dialysis; again to determine the intake of nitrogen. The calculations required for a nitrogen balance are quite straightforward. The intake of protein or amino acids is converted to grams of nitrogen. The nitrogen in the urine can be measured in the laboratory or

Table 4.12 Corrections applied to metabolic balance for insensible water loss and fever (From *Essential Intensive Care*, with permission)

	Water (litres)	Sodium (mmol)	Potassium (mmol)	Nitrogen (g)
Lungs, skin and formed stools	0.79	11	18	1.07
Additional losses for each degree (°C) rise in temperature	0.90	52	9	0.27

a useful approximation obtained by measuring the urinary urea. The nitrogen balance is then charted. When the blood urea changes during a 24 h balance period then an allowance must be made. This is quickly calculated by the equations below.

Urinary urea (X) in g/24 h
$X \times 0.56 = (a)$
Proteinuria (Y) in g/24 h
$Y \times 0.16 = (b)$
Rise in blood urea (Z) in mg/100 ml
$Z \times$ body weight (kg) $\times 2.8 = (c)$.
Nitrogen catabolism (g/day) $= (a) + (b) + (c)$

Corrections can be used to give more accurate interpretation and when it is wished to compare the data with results published in the literature. The losses other than those in the urine are given in Table 4.12. It will be seen that fever causes a marked increase in the output of water and electrolyte. The results of the day-to-day balance and of the trends over several days can only be interpreted in the light of the history, physical signs and the blood chemistry. The interpretation should proceed in a logical manner and this is best illustrated by referring to three examples; these illustrate saline depletion, potassium depletion and the metabolic response to injury. In Figure 4.5 'A' indicates the onset of acute illness and 'B' the start of a balance. Intake and output are started above and below the line respectively. To keep things simple, the daily intake and output of water and sodium have been charted as saline; in practice these are recorded separately. In the first example the balance is commenced on day 5 and shows an initial positive balance for saline. Was this due to a preceding deficit or is the kidney unable to excrete saline in the normal manner? The answer is obtained from a knowledge of the events during days 1 to 4. There was a history of negligible

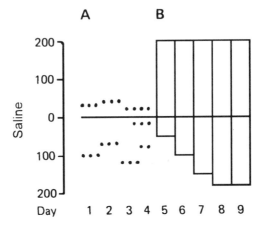

Figure 4.5 Balance results on a patient with saline depletion. Intake is shown above the horizontal line and output below. The bold dots represent probable values before balance data were obtained (From *Essental Intensive Care*, with permission)

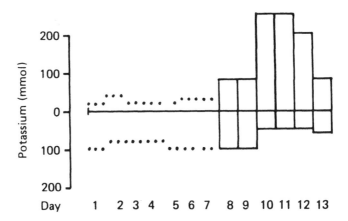

Figure 4.6 Balance results on a patient with potassium depletion. Intake is shown above the horizontal line and output below. The bold dots represent probable values before balance data were obtained (From *Essential Intensive Care*, with permission)

intake and intermittent vomiting. The mouth and skin showed signs of saline depletion. The Nap and Kp were normal but the blood urea was 10.0 mmol/l. The composition of the urine was sodium 15 mmol/l, potassium 100 mmol/l and urea 17.0 mmol/l (1000 mg/100 ml); findings strongly pointing to saline depletion. The patient was given 1.3 litres of normal saline per day and the state of balance was reached by day 9, by which time the blood urea was normal.

The second example (Figure 4.6), is a patient with paralytic ileus who was kept in balance for saline but the intakes of energy and potassium were negligible for the week preceding the balance. The blood shows a raised urea and hypokalaemia. An intake of 80 mmol of potassium was started on day 8 and later increased to 250 mmol per day. On days 8 and 9, the balance was negative despite the normal intake. During the 10th to13th days, the loss of potassium fell because the paralytic ileus resolved, and this together with an increased intake of potassium resulted in the positive balance. By day 13 the Kp had risen to normal and an intake of 84 mmol was matched by a urinary output of 70 mmol. Unfortunately, the data obtained during rapid changes in metabolism over short periods cannot be used to calculate the cumulative balance, for example the total potassium deficit in the above case. We can however deduce that over 1000 mmol of potassium were given intravenously before a state of balance was reached.

In the third example (Figure 4.7) the balance data for single days has been selected to illustrate the changes for saline, potassium and nitrogen. The patient's blood urea was measured at the start and end of each 'day' and the result is inserted below the balance results. Starting with 'A' which shows the data for a healthy subject; the outputs in the urine only are shown and there is a state of balance for saline, potassium and nitrogen. The balance data at 'B' were obtained 5 days after a cholecystectomy. Fluid therapy consisted of 'two of dextrose and one of saline' and hence the intake of potassium, energy and nitrogen were non-existent. On the day selected the observations show: a positive balance for saline; a negative balance for potassium and nitrogen. Because the patient was starved the energy balance would have been negative. The results of 'B' illustrate a disturbed balance caused by such an operation and the desirability of giving potassium, if not energy and nitrogen as well. The blood urea of this patient remained normal. The metabolic response to multiple injuries and the effects of nutrition are illustrated in 'C'. The data at 'C' were obtained 5 days following multiple injuries. Again the intake was dextrose/saline. There is a positive balance for saline. Is this due to a preceding depletion or is there a state of saline excess? A study of the balance for the preceding 4 days and examination of the patient concluded quite definitely that there was a

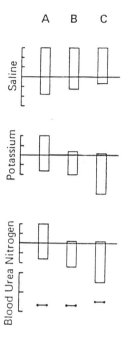

Figure 4.7 Balance data for saline, potassium, nitrogen and blood urea. A, control; B, following cholecystectomy; C, following multiple injuries. Details are given in the text (From *Essential Intensive Care*, with permission)

dangerous excess of saline. There was a negative potassium balance. The state for nitrogen was 20 g negative for the day; 2 weeks of this would consume three-quarters of the patient's body protein which is incompatible with survival; the blood urea showed a progressive increase

The aim of this chapter is to provide the beginner with background knowledge of the body fluids. The reader should then be better able to follow the organ or system failure described in later chapters. The assessment of the body fluid is necessary in all intensive care patients, but its priority is variable. For example, for resuscitation (Chapter 21) the body fluids would commonly be about fourth on the list. In contrast, severe hypoglycaemia might top the list. The weighing of priorities in this way is called 'triage'.

5
Disorders of acid–base balance

Scientists who introduce new terminology should, by law, be required
to post a $ 1,000 bond, to be forfeited if the terminology is both
misleading and used.   Julius H Comroe, 1965.

The condition known as acidosis is today hardly less familiar than
anaemia.   L.J. Henderson, 1928.

I   INTRODUCTION
II   ACID–BASE BALANCE OF THE BLOOD
III   DISEASES OR SYNDROMES CAUSING DISTURBED
      BALANCE
IV   INTERPRETATION

I INTRODUCTION

In everyday practice the term acid–base balance refers to the state of the
arterial blood. The term is quite different when the term balance relates to
water, sodium or potassium; in this sense balance means the difference
between the intake in food or drink and the output in the urine, faeces, sweat
or expired air. The acid–base balance of the blood is the only measure of
acid–base balance available during intensive care and resuscitation. The
measurements are used as a guide to the acid–base state of the internal
medium or ECF. Severe changes in the acid–base balance of the internal
medium disrupts the functioning of cells and organs and the patient dies.
The more rapidly the change occurs the greater the disruption of cell
function, since there is then less time for the body to defend the change by
compensatory mechanisms. Before analysing the acid–base balance of the
blood, that of the body as a whole is described, to enable the reader to make
comparisons with the balances of fluid and nitrogen (Chapter 4). In Figure
5.1 the normal balance for sodium is shown at 'A'; a daily intake of food or
beverages of 100 mmol, and the same amount lost in the urine, faeces, etc.;
none is made in the body! At 'B' is the normal acid balance. A conventional
western diet contains a few mmol of acid, and about 60 mmol of acid is
excreted in the urine. But a healthy subject at rest produces about
15 000 mmol of carbon dioxide a day. Carbon dioxide is not an acid, but a
potential acid; that is when dissolved in water or the body fluids it forms
carbonic acid. Unless removed from the body at the same rate as produced,

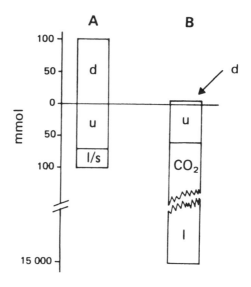

Figure 5.1 Diagram showing metabolic balance for sodium (A) and hydrion (B). d, intake in the diet; u, output in the urine; 1, loss through the lungs; s, loss via the skin (From *Essential Intensive Care*, with permission)

the carbon dioxide can lead to an intolerable positive balance of acid. It will be recalled that the carbon dioxide in the arterial blood and ECF represents the balance between the production of carbon dioxide and its elimination by the lungs. The output of carbon dioxide (B) below the horizontal baseline is therefore proportional to alveolar ventilation. So much for the body balance of acid. What is the state of affairs for base? The intake in food is again negligible and in health that lost in the urine is small.

II ACID–BASE BALANCE OF THE BLOOD

1. Applied physiology

In intensive care, acid–base balance centres on that of the arterial blood. The balance between acid and base is expressed as the concentration of hydrion (cH), expressed in nanomoles per litre of the plasma. Although this is by far the most appropriate unit, tradition has decreed the use of the alternative unit pH, which is related to cH as follows:

$$pH = \log \frac{1}{cH} \qquad [1]$$

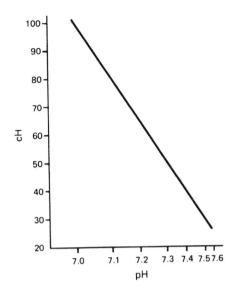

Figure 5.2 Diagram showing the relationship between hydrion concentration cH (nanomoles/litre) and pH units (From *Essential Intensive Care*, with permission)

The relationship is shown graphically in Figure 5.2, when it can be seen that as the concentration of hydrion (cH) increases the pH falls, and vice versa. The pH of the arterial blood of healthy subjects at rest lies between 7.35 and 7.45 units; neutrality is 7.00. The limits compatible with life are 6.8 (severe acidosis) to 7.8 (severe alkalosis). In health the principal acid of the plasma is carbonic, and sodium bicarbonate the base; the ratio of their concentrations is about 1 : 20. Now the concentration of carbonic acid is directly proportional to the partial pressure of CO_2 (PCO_2). There is a good reason for using PCO_2 rather than carbonic acid, as explained in Chapter 6; the PCO_2 is the most useful measurement of alveolar ventilation. The three components of the acid–base state of the plasma are therefore the pH, the amount of carbonic acid or PCO_2, and the concentration of sodium bicarbonate (or more precisely the sum of the bicarbonates of sodium, potassium, calcium and magnesium). Normal values for a healthy subject at rest are given in Table 5.1. In 1880 it was shown that the three variables were related mathematically by an equation (Henderson-Hasselbalch). For our purpose this can be written:

$$pH \propto \log \frac{HCO_3}{PCO_2} \qquad [2]$$

Table 5.1 Acid–base balance of arterial blood of healthy subjects at rest (From *Essential Intensive Care*, with permission)

pH (units)	7.35 to 7.45
$PaCO_2$ (kPa)	4.7 to 6.0
(mmHg)	35 to 45
Plasma bicarbonate (mmol/l)	19 to 26

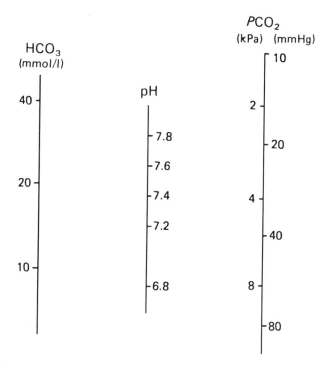

Figure 5.3 Nomogram relating pH, PCO_2 and HCO_3. A straight edge placed against any two variables will give the third variable (From *Essential Intensive Care*, with permission)

The only relevance of this mathematics to intensive care is that it provides a useful short cut to the assessment of the acid–base balance of the blood. This is quickly appreciated by referring to Figure 5.3 which is the H-H equation in a graphical form, and known as an alignment chart or nomogram. If the pH and PCO_2 are measured and a straight edge set against the results, then the plasma bicarbonate can be read off; in everyday practice the bicarbonate is calculated by the blood gas machine, but it is satisfying to understand how these figures were obtained. To return to the equation [2]

$$pH \propto \log \frac{HCO_3}{PCO_2}$$

the relationship is an easy one to manipulate. If the PCO_2 falls due to increased alveolar ventilation and the base remains unaltered, then the pH will rise; the converse holds. If on the other hand the plasma bicarbonate increases and the PCO_2 remains steady, then the pH will again increase. Before turning to the terminology and interpretation of acid–base disturbances, it is necessary to digress briefly to describe the relationship in the body between PCO_2, pH and plasma bicarbonate. The PCO_2/bicarbonate relationship is the familiar carbon dioxide titration curve. To obtain this curve for healthy subjects the PCO_2 and HCO_3 of the blood are measured at rest; the results will lie in the area bounded by PCO_2 values of 4.7–6.0 kPa (35–45 mmHg) and HCO_3 values of 19–26 mmol/l. To construct the curve

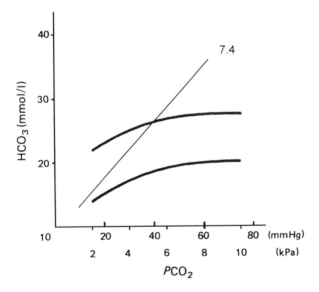

Figure 5.4 Carbon dioxide titration curves obtained *in vivo* on healthy subjects. Normal values lie within the two curves and pH 7.4 lies along the oblique straight line

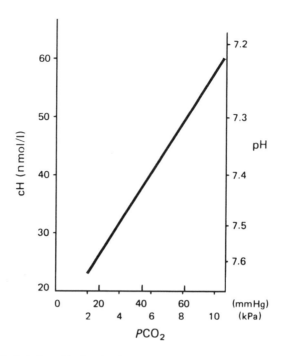

Figure 5.5 Relationship *in vivo* between PCO_2, cH and pH in healthy subjects. (From *Essential Intensive Care*, with permission)

(or rather curves) the PCO_2 is first lowered by hyperventilation and subsequently raised by breathing 7.0% carbon dioxide. The results are shown in Figure 5.4. The important points are as follows; the normal values occupy a wide band, approximately 7.5 mol in width; a large change in PCO_2 causes only a small change in bicarbonate. The relationship of PCO_2,/cH in our experiments is shown in Figure 5.5. It will be seen that the results of PCO_2,/cH fit closely to a straight line, that is the concentration of hydrion (cH) is directly proportional to the PCO_2. The pH scale, which is logarithmic, is also shown.

2. Terminology

Most of the disturbances of acid–base balance and certainly those relevant to intensive care were defined by 1928. The pioneers introduced a clear terminology, which is easy to learn, easy to teach, and of equal importance, relates directly to treatment. Since 1948 other terminologies have been invented, each with a good intention of making interpretation simpler.

Unfortunately this intention has not been achieved, and if anything various terminologies (alkali reserve, buffer base, standard bicarbonate, base excess) have confused rather than aided the clinician. In the manner used to classify changes in the blood sugar or urea, each of the three components of acid–base balance can be classified as normal, low or high. Indeed this straightforward method was the one recommended by an International Committee (Nahas, 1967). Giving a label to an abnormal pH or an abnormal PCO_2 is helpful in interpreting and treatment provided the terms* are clearly defined. We use the term acidosis (acidaemia) to describe the balance when the pH is below 7.35, and alkalosis when the pH is greater than 7.45. The terminology is just as simple as that of testing the urine with litmus paper; the urine can be neutral, acid or alkaline. An acidosis and alkalosis can be graded as moderate or severe and this helps to decide the priority of one treatment over another. A fall in $PaCO_2$ below 4.7 kPa (35 mmHg) is labelled hypocapnia, and a rise above 6.0 kPa (45 mmHg) hypercapnia. The plasma concentration of bicarbonate (HCO_3p) is simply described as normal. (19–26 mmol/l), increased or decreased.

Effects of disturbed acid–base balance on body functions. It seems probable that the harmful effects of acidosis or alkalosis are brought about directly by the pH effect on cell metabolism, rather than by a direct action of carbonic acid or bicarbonate. This would mean that a raised PCO_2 disturbs cell metabolism because it leads to an acidosis. What is certain is that a patient dies when the arterial pH falls below 6.8 or rises above 7.8. It should be recalled that such shifts represent enormous changes in cH. Acidosis or alkalosis does more harm when it develops rapidly over minutes or hours, than when the disturbance develops slowly over days or weeks. As might be anticipated, an imbalance is a greater threat to life when compounded with other changes in the ECF; examples are acidosis and hypoxia; acidosis and hyperkalaemia. A list of harmful effects of acidosis and alkalosis are given in Table 5.2

3. Blood samples

In adults, arterial puncture is simple but causes pain. In common with all investigations, arterial puncture is carried out when the indications are clear. Only 1.0 or 2.0 ml of blood is required to measure the pH and $PaCO_2$, in the 'blood gas machine'. We use plastic 2.0 ml syringes and fill the dead space of the syringe and needle with heparin solution (1000 units/ml). The

---

* 'When I use a word', Humpty Dumpty said in a rather scornful tone, 'it means just what I choose it to mean – neither more nor less'.

Table 5.2   Harmful effects of acidosis and alkalosis (From *Essential Intensive Care*, with permission)

Acidosis	Decreased cardiac output
	Pulmonary hypertension
	Cardiac dysrhythmias and arrest
	Oliguria
	Mental changes
	Loss of potassium from ICF to ECF
Alkalosis	Tetany
	Hypocapnoeic vasoconstriction
	Unfavourable shift in oxygen dissociation curve
	Mental changes
	Hypokalaemia

radial or femoral are the arteries commonly chosen. Except in emergencies the procedure is explained to the patient who is then prepared for momentary pain. When the blood sample has been drawn up into the syringe and the needle withdrawn, firm pressure is quickly applied with a pad of gauze. The pressure is maintained for several minutes to avoid a haematoma. If an air bubble has entered the syringe, this is quickly expelled. The pH and $PaCO_2$ of the sample at 37°C are now measured in the blood gas machine. When delay cannot be avoided, the syringe containing the blood is kept at 4°C to minimize changes which occur in shed blood. The largest portion of the blood sample is then centrifuged without contact with air. The results of pH and $PaCO_2$ are available almost instantly unless the machine has to be calibrated, which doubles the time. To facilitate interpretation of the pH and $PaCO_2$ a few simple measurements are recorded a few minutes before blood sampling. These are the body temperature (°C), the minute volume ventilation ($\dot{V_E}$), respiratory frequency, and the time from taking the blood to making the measurements (elapsed time). A printed label (Table 5.3) has been found useful.

4. Measurements

For general intensive care, most acid–base disturbances can be diagnosed and treated by measuring the pH and $PaCO_2$, and then calculating the plasma bicarbonate. The modern blood gas machine can perform this calculation automatically, but alternatively the HCO_3p is quickly obtained from an alignment chart (Figure 5.3). The three variables are then studied in relation to the pathological processes and preceding therapy. In a few instances, the interpretation is uncertain, or even impossible. The next step

Table 5.3 Facsimile of the label (70 × 75 mm) for recording blood gas results in the case notes (From *Essential Intensive Care*, with permission)

Date	Time.........................
$\dot{V}_E$	....
f	....
F_IO_2	...............................%
pH (normal 7.35–7.45)	....
$PaCO_2$ (normal 4.66–6.0)	.... kPa
HCO_3　measured　　calculated (normal 18.6–25.9 mmol/l)	.......................mmol/l ....mmol/l
PaO_2	.... kPa
$t°$	....
Elapsed time	.... mins
Hb	.... g/dl

Table 5.4 Laboratory investigation of acid–base balance in acute illness (From *Essential Intensive Care*, with permission)

Stage	Tests	Comment
I	Measure pH and PCO_2 Calculate HCO_3p	Adequate for most intensive care
II	Measure HCO_3p	Will usually unravel 'mixed' disorders
III	Measure blood acids Potassium balance Measure urine titratable acidity, ammonium, bicarbonate	Will determine 'cause' of acidosis or alkalosis

is to repeat the pH and $PaCO_2$ and also to measure the HCO_3p. The disturbances then defying an explanation will be few and far between. For research, or trials of new treatments, a much more comprehensive laboratory investigation is necessary; some of these measurements are given in Table 5.4.

III DISEASES OR SYNDROMES CAUSING DISTURBED BALANCE

The acid–base variables of arterial blood can only be interpreted in relation to the natural history of the disease and the signs, clinical and biochemical. The beginner may not as yet be familiar with the pathological processes underlying the intensive care patient, so that this brief review may prove helpful.

Most metabolic processes in the body lead to the production of acid rather than of base; 'the body is constantly fighting off an acidosis'.

1. Respiratory failure

For the present purpose we can group respiratory failure according to alveolar ventilation ($\dot{V}_A$). During hyperventilation the PCO_2 and carbonic acid are reduced, so that the pH will rise – an alkalosis. The relationships are readily appreciated by referring to Figure 5.5. Such a respiratory alkalosis is common in many patients with acute respiratory failure; pulmonary embolism, pulmonary oedema, chest injury. The same acid–base picture will be found when IPPV causes hyperventilation. It should be remembered that the pain of arterial puncture will cause hyperventilation and a consequent fall in $PaCO_2$ and a rise in pH. When alveolar ventilation is reduced, the carbonic acid and $PaCO_2$ are increased. If the respiratory failure develops acutely, for example in self-poisoning, the pH will fall according to the relationship shown in Figure 5.5; this disturbance is a respiratory acidosis. In chronic respiratory failure due to advanced chronic bronchitis – the 'blue bloater' picture – the $PaCO_2$ is raised for weeks or months, and the kidney compensates by raising the HCO_3p; the pH is therefore normal. This is a compensated respiratory acidosis. The acid–base disturbances in severe asthma illustrate how the balance can swing from alkalosis to acidosis over some hours. At first the $PaCO_2$ is low with a respiratory alkalosis. In worsening asthma, alveolar ventilation falls to normal and then decreases, so that the blood then shows a respiratory acidosis. In the moribund asthmatic tissue hypoxia can superimpose a metabolic acidosis.

2. Circulatory failure

Shock following haemorrhage, injury, burns saline depletion is associated with a low cardiac output, vasoconstriction and poor tissue perfusion. Tissue hypoxia, and possibly the high concentrations of catecholamines, lead to an increase in the concentration of lactic acid in the blood. The normal value for arterial blood is 0.4–1.4 mmol/l and in severe shock this can rise to over 5.0 mmol/l. Lactic acid is buffered by the ECF and ICF and the HCO_3p falls. This will cause a drop in pH (equation 2), unless the body compensates by increasing ventilation and so reducing the $PaCO_2$. The net result is a normal pH with low HCO_3p and a low $PaCO_2$ a compensated metabolic acidosis; or a low pH – a metabolic acidosis. The acidosis itself further reduces the cardiac output and thus establishes a vicious circle. A severe metabolic acidosis will follow cardiac arrest, unless the heart is quickly restarted or the circulation maintained by external cardiac compression. The acidosis makes defibrillation of the heart more difficult.

3. Diabetic keto-acidosis

The metabolic acidosis of diabetes mellitus was described in 1884, and alkali therapy was successfully used 25 years before the discovery of insulin in 1926. In severe uncontrolled diabetes, large quantities of aceto-acetic acid and 3-hydroxybutyric acid are produced, and the blood levels can rise to 1.0–7.0 and 4.0–20.0 mmol/l respectively. The result is a metabolic acidosis, at first compensated and then overt. The respiratory compensation can be extreme, with $\dot{V}_E$ of 20–30 litres and $PaCO_2$ values of 0.67–2.0 kPa (5–15 mmHg). The acidosis itself is an important factor in the pathogenesis of the coma, shock and eventual cardiac arrest. In the less acute case the kidney contributes to the compensation by an increased production of ammonia.

4. Gastrointestinal diseases

These are potent causes of acid–base disturbances, but the patterns are very varied. Patients with the same disease can show contrasting distur-bances or mixed disturbances. Examples of the acid–base disturbances and the pathological processes are shown in Table 5.5. Some of the patho-physi-ology is common to the patients in this group. The increased metabolism increases the production of carbon dioxide, which is readily eliminated by a proportional increase in alveolar ventilation. But the catabolism induced by sepsis (e.g. peritonitis), inflammation (e.g. ulcerative colitis) or surgery, causes an increased production of keto-acids, sulphuric, phosphoric and lactic acids and a metabolic acidosis can result. The second pathological process is semi-starvation; in particular a failure to match the increased demands for energy. In turn this accelerates the catabolism of fat and muscle, and again leads to a metabolic acidosis. Two other pathological processes tend to move the acid–base balance in the opposite direction.

Table 5.5 Gastrointestinal disease which can disturb acid–base balance. Hypercatabolism is common to many conditions (From *Essential Intensive Care*, with permission)

Disease	Disturbance	Pathological process
Pyloric stenosis	Metabolic alkalosis	Loss of gastric HCl Potassium depletion
Intestinal obstruction/ Paralytic ileus	Metabolic acidosis Metabolic alkalosis Respiratory alkalosis	Inadequate energy Potassium depletion Respiratory failure
Ulcerative colitis/ Crohn's colitis in relapse	Metabolic acidosis Metabolic alkalosis	Inadequate energy Potassium depletion
Pancreatic fistula	Metabolic acidosis	Loss of $NaHCO_3$, from the fistula
*Cholera	Metabolic acidosis	Loss of $NaHCO_3$ in the stools

*Will not be encountered in the western world, but was included because the study of cases in the UK was so important to fluid therapy (Nahas, 1966)

Gastric suction (e.g. intestinal obstruction) or diarrhoea (e.g. ulcerative colitis) can quickly lead to potassium depletion, which itself causes a metabolic alkalosis. The sequence of events is as follows: loss of potassium from the ICF leads to secondary shifts between ICF and ECF. This results in an increase in HCO_3p. The ensuing metabolic alkalosis is usually uncompensated; the pH and the HCO_3p are increased, the $PaCO_2$ normal. Most organs of the body are affected by potassium depletion. The kidney excretes an excess of acid (ammonium), and this acid wasting worsens the metabolic alkalosis. In pyloric obstruction or pancreatic fistula the acid–base balance is disturbed by the loss of acid or base from the body. Following chronic pyloric obstruction large quantities of HCl are lost in the vomit or gastric aspirate. This can amount to 500 mmol per day. Together with potassium depletion, this leads to a metabolic alkalosis. As a rule the pH is high, the HCO_3p is raised and the $PaCO_2$ is normal. In contrast, the fluid lost from a pancreatic fistula contains 100 mmol/l of HCO_3p, and this can quickly lead to a metabolic acidosis. Respiratory failure is commonly seen in the surgical patient with generalized peritonitis, intestinal obstruction: ventilation increases, the PCO_2 falls and the result is a respiratory alkalosis. The interaction of the various processes (Table 5.5) means that it is difficult or impossible to predict the acid–base balance in the individual patient;

measurement is the answer. In this group of patients it is often necessary to measure the HCO_3p in order to interpret the disturbance.

5.   Renal failure

As seen in the general intensive care unit, this can be classified as acute or chronic, and the disturbances of acid–base balance show distinctive patterns. In acute oliguric renal failure the body rapidly loses a normal daily output of about 60 mmol of acid in the urine; so a positive balance for acid occurs. In the case without hypercatabolism, the ICF is quite able to cope with this load and the acid–base balance of the arterial blood is normal or neatly so, especially when nutrition is given properly. Commonly found results would be: pH = 7.33, $PaCO_2$ = 4.0 kPa (30 mmHg), HCO_3p = 15 mmol/l; a partly compensated metabolic acidosis. In contrast, when the acute renal failure is associated with the hypercatabolic state (sepsis, burns, etc.) a metabolic acidosis quickly develops, and unless treated, endangers life. There is a high risk of cardiac arrest because of a concomitant hyperkalaemia. The acids which accumulate in the ECF are keto-acids, phosphoric, sulphuric and lactic. The body attempts to compensate by an increase in alveolar ventilation, but the compensation is quite inadequate to restore the pH to safe values. In these patients the acid–base balance can be preserved by intensive dialysis. In chronic renal failure a metabolic acidosis occurs slowly over months. The mechanisms are three-fold: failure of the kidney to excrete phosphoric or sulphuric acids; decreased ability to synthesize ammonia; a wasting of bicarbonate in the urine. The acidosis, like the concomitant uraemia can be aggravated by starvation. This pathophysiology was discovered some 60 years ago. In the past ten years an additional mechanism has been described; the overproduction of hydrion by the liver. The net result in the blood is a compensated or uncompensated metabolic acidosis. The ventilatory compensation can reach extreme levels, comparable to those seen in diabetic keto-acidosis.

6.   Caused by treatment

Infusions used during intensive care can influence the acid–base balance. To start with the simplest group (Table 5.6), the antacids. Peptic ulcer patients may abuse antacids and this is an additional cause of a metabolic alkalosis in pyloric obstruction. Solutions of sodium bicarbonate are necessary for the treatment of severe metabolic acidosis and for a forced alkaline diuresis, but if misused can lead to a metabolic alkalosis with distressing or dangerous tetany. The fluids used in haemodialysis or peritoneal dialysis

Table 5.6 Infusions or drugs disturbing acid–base balance
(From *Essential Intensive Care*, with permission)

BASES	
Antacids: sodium bicarbonate,	
calcium carbonate (Rennies, Nulacin)	mmol base/l
Sodium bicarbonate solutions, 1.26–8.4%	150–1000
POTENTIAL BASES	
Citrate in whole blood	105
Acetate in dialysate	40
	Titratable acidity, mmol hydrion/l
ACIDS	
Amino-acid solutions	70
50% glucose	5
Lactic acid in banked blood	20–200
POTENTIAL ACID	
Intralipid	

are designed to maintain metabolic balance and this includes acid–base balance. Dialysate containing bicarbonate or acetate – which is rapidly converted to bicarbonate – will achieve this objective. A commonly used peritoneal dialysate contains lactate in place of bicarbonate or acetate. In patients with a metabolic acidosis due to a high blood level of lactic acid (say 5.0 mmol/l), the lactate which enters the body cannot be metabolized, and the acidosis will increase. Banked blood or plasma can affect the acid–base balance in either direction. Blood stored at 4°C produces lactic acid by glycolysis and the concentration increases with the duration of storage. The shocked patient cannot metabolize the lactic acid in large blood transfusions, and the lactic acidosis already present is aggravated. The consequences can be serious. Banked whole blood contains citrate anti-coagulant and this is a potential alkali. Hence, large infusions can cause a metabolic alkalosis, provided the lactic acid can be metabolized.

The remaining infusions which can influence acid–base balance are the intravenous nutrients. This is rather ironical in that, unless they are used appropriately, the resulting starvation also disturbs this balance! Intravenous nutrition by means of sugars, amino-acids and fat emulsion differs in the acid–base aspect from conventional food or a liquid diet. The latter give a net intake of a few mmol of acid or base. In contrast, intravenous amino-acids contribute a clinically significant acid load, which can cause a metabolic acidosis. Similarly, strong solutions of dextrose constitute an acid load to the body. Finally, intravenous fat emulsions, like the endogenous fat, unless it is metabolized properly will cause an acidosis from an excess of keto-acids or free fatty acids.

IV INTERPRETATION

Our system is based on our long experience in the teaching of post-basic nurses and junior doctors, who find acid–base terminology confusing. Deductions during emergency resuscitation must be made quickly, and this problem is dealt with before describing a more leisurely interpretation.

The pH, $PaCO_2$ and calculated HCO_3p are examined in that order. A normal pH means that the treatments are highly successful. If the pH is less than 7.0, give 100 mmol of sodium bicarbonate intravenously (100 ml of 8.4% sodium bicarbonate). If the pH is low, but above 7.0 examine the $PaCO_2$. If the latter is normal or low give intravenous alkali according to the pH value and at the same time quickly assess the treatment being given to the patient. If the $PaCO_2$ is high, IPPV should be started, or if in use, the ventilation should be increased; the acid–base is measured again in 10 minutes. Following cardiac arrest or the pulseless state (extreme hypotension), 100 mmol of sodium bicarbonate should be given without waiting for acid–base measurements to be made. When decisions are less hurried, a more thorough system of interpretation can be used. The results are listed in the order pH, $PaCO_2$, and HCO_3p; the respiratory measurements should also be available.

1. pH normal

The acid–base balance is normal, or an acidosis or alkalosis are compensated. Examine the $PaCO_2$.

(1) $PaCO_2$ also normal; the acid–base balance of the blood is normal.
(2) $PaCO_2$ low; a compensated metabolic acidosis is probable.
     Follow the pattern for metabolic acidosis.
(3) $PaCO_2$ raised; a compensated respiratory acidosis is probable.
     Ascertain why pulmonary ventilation is decreased; advanced chronic bronchitis? patient on a ventilator with chronic lung disease or interstitial oedema?
(4) $PaCO_2$ raised; a compensated metabolic alkalosis possible, but very rare; ascertain the possible cause of a metabolic alkalosis – potassium depletion or vomiting of gastric HCl.

2. pH low

Acidosis, which can be respiratory, metabolic or combined.

(1) $PaCO_2$ low; acidosis is metabolic due to an excess of an acid (other than carbonic) or a deficit of base (bicarbonate), which is rare. Diseases or syndromes should give a clue to an excess of acid – diabetes mellitus, chronic renal failure, shock. Loss of bicarbonate leading to acidosis is rare, and the cause is obvious – pancreatic fistula.

(2) $PaCO_2$ raised; pure respiratory acidosis or mixed respiratory and metabolic. It is certain that the patient has respiratory failure, and before the balance is investigated further, the decision is made whether or not to start IPPV. The pH and $PaCO_2$ results are next fitted to Figure 5.5. If the results lie close to the normal, then the acidosis is probably respiratory. On the other hand, a discrepancy suggests a mixed acidosis. In general intensive care the commonest cause of such a mixed acidosis is sedative poisoning, with respiratory and circulatory failure; a combined carbonic acid and lactic acidosis. The same acid–base disturbance is sometimes seen in the moribund asthmatic. Further investigation of the balance does not help in the treatment of either condition. For the sake of curiosity or research, the physician may decide to decipher the acidosis. To do this the HCO_3p is measured. Using Figure 5.4 one can quickly determine whether the measured HCO_3p lies within the normal CO_2 titration curve. If the result does so, then the acidosis is respiratory; if the HCO_3p lies below the lower limit, then the acidosis is a mixed one. The investigation can be extended by measuring the concentration of lactic and other metabolic acids in the arterial blood.

3. pH high

Alkalosis, which can either be respiratory, metabolic or combined. Alkalosis means too little carbonic acid or an excess of bicarbonate. Examine the $PaCO_2$.

(1) $PaCO_2$ low: a respiratory alkalosis; search for the cause of the increased alveolar ventilation – pain, fear, hypoxaemia, head injury, encephalitis, etc. Of course, the $PaCO_2$ may have been lowered deliberately during IPPV. The two measured variables, pH and $PaCO_2$ should be a close fit to the line in Figure 5.5.

(2) $PaCO_2$ normal: a metabolic alkalosis, without respiratory compensation. The cause of the alkalosis will be found by asking the following questions: has the patient been given alkali or potential base? Is the

patient's potassium depleted? Has there been chronic loss of HCl by vomiting or gastric suction? Unless one of these causes is found, the alkalosis may be of the combined variety. The clinical picture will solve the problem; alkali given during resuscitation which includes IPPV; respiratory failure with hypoxaemia in the potassium depleted surgical patient.

The foregoing introduction to acid–base balance should be digested and then integrated into the wider knowledge of the body fluids. In particular the beginner should think of an acid–base, disturbance in terms of the internal medium (Chapter 4). Why is electrical neutrality Important to cell function. How is this constantly maintained? How is the balance defended?

The interpretation of acid–base balance used in this chapter is based on the system of teaching used since 1970. Our experience showed that the system adopted was soon learnt and applied by beginners. Our view of the numerous alternative methods was crystallized by the late Julius Comroe in the quote on page 67.

6
Respiratory failure

Anoxaemia not only stops the machine,
but wrecks the machinery. J.S. Haldane

I   INTRODUCTION
II   DEFINITIONS
III   CAUSES
IV   DIAGNOSIS AND ASSESSMENT

I INTRODUCTION

Respiratory failure, which is defective gas exchange in the lung, is frequently seen in the casualty department and the medical and surgical wards of the district general hospital. The respiratory failure may be the dominating factor of the patient's illness and the primary reason for hospital admission. On the other hand acute respiratory failure may not be obvious and is diagnosed only after systematic examination and investigation of a surgical or injured patient. The natural history of acute respiratory failure is very variable; from a transient disturbance of gas exchange without symptoms to a progressive and life-threatening illness. The role of the intensive care unit is three-fold. Firstly, to investigate and treat selected patients; secondly, to provide intensive observation of patients who have a high risk of developing acute respiratory failure; lastly, the educational role of teaching the early recognition, treatment and prevention. Since the majority of patients admitted to an ICU have acute respiratory failure of some degree, the causes and diagnosis are outlined in this early chapter.

The inexperienced for whom this book was written should revise their knowledge of the mechanics and the control of respiration. There follows a synopsis on ventilation and perfusion. Ventilation of the lung is no different from that of a room when the ventilation is expressed as changes of air per hour. For the total ventilation of the lungs, the term applied is called minute volume ventilation. This is the volume of gas which is either inspired ($\dot{V_I}$) or expired ($\dot{V_E}$) in unit time of one minute. Minute volume ventilation is the sum of alveolar ventilation ($\dot{V_A}$) plus dead space ventilation ($\dot{V_D}$). Thus:

$$\dot{V_I} \text{ or } \dot{V_E} = \dot{V_A} + \dot{V_D}$$

Values for a normal adult would be as follows:

$$\dot{V}_E = 6.0, \ \dot{V}_A = 4.2, \ \dot{V}_D = 1.8$$

In healthy subjects the dead space ventilation remains constant and the $\dot{V}_A$ can be calculated from $\dot{V}_E$, but this does not apply in disease when $\dot{V}_D$ can increase dramatically. To return to the analogy of room ventilation. Imagine a room with the windows and doors closed and a group of people (not of course nurses or doctors!) smoking. The concentration of tobacco smoke will increase with time. If the windows and doors are now opened, ventilation will rapidly increase and the concentration of smoke will fall; the one is inversely proportional to the other. A state could be arranged in which the occupants of the room smoked at a constant rate and the ventilation was adjusted to a constant rate; production will then match removal and the concentration of smoke would be constant. These simple facts can now be applied to a lung unit (Figure 6.1).

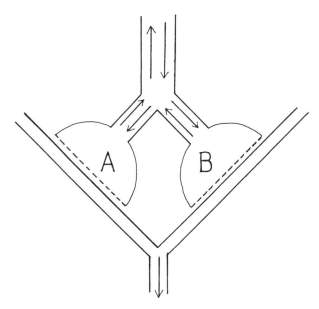

Figure 6.1 A model of the normal lung, showing two lung units (A,B) and their pulmonary veins. The broken line represents the alveolar-capillary membrane

The CO_2 produced by metabolism is carried in the blood to the lung unit where it diffuses into the air space, from which it is removed by ventilation. For intensive care we can use CO_2 as the marker for alveolar ventilation.

Thus, a decrease in alveolar ventilation will result in an increase in alveolar CO_2. Rather than use the concentration of CO_2 in the alveolar gas, the pressure of CO_2 ($PACO_2$) is more convenient. The relationship of alveolar CO_2 to alveolar ventilation can now be written as an equation:

$$\dot{V}_A \propto \frac{1}{PACO_2} \quad \text{or} \quad PACO_2 \propto \frac{1}{\dot{V}_A}$$

For routine clinical practice we do not attempt to measure the $PACO_2$; instead the arterial carbon dioxide tension ($PaCO_2$) is measured and the $PACO_2$ assumed to be the same. Hence, $PaCO_2$ can be substituted for $PACO_2$ in the above equation. So far we have described ventilation, of the lung as a whole rather than the sum of its parts. To understand the respiratory failure of the intensive care patient it is essential to grasp the distribution of gas (and of blood) in different parts of the lung, referred to as regions. Figure 6.1 shows one lung unit in each of two regions. The unit A is better ventilated than B and this clearly effects the removal of CO_2. In this example the blood flow (perfusion) to each unit is similar. The distribution of ventilation to the two regions of this lung is determined by two factors, the anatomy of the airways and by gravity. It follows that changing posture from the upright to lying has considerable effects on regional ventilation. Similar facts apply to perfusion, which is considered next. The total blood flow through the lung is the cardiac output, about 5 litres per minute. As with the inspired air and for the same reasons. this total is not uniformly distributed to the regions of the lung. In health, however, there is a remarkable efficient matching of air and blood referred to as ventilation perfusion (V/Q) regional balance. Precise matching of air and blood is one of the mechanisms which maintains a constant amount of carbon dioxide and oxygen in the arterial blood at rest.

II DEFINITIONS

Acute respiratory failure means defective gas exchange in the lung. The physiological diagnosis depends on finding a reduced amount of oxygen in the arterial blood (hypoxaemia), the carbon dioxide being normal, high or low. For emergency medicine it is advantageous to express the oxygen and carbon dioxide in the arterial blood as partial pressures. The pressure is measured in one of two units; the kilopascal (kPa) or millimetres of mercury (mmHg) and these are related. as follows:

$$kPa = mmHg \times 0.133 \text{ or } mmHg = kPa \times 7.52$$

Fortunately there is international agreement on the diagnostic criteria. Respiratory failure is diagnosed when a patient breathing room air has an arterial oxygen (PaO_2) or less than 8.0 kPa (60 mmHg) or the CO_2 tension ($PaCO_2$) is above 6.5 kPa (49 mmHg) Thus a low PaO_2 is always present but it is important to understand that the $PaCO_2$ may be low, normal or raised. Another fact needs emphasis; when a patient is breathing room air and the $PaCO_2$ is found to be raised, then hypoxaemia is invariably present. The defective gas exchange in the lung fits one of two patterns. To understand these patterns it is necessary to recall the following facts. The arterial PCO_2 and the alveolar PCO_2 are the same and each is inversely equated to alveolar ventilation. Indeed, in the intensive care patient we measure the $PaCO_2$ in order to assess alveolar ventilation. A patient with a raised PCO_2 has ventilatory failure. The second pattern is known as hypoxaemic failure, the blood then shows a reduced PaO_2 but a normal or low PCO_2. To recapitulate, in hypoxaemic failure alveolar ventilation is normal or increased, in contrast to ventilatory failure. When some disease causes a fall in alveolar ventilation and the patient is breathing room air then it is easy to understand that hypoxaemia will inevitably occur, even though the lunge are capable of normal function. But in many cases of acute respiratory failure the $PaCO_2$ is normal or reduced, i.e. alveolar ventilation is normal or excessive and the physiology of the hypoxaemia is more difficult to understand. In these patients the hypoxaemia results from a disturbed balance between ventilation (V) and perfusion (Q), referred to as a disturbed ventilation/perfusion (V/Q) ratio. This pathophysiology is easier to understand by referring to the lung unit of the Introduction. Compare the Figures 6.1 and 6.2. The lung units shown in Figure 6.2 are examples of disturbed V/Q balance. At C the lung is ventilated in a normal manner, but underperfused; at D the converse exist due to a narrowed airway. The blood leaving the units mixes to become arterial blood. At this stage of learning we have to be didactic and write that the chief consequence of the V/Q imbalance is hypoxaemia.

III CAUSES

The causes of acute respiratory failure are legion and at first sight some of them seem very unlikely! An important starting point and an obvious cause is obstruction of the upper airway. This usually caused by the tongue falling backwards against the pharynx. This commonly occurs during coma or semi-coma and is more likely when the head is flexed at the neck. Incomplete obstruction caused by the tongue can be worsened by the presence of blood, vomit or denture. Following complete obstruction of the upper airway there is a transient Increase in respiratory movements followed by apnoea; gas exchange ceases at once and the heart arrests. Consider next the structure of the lung in acute respiratory failure, as outlined in Table 6.1.

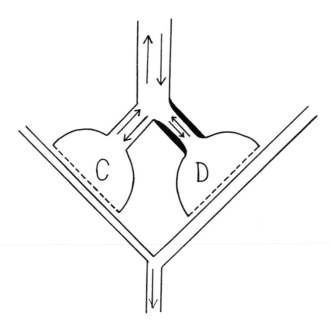

Figure 6.2 A model of a diseased lung showing ventilation–perfusion imbalance

Perhaps surprisingly the lung can be normal, but by definition gas exchange is defective. This situation is seen in the overdose patient or when the respiratory muscles are paralysed. In contrast the lung can be diseased. Changes in pulmonary structure may be due to a clearly defined lung disease, such as asthma or bacterial pneumonia. In these cases the relationship between disordered structure and gas exchange is straightforward, but in many cases of acute respiratory failure the lung disease cannot be categorized as a clearly defined entity and is 'secondary' to a disease elsewhere in the body. Examples are acute myocardial infarction or generalized peritonitis. In this important group of patients the changes in lung structure are non-specific; pulmonary oedema and absorption collapse are especially important. The diversity of the causes of acute respiratory failure can be appreciated by examining the sites of the primary disease. These are shown in Table 6.2. From this abbreviated list of causes it will be clear that acute respiratory failure can be a facet of almost any illness – 'medical', 'surgical', 'traumatic' and so on. Some of the causes and the resulting changes in lung structure and function will be considered in later chapters. At this stage it is important to acquire background knowledge on the non-specific changes in lung structure commonly seen in the intensive care

Table 6.1 The structure of the lung in acute respiratory failure (From *Essential Intensive Care*, with permission)

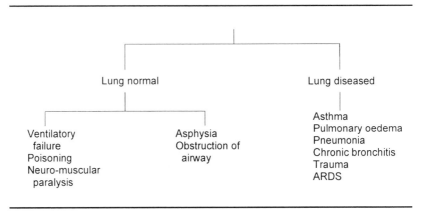

Table 6.2 Causes of respiratory failure according to the site of the primary disease (From *Essential Intensive Care*, with permission)

1. Brain
   Sedative poisoning
   Epilepsy
   Head injury
   Cerebro-vascular accident
   Encephalitis

2. Spinal cord, motor neurone,
   neuromuscular junction,
   peripheral nerve,
   respiratory muscles
   Spinal injury
   Poliomyelitis
   Tetanus
   Myasthenia gravis
   Polyneuritis

3. Thoracic cage and diaphragm
   Crushed chest
   Thoracotomy
   Ruptured diaphragm
   Extreme kyphoscoliosis

4. Heart and circulation
   Acute heart failure
   Shock
   Pulmonary embolism

5. Lung
   Asthma
   Chronic bronchitis
   Pneumothorax
   Pulmonary aspiration
   Injury to the lungs

6. Gastrointestinal
   Intra-abdominal sepsis
   Acute pancreatitis
   Inflammatory bowel disease

patient. Brief consideration is next given to generalized airway obstruction, absorption collapse (atelectasis), consolidation, pulmonary oedema and lastly the Adult Respiratory Distress Syndrome.

1. Generalized airway obstruction

This label will be familiar in relation to chronic bronchitis, widespread emphysema or asthma. In these diseases there is widespread or generalized narrowing of the airways. But there are other important causes. Acute bacterial or viral infections of the lung lead to airways obstruction; bronchospasm can follow pulmonary embolism or the inhalation of vomit. Bronchospasm also occurs in cardiac asthma (chronic left ventricular failure) as well as the bronchial variety. Pulmonary oedema due to any cause leads to widespread narrowing of the bronchi. This is because the oedema of the interstitial tissue surrounding the bronchi compresses them. The degree of obstruction can be assessed by auscultation of the chest and by simple bedside tests to be considered later.

2. Absorption collapse

This pathological process must be distinguished from widespread obstruction. Absorption collapse or atelectasis occurs when a bronchus or bronchiole is occluded by mucus, pus, blood or inhaled vomit. Clearly the smaller the bronchus the smaller the volume of lung which collapses. The volume of the affected lung falls markedly and the alveoli are airless. Thus the lesion varies from a whole lung down to a small lobule. In health a combination of mechanisms prevents absorption collapse; these are the action of the bronchial cilia, the cough reflex and an expulsive cough mechanism. In many critically ill patients one or more of these defence mechanisms is defective and the scene is set for absorption collapse to occur. The newcomer to intensive care will soon gain familiarity with bilateral basal atelectasis (labelled 'plate' atelectasis, the plate being edge on) in patients who do not have primary lung disease. The primary diagnosis is very varied, for example paralytic ileus, inflammatory bowel disease. This secondary lung pathology is so common that we call it the syndrome of the lower lobes. Recognition is based on a change in the pattern of breathing and frequent portable chest radiographs.

3. Consolidation

This means that the alveoli are filled with fluid, with or without blood cells, but the airways are patent. The consolidated lung is airless. When the fluid is caused by an inflammatory process (an exudate) the term pneumonia may be applied. On the other hand the consolidation can be caused by oedema fluid (transudate) rather than inflammatory exudate. This is an important reason for using the term consolidation rather than pneumonia. The recognition of consolidation in the intensive care patient is almost wholly dependent on the chest radiograph.

4. Pulmonary oedema

The new recruit to intensive care will quickly realize that pulmonary oedema is a frequent and important facet of a patient's illness. Such patients show a bewildering variety of diseases or illnesses and to complicate things further, in the individual patient, the pulmonary oedema can be due to more than one cause. It Is thought likely that pulmonary oedema starts in the interstitial tissue of the lung and may then extend to become alveolar oedema. The mechanisms of pulmonary oedema can be grouped under three headings as shown in Table 6.3. When the pulmonary capillary pressure rises above 24 mmHg (3.2 kPa) from the normal value of 15 mmHg, then oedema will develop. The commonest cause in the ICU is left ventricular failure due to acute myocardial infarction. An alternative mechanism occurs when the permeability of the capillary is increased – capillary leak – oedema can then occur with a normal pressure in the capillary. It is probable the capillary leak occurs in a wide variety of syndromes (Table 6.3).

5. Adult Respiratory Distress Syndrome (ARDS)

Allied to pulmonary oedema is the Adult Respiratory Distress Syndrome.* This condition still lacks a sound definition and the early structural changes in the lung are unknown. By the time the diagnosis is made a lung biopsy shows interstitial oedema. This can recover or progress to cellular infiltration and hyaline membranes, alveolar oedema and haemorrhage. The histology in a fatal case is the same as that of the Respiratory Distress Syndrome of the new-born and in turn similar to pulmonary oxygen toxicity in animals. In all three instances the lung is deficient in surfactant. It seems probable

---

*   Post-traumatic pulmonary insufficiency, shock lung, respirator lung, high output respiratory failure, diffuse interstitial pulmonary oedema, wet lung, congestive atelectasis.

Table 6.3 Mechanisms of pulmonary oedema in the intensive care patient (From *Essential Intensive Care*, with permission)

Mechanism	Examples
Increased capillary pressure	Acute heart failure
Capillary leak	Endotoxaemia Anaphylaxis Renal failure Hepatic failure Inhalation of irritant gases or vomit Pulmonary embolism Blast injury Bruising of the lung Paraquat poisoning Salicylate poisoning Oxygen toxicity Amniotic fluid embolism
Unknown	Fat embolism 'Neurogenic' (head injury, subarachnoid haemorrhage)

that the lung oedema can result from many causes and it is probable that two or more must operate in the same patient. Most of the patients who develop ARDS can pass through a state of shock (hence one synonym – shock lung). One of the important and puzzling features of ARDS is that the associated disease or condition is often sited in an organ remote from the lung. The recognition of ARDS depends on bedside observations of the respirations (breathing pattern), the blood gases and chest X-ray.

IV DIAGNOSIS AND ASSESSMENT

From the scientific point of view the diagnosis of respiratory failure requires measurement of the arterial blood gases. In the writer's opinion far too much stress is placed on the 'blood gases' and far too little attention given to the patient! A clinical diagnosis of acute respiratory failure can sometimes be made in a matter of seconds. Respiratory failure is present when the upper airway is obstructed or there is apnoea; in these situations analysis of the arterial blood is absurd. In other patients – and the instances are numerous – acute respiratory failure can pass unnoticed. For example, a patient can show increased breathing (hyperventilation) but deny dyspnoea, the chest

Table 6.4 Assessment of the patient (From *Essential Intensive Care*, with permission)

1. Breathlessness	5. Clinical signs of gas exchange
2. Cough and sputum	6. Arterial blood analysis
3. Breathing patterns	Oxygen
Decreased	Carbon dioxide
Increased	pH
Obesity or abdominal	7. Circulation
distension	Pulse and blood pressure
Paradoxical	Signs in the heart
Fatigue	CVP
	ECG
4. Respiratory measurements	
Frequency	8. Chest radiograph
Minute volume ventilation	
FVC, FEV_1	
PEF	

radiograph might be normal but nevertheless blood gas analysis reveals that gas exchange is defective. Clearly then, it is important to be constantly on the look out for acute respiratory failure and this is especially so in the intensive care patient. Whether the diagnosis is clear cut or still in the realms of a possibility, the assessment of a patient must be both thorough and systematic. Such an assessment is set out in the next section and summarized in Table 6.4. It should be appreciated that in any one disease causing acute respiratory failure, or in the individual patient, only one or two of the eight components may be relevant. A systematic assessment is especially important for the early recognition of acute respiratory failure and after a little experience can be carried out in a much shorter time than is required to read the section below.

1. Breathlessness or dyspnoea

It might be thought superfluous to have to define breathlessness, but the term is often used in a loose manner and confused with rapid breathing (tachypnoea), overbreathing (hyperpnoea) or excessive ventilation (hyperventilation). 'Dyspnoea is difficult, laboured, uncomfortable breathing; it is an unpleasant type of breathing though it is not painful in the usual sense of the word' (J.R. Comroe, 1966). Dyspnoea is of value in the assessment provided that certain limitations are understood. To start with the obvious: a drowsy patient or one in a coma cannot have symptoms; a patient can

Table 6.5 The grading of breathlessness due to disease of the heart or lungs (From *Essential Intensive Care*, with permission)

Grade 1	Dyspnoea on severe exertion such as running up two flights of stairs
Grade 2A	Dyspnoea on moderate exertion such as walking normally up two flights of stairs
Grade 2B	Dyspnoea on mild exertion such as walking slowly up one flight of stairs
Grade 3	Dyspnoea on minimal exertion such as walking from room to room
Grade 4	Dyspnoea at rest

complain of dyspnoea without having acute respiratory failure. Nevertheless dyspnoea in a patient in a surgical or trauma ward is an important pointer to the recognition of acute respiratory failure. Unfortunately the converse does not hold; such a patient can have acute respiratory failure without dyspnoea. To recapitulate, dyspnoea in the patient without known disease of the heart or lungs should alert the ward team to the development of acute respiratory failure, whether the patient has peritonitis or renal failure, a fractured pelvis or acute pancreatitis. When dyspnoea is present then its severity should be determined. The grade of dyspnoea is of value in the intensive care of the asthmatic and the patient with chronic lung disease. Breathlessness is a cardinal feature of this disease and the resulting disability can be used to grade the severity of an attack. Such grading avoids the difficulties in using ill-defined terms such as 'severe asthma' (how severe is severe?) or status asthmaticus. The grading developed in this unit helps to decide the need for hospital admission or intensive care. When a patient with advanced chronic lung disease develops an 'exacerbation' requiring admission to hospital, then dyspnoea is invariably severe; the rare exception is the patient in semi-coma or coma. The dyspnoea cannot be used to determine the severity of the respiratory failure. The grade of dyspnoea (Table 6.5) prior to the acute illness is decidedly relevant to the assessment because this will guide the therapy. When a patient has grade 3 dyspnoea prior to the acute illness then he runs a high risk of life-threatening acute respiratory failure and the therapy can be planned with the aim of survival. On the other hand a totally disabled man with long-standing grade 4 dyspnoea is unlikely to survive an acute and severe illness with or without intensive therapy. Indeed in many cases intensive therapy would be inappropriate.

Table 6.6 Causes of ineffective cough
(From *Essential Intensive Care*, with permission)

Suppression of painful cough
    Surgery   – thoracic
              – abdominal
    Pleurisy
    Tracheal pain

Cough reflex depressed or absent
    Semi-coma or coma
    Potent sedatives and analgesics
Insensitive mucosa (cigarette smokers)

Defective mechanics
    Chronic bronchitis
    Chest injury
    Neuro-muscular paralysis
    Laryngeal paralysis

---

2. Cough and sputum

In health important processes keep the airway clear of excess mucus or inhaled foreign material. Failure of these defences can lead to narrowed or blocked airways which cause absorption collapse. The first process is the normal working of the ciliated mucous membranes which is inhibited by hypoxia, anaesthetic gases, dry inhaled gas, and general dehydration of the body. Endotracheal suction also damages the cilia of the trachea and main bronchi. The functioning of the ciliated mucosa cannot be assessed at the bedside. Defective cilial activity should be suspected when the patient is dehydrated, has suffered hypoxia or has been allowed to breath dry gases for a long period.

A second defence is the cough mechanism (Table 6.6) which is a complex mixture of mechanics and reflex arcs. An effective cough can expel (raise) excess bronchial mucus or inhaled saliva or blood. The bedside investigation of coughing, often repeated at intervals, is an integral part of any assessment of respiratory failure either suspected or overt. The first question to ask oneself is, should this patient have a productive cough? For example does the patient have chronic bronchitis or bronchiectasis? Likewise during a severe attacks of asthma the physician will expect the patient to raise sputum* and failure to do so is a danger sign. When assessing a patient with

---

*   The appearance and consistency of a thick cellulose wallpaper paste, containing little grey plugs.

a chest injury or a recent abdominal or thoracic operation, but who denies the symptoms of chronic lung disease, it is equally important to test out the cough mechanics. The test is made by asking the patient to give a powerful cough and to try and raise sputum. When it is evident that this will cause severe pain an analgesic is given before making the assessment. In addition, the patient or a physiotherapist supports the injured chest or abdominal wall. Repeated trials should be made before concluding that the airways are free from sputum or the patient is unable to cough effectively. Various techniques of the physiotherapist can also be employed; these are percussion and assisted expiration (vibrations). An assessment of the cough mechanics in the drowsy subject requires a different approach. The cough reflex is stimulated with a suction catheter passed into the pharynx. This can either be carried out by the use of the laryngoscope or alternatively by passing the suction catheter through the nose and into the pharynx. During coma, the patient will have an artificial airway, either an endotracheal tube or a tracheostomy tube. In such instances the cough mechanics is tested by carrying out endotracheal suction. This procedure is described in Chapter 18. It should be mentioned here that during prolonged artificial ventilation testing the cough 'power' is an essential day-to-day assessment of progress.

An examination of the sputum is an obvious part of the assessment. The volume, colour and consistency are noted and a specimen is quickly despatched to the bacteriological laboratory. The results of Gram staining can be made available within the hour and bacterial pathogens can be identified within the next 24 hours.

3. Breathing patterns

The experienced observer can learn much from observing the respiratory movements of the chest and abdomen, i.e. the pattern of breathing. The observations should be made both during the traditional examination of the heart and lungs, i.e. at the side of the patient. and also from the foot or head of the bed. In the first instance the pattern should be classified as normal, decreased breathing or increased breathing. Observation of the breathing pattern is of value in all critically ill patients and during preoperative and post-operative assessments. The following are examples of abnormal breathing patterns. (i) In the first group respiratory movements are feeble or even difficult to detect. The first essential in such a patient is to ensure that the airway is clear and protected. The respiratory failure can then be confirmed or refuted by measurements. Some causes of the respiratory failure in this decreased breathing group are listed in Table 6.7. (ii) The trainee working in intensive care will at first, be surprised to learn that many

Table 6.7 Patterns of breathing in the intensive care patient (From *Essential Intensive Care*, with permission)

Cause	Associated symptoms
Group 1 Decreased breathing	
Self poisoning	Coma, circumstantial evidence
Potent sedatives or analgesics	
Following anaesthesia	
Brain damage	Head injury, hypertension, source of emboli
Polyneuritis Myasthenia gravis	Conscious, specific CNS signs
Chronic bronchitis	Natural history
Group 2 Increased breathing	
Pneumothorax Asthma Pneumonia	Natural history
Pulmonary embolism	DVT, surgery, trauma
Pulmonary aspiration	Coma, fits, vomit in the mouth or pharynx
Pulmonary oedema	Those of the cause (Table 6.3)
ARDS	Those of the preceding illness
Intra-abdominal sepsis Inflammatory bowel disease	Natural history

patients with acute respiratory failure show increased breathing. This purely descriptive term means that the breathing is excessive, either in frequency or depth, or in the muscular effort expended. The patient may or may not admit to dyspnoea. The label of increased breathing is preferred to hyperventilation because the latter implies that ventilation can be assessed without measurement, which is not the case. Blood gas analysis of this group of patients shows that, in the main, the failure is of the hypoxaemic variety. The lung pathology is either that of specific pathological process, e.g. asthma, or is one of the non-specific changes, such as oedema, already referred to. Such non-specific changes can be brought about by very varied diseases, some of which are listed in Table 6.7. It should be emphasized here that not all patients who show increased breathing, with or without dyspnoea, have respiratory failure. Important exceptions are the acidosis of diabetes or uraemia and, more rarely, following a head injury. (iii) Obesity or abdominal distension due to gas or fluid. Obesity restricts breathing and can reduce cough power. When the disease is advanced the patient shows reduced breathing and 'belly-breathes'. Obesity alone rarely causes respiratory failure but there is a high risk of failure following respiratory infection, surgery or trauma. The abdominal distension caused by intestinal ileus or ascites also restricts breathing by exerting pressure on the diaphragm. This is compensated by increased thoracic movements. (iv) See-saw breathing. This pattern of inco-ordinate breathing is readily recognised. The chest and abdomen see-saw in an alarming manner. During inspiration the chest expands and the abdomen becomes indrawn and these movements are reversed during expiration. See-saw breathing is found during states of impaired consciousness, but the pathophysiology is obscure. (v) Paradoxical breathing. During normal inspiration the thoracic cage expands in a symmetrical fashion. Paradoxical breathing refers to a state in which the thoracic cage moves inward during inspiration. This state is quite distinct from the indrawing of the lower ribs or intercostal spaces seen when infants have airway obstruction. The paradoxical breathing is usually limited to a segment of the thorax or hemithorax, the reason being that the paradox of the entire thorax, unless promptly detected and treated, is rapidly fatal. Paradoxical breathing due to multiple fractures of the ribs, sternum or costal cartilages is often caused by the impact of the steering wheel or seat belt of a motor vehicle. A segment of the thoracic cage is then rendered flail and moves inwards during inspiration. This in turn disrupts the mechanics of breathing and acute respiratory failure can follow. In some causes the paradox is difficult to detect and repeated examinations may be required. Obesity, oedema or surgical emphysema can conceal the paradox. (vi) Respiratory fatigue. There are many conditions which make it necessary for a patient to work hard to breathe and this can lead to fatigue of the respiratory muscles. Examples of conditions leading to respiratory fatigue are severe asthma, chronic bronchitis, advanced mitral valve disease, or the Adult Respiratory Distress Syndrome. During some of these diseases the continuous muscular work of breathing tires the patient and in all probability a state can be reached of true muscle weakness and fatigue, which seriously worsens the respiratory failure. At the present time the diagnosis of fatigue of the respiratory muscles is a clinical one. The respiratory pattern is that of increased breathing; the accessory muscles are in action continuously. When the load imposed on the muscles is both severe and prolonged the increased breathing gives way to decreased breathing and hypoxic cardiac arrest follows.

4. Clinical signs of gas exchange

The accurate recognition and practical management of respiratory failure were greatly aided by the invention of methods for measuring the tensions of carbon dioxide and oxygen in arterial or capillary blood. These measurements are now part of routine practice in the general intensive care unit but cannot supplant an informed clinical assessment. Unless the observer is aware of the signs of acute hypoxaemia and hypercapnia the diagnosis of acute respiratory failure may never be suspected and it is then unlikely that blood gas tensions will be measured! Acute and especially progressive hypoxaemia leads to generalized hypoxia and the brain is by far the most sensitive organ. The resulting brain failure (Chapter 10) leads initially to diminished cognition, conveniently labelled delirium. The manifestations are restlessness, irritability and disorientation in time. Should the gas exchange worsen and the PaO_2 fall to 2.7 kPa (20 mmHg) then consciousness is impaired; severe hypoxia causes brain death. The error in using cyanosis of the inside of the lip as an assessment of acute hypoxaemia is so great that no important therapeutic decisions should depend on this sign. The same criticism does not apply to the crude estimation of the oxygen saturation of a sample of arterial blood contained in a syringe. Pink blood has a PaO_2 above 7.0 kPa (53 mmHg), blood which shows detectable cyanosis has a PaO_2 of about 5.0 kPa (38 mmHg) and the blue-black blood has a PaO_2 of less than 4.0 kPa (30 mmHg).

Hypercapnia adversely affects all organ function but clinically brain failure is the most obvious. There is depression of the nervous system with somnolence, impaired consciousness and convulsions. Consciousness is rarely lost below $PaCO_2$ values of 10.0 kPa (75 mmHg). Hypercapnia can also cause tremor, headache, sweating, dilated veins and warm extremities.

5. Respiratory measurements

The pulmonary function laboratory of the hospital possess many techniques with which to investigate lung function, but only a few of these are helpful during intensive care. The reason for this is that many of the tests require the patient to carry out manoeuvres which, the critically ill cannot perform. The measurements of value during intensive care are as follows: respiratory frequency (f), Expired Minute Volume Ventilation ($\dot{V}_E$), Forced Vital Capacity (FVC), Forced Expiratory Volume in the first second (FEV_1) and Peak Expiratory Flow (PEF). The equipment required to make these measurements at the bedside is portable and should be readily available in the unit. These four measurements can be used in the detection of respiratory failure and in recording progress, that is monitoring. A particular measurement is chosen according to the clinical problem and should relate to the natural history of the respiratory failure.

(i) *Respiratory frequency.* When rapid breathing (tachypnoea) is found in a surgical, orthopaedic or trauma patient it draws attention to disordered lung function and to the possibility that the patient has developed acute respiratory failure. The observer should consider pulmonary embolism, oedema, or segmental collapse and make a search for these. Alternative explanations are shock or bacteraemia. Should rapid breathing or abnormally slow respiration follow a head injury then severe brain damage is probable. When the respiratory frequency is low and the breathing decreased, then depression of the respiratory centre should be suspected. Causes seen in the ICU are sedative poisoning, subarachnoid haemorrhage or encephalitis.

(ii) *Minute Volume Ventilation* ($\dot{V}_E$). It will be recalled that in the healthy subject total ventilation is the sum of alveolar ventilation and dead-space ventilation. In normal subjects the dead-space ventilation can be predicted with reasonable accuracy on the basis of previous measurements. From this information it follows that measurements of the total ventilation provide a measure of alveolar ventilation. This relationship does not hold in the intensive care patient and so alveolar ventilation cannot be calculated from the total ventilation. This does not mean that measurements of total ventilation have no place in the assessment. Measurements, especially serial ones, are of value both in the detection of respiratory failure and in monitoring its course. In day-to-day practice total ventilation is expressed as a volume of gas exhaled over one minute. This volume is conveniently measured by a Wright's spirometer. The instrument is fitted to a moulded rubber face-piece or connected to the endotracheal tube. In the conscious patient the nature of the test is explained and the face-piece kept in position. A few minutes are allowed to pass before taking a reading. The result is the minute volume ventilation expressed in litres. In healthy adults at rest the normal range varies according to body weight (or surface area), sex and metabolic rate; a rough guide is 5.0–7.0 l/min and a more accurate value is quickly obtained from tables. The chief $\dot{V}_E$ use of in the ICU is to assess total ventilation in the patient who shows decreased breathing, for example acute sedative poisoning without shock or pulmonary complications. In the adult patient, a $\dot{V}_E$ below 5.0 litres indicates that respiratory failure is a probability and artificial respiration should be started. Ideally the blood gases should be measured before starting artificial respiration but this analysis should not be allowed to delay treatment beyond a few minutes. Similar principles apply to other causes of decreased breathing, for example head injury or polyneuropathy. In the patients referred to, there are invariably signs of respiratory failure and the $\dot{V}_E$ is used to confirm the diagnosis or to monitor total ventilation. Measurements of $\dot{V}_E$ are also of value in the recognition of respiratory failure in the patient showing increased breathing (high output). In these patients the respiratory failure develops after non-thoracic trauma, bacterial infection, acute upper gastrointestinal haemorrhage, etc. Most of the patients have been treated for shock and the circulation is stable when the increased breathing is observed. The $\dot{V}_E$ is greatly increased (14–25 l) and the result is of value in confirming that all is not well with lung function. The arterial blood at this stage of the respiratory failure shows hypocapnia and hypoxaemia.

(iii)   *Forced Vital Capacity (FVC)* is the volume of air which the subject can force from the lungs following a maximum inspiration. The normal values vary according to age, sex and height. For intensive care the test is carried out at the bedside by using a dry spirometer and mouth-piece. The spirometer should have a device to enable the FEV₁ to be obtained at the same time. The FVC is of value in the following situations. Firstly in the reduced breathing group of diseases, polyneuropathy, myasthenia, the FVC can help to confirm or monitor respiratory failure. When the FVC is 25% of the predicted value then the patient is likely to need assisted ventilation. On the other hand daily readings which show an improving trend would indicate recovery from paralytic respiratory failure. The second use of the FVC is to help in the pre-operative assessment of the patient with chronic lung disease. When the FVC is greatly reduced to say one-third of the normal value, then there is a considerable risk of 'chest complications' developing in the immediate post-operative period. After-care in the ICU may help to reduce this risk of acute respiratory failure.

(iv)   *Forced Vital Capacity one second (FEV₁).*   In health over 70% of the FVC can be forced out in the first second. In contrast when the bronchi or bronchioles are narrowed due to chronic bronchitis, emphysema or asthma (generalized obstruction to air flow) this value falls to below 50%. In a patient with acute-on-chronic respiratory failure due to chronic lung disease, measurements of FEV₁ taken prior to the acute illness are of value in planning the therapy. Thus, if the preceding FEV₁ was in the range of 0.5–0.7 litre then acute respiratory failure will probably threaten life. The FEV₁ therefore serves as a warning to the therapeutic team, who may decide on a plan of intensive observation including blood gas analysis. On the other hand the greatly reduced FEV₁, when interpreted together with the patient's age, respiratory disability and his attitude to the disease, may cause the physician to decide not to recommend intensive care. During acute-on-chronic respi-

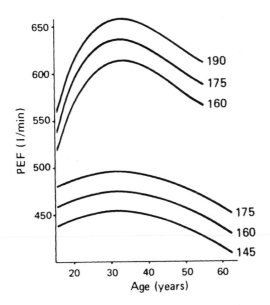

Figure 6.3 Peak expiratory flow (PEF, l/min) for healthy subjects. The upper three curves are for males and the lower curves for females; heights in cm. (From *Essential Intensive Care*, with permission)

ratory failure the patient is rarely able to perform tests of FVC and FVC_1; consequently they cannot be used in assessment.

(v) *The Peak Expiratory Flow (PEF)* is a quantitative version of the candle test in which, after a maximum inspiration, the subject blows out as rapidly as possible through the open mouth in the direction of a lighted candle placed at 200 mm. In using the PEF meter the subject 'gives a great puff' through the mouth-piece and the meter records the PEF in litres per minute. Normal values are shown in Figure 6.3. The meter has the merits of compactness and portability, weighing only 1.8 kg. Readings of PEF are of considerable help in assessing an attack of asthma. As with the FEV_1, it is of additional value if determinations have been made when the asthmatic patient is at her best; trends are of more value than absolute figures. An unexpected decrease from 450 to 250 l/min is a warning sign and especially so if the reading is unchanged by a bronchodilator. During the asthmatic attack, 4-hourly readings contribute to the plan of intensive observation.

6. Arterial blood analysis

For intensive care, gas exchange between the lungs and blood can be quantified by measuring the 'blood gases'. Strictly speaking these are carbon dioxide and oxygen, but the pH is always measured at the same time and the result used in the assessment of respiratory failure. The pH is not a blood gas but is a measure of the acid-base balance of the blood. The three variables, blood oxygen, carbon dioxide and pH are of value in confirming the diagnosis. judging the severity and progress, and guiding or monitoring the therapy. It should again be explained that these measurements cannot replace knowledge and experience of the natural histories of respiratory failure. Also, even in skilled hands there are considerable errors in the measurements of these variables. In common with many measurements made in the hospital laboratory the blood gases are frequently misused and incorrectly interpreted.

In the brief review of the blood gases which follows it is assumed that the reader possesses an elementary knowledge of the carriage of oxygen and carbon dioxide by the blood.

(i) The blood sample is commonly taken from the femoral, brachial or radial artery, the choice depending on the routine procedure or build of the patient. In very obese subjects it can be nearly impossible to take the sample from the femoral artery. When frequent samples are necessary over a period of a few hours then it is customary to leave a plastic cannula in the radial or brachial artery, for this will reduce the discomfort caused by repeated punctures. Unless the patient is heavily sedated the procedure is explained to the patient who must anticipate momentary pain. A fine needle will help to reduce the discomfort and most blood-gas machines require only a small sample. A small volume of heparin solution (5000 units per ml) is drawn up in a 2.0 ml syringe and the air expelled, leaving the dead-space of the syringe filled with heparin. The skin over an artery is sterilized with hibitane in ethanol and the sample withdrawn. Firm pressure is applied immediately with a gauze pad to prevent haematoma. The sample of arterial blood is next analysed as quickly as possible. When some delay is unavoidable the syringe containing the blood is immersed in iced water or stored in a refrigerator at $4°C$ to minimize the changes which occur when blood is removed from the circulation. The time elapsed from the taking of the sample to the analysis is noted. In addition to the following measurements: core temperature, $\dot{V}_E$, frequency of breathing and the inspired concentration of oxygen.

(ii) *Oxygen in the blood.* The oxygen in a sample of blood can be expressed in one of three ways. Firstly as the content (concentration) expressed in ml of oxygen per 100 ml. The second approach is to obtain the percentage saturation of the haemoglobin ($HbO_2\%$); for example the arterial blood of a resting healthy subject is 95% saturated. The third method is to measure the partial pressure of oxygen in the sample (PaO_2) expressed in mmHg or the SI unit the kilopascal (kPa). In healthy subjects the PaO_2 varies considerably with age but in day-to-day therapy this variation can be ignored and the normal range of PaO_2, when breathing air taken as 12.0–13.0 kPa (90–100 mmHg). When greater precision is required an equation can be used to calculate the predicted value for a healthy subject:

$$PaO_2 \text{ (kPa)} = 14.1 - 0.3 \times \text{age (years)}$$

Values below the predicted normal are referred to as hypoxaemia and this can be graded as moderate, 6.5–9.5 kPa (50–70 mmHg), or severe, 4.0–6.5 kPa (30–50 mmHg).

So far the results were obtained on samples of arterial blood and monitoring was intermittent, continuous monitoring of the blood oxygen would benefit some patients when there are rapid fluctuations in gas exchange. A continuous reading of the oxygen saturation can be obtained by means of the oximeter. A brief description of the essentials is given next. Blood at 37°C flows rapidly through the capillaries of the inside of the lower lip. This is a good place to look for cyanosis, a valuable but crude guide to severe hypoxaemia. The lobe of the ear or finger can also be used, provided that the blood flow is rapid. The degree of oxygenation of the blood is expressed as the percentage saturation (SaO_2) which closely mirrors the haemoglobin saturation (HbO_2). The SaO_2 can be measured on a blood sample or through the skin; the latter is called transcutaneous oximetry. A tiny lamp illuminates the skin with red light of a specified wave length. At this particular wave-length the amount of light absorbed or reflected is very different for oxygenated or reduced haemoglobin; this is the key to the technology. The light reflected from the capillary blood is collected and the amount of light can be used as a measure of the oxygen saturation. The SaO_2 is displayed and the result is correct to about 2%. The same instrument will count the pulsations in the small blood vessels and display the pulse rate; hence the name pulse-oximeter.

(iii) *Alveolar/arterial pressure gradient.* Having measured the PaO_2 the next step is to obtain an estimate of the pressure gradient for oxygen between the alveolus and arterial blood; the alveolar/arterial gradient: $PAO_2 - PaO_2$. The calculation is quite straightforward but requires measurement of the arterial PCO_2 (which is taken to be the same as the $PACO_2$) and inspired oxygen tension (PIO_2). The equations are as follows:

$$PAO_2 = PIO_2 - \frac{PaCO_2}{0.8} \qquad [1]$$

Alveolar/arterial gradient $= PAO_2 - PaO_2$ $\qquad$ [2]

In healthy subjects the pressure gradient is quite small (Table 6.8) but varies with age and during oxygen therapy. The variation in the oxygen gradient with age during oxygen breathing cannot be ignored because the gradient increases considerably with age. It is also useful to have available normal values for the oxygen gradient when breathing 40% to 60% oxygen since these concentrations correspond with those used during oxygen therapy. Such normal values are given in Table 6.8. The use of this information is best illustrated by an example. A patient aged 40 years is breathing 40% oxygen; the barometer reads 106 kPa. The blood gases are found to be: $PaO_2 = 15.0$ kPa, $PaCO_2 = 4.0$ kPa. How does the alveolar/arterial gradient compare with the normal? The first step is to calculate the PIO_2 from

$$PIO_2 = \text{(atmospheric pressure} - \text{water vapour pressure at } 37°C)}$$
$$\times FIO_2$$

$$= (106 - 6.0) \times \frac{40}{100} = 40 \text{ kPa}$$

The PAO_2 is now calculated by using equation [1] above

$$PAO_2 = 40 - \frac{4.0}{0.8} = 35 \text{ kPa}$$

Finally the gradient is obtained from equation [2]

Alveolar/arterial gradient $= 35 - 15 = 20$ kPa

This can now be compared with the normal of 2.5–7.9 kPa obtained from Table 6.8. The end result is that our patient has a four-fold increase in the gradient. Unfortunately, the complexity of the alveolar/oxygen gradient in healthy subjects also requires information on the gradient during artificial respiration. Clearly this information is difficult to obtain, since healthy conscious subjects rarely want to be treated to a spell of IPPV! The nearest to the ideal experiment is general anaesthesia with IPPV controlled by means of a muscle relaxant. Under these circumstances the gradient is similar to that found during spontaneous respiration and the values in Table 6.8 can therefore be used.

(iv) Carbon dioxide in the blood is present in three forms: As the bicarbonates of sodium and potassium, as carbonic acid, and carbamino-haemoglobin. For day-to-day patient care we calculate the total carbon dioxide (bicarbonate + carbonic acid), and the partial pressure of carbon dioxide is measured in the blood-gas machine. To interpret the results obtained in disease certain physiological relationships are required. In the arterial blood of healthy subjects at rest the PCO_2 ($PaCO_2$) lies within the range of 4.7–6.0 kPa (35–45 mmHg). The first relationship is that the PCO_2 of blood is proportional to the carbonic acid in the blood. When, due to disease, the PCO_2 rises or falls the concentration of carbonic acid of the blood causes a change in the acid-base balance of the blood and other body fluids. The next relationship is that between the PCO_2 of arterial blood and the PCO_2 of the alveolar gas ($PACO_2$); for our purposes they are the same. The $PaCO_2$ is related to the balance between the removal of carbon dioxide by the lung, that is alveolar ventilation, and the production of CO_2 by the tissues according to:

$$PaCO_2 = \frac{CO_2 \ production}{alveolar \ ventilation} \times 0.86$$

For routine intensive care, a change in the CO_2 production is ignored and the $PaCO_2$ is then used as a measure – the most important measure – of alveolar ventilation. Thus when the $PaCO_2$ is found to be raised, a state referred to as hypercapnia, it is deduced that alveolar ventilation is reduced, and vice versa. The relationship between the PCO_2 (and therefore carbonic acid) of the blood to the concentration of bicarbonate takes the form of the familiar carbon dioxide association curve. Results obtained in this unit for healthy subjects are shown in Figure 6.4. At rest the PCO_2 usually lay within the quoted range of 4.7–6.0 kPa (35–45 mmHg) and the corresponding bicarbonate was 19–26 mmol/l. The PCO_2 was lowered by positive pressure breathing by a respirator, the subjects own respiration being assisted by the machine. This procedure quickly lowered the PCO_2 to approximately 2.7 kPa (20 mmHg), but there was only a small decrease in the plasma bicarbonate. When the healthy volunteers breathed 9.0% carbon dioxide the PCO_2 rose to about 9.0 kPa (67 mmHg), but again there was little change in the bicarbonate. In this study the plasma bicarbonate was measured and not calculated by the method described later. From the results shown in Figure 6.4 we can see that large changes in PCO_2 cause only minor changes in bicarbonate. This relationship is equally valid for acute changes in PCO_2 occurring in disease. If the reader compares this association curve with that in most textbooks of physiology, a striking difference will be evident. The reason is that the 'classical' association curve was obtained by experiments

Table 6.8 Alveolar arterial oxygen pressure gradients in healthy subjects: variations with inspired oxygen concentration (F_IO_2) and age (From *Essential Intensive Care*, with permission)

Age (years)	F_IO_2 (%)	Gradient (kPa)	(mmHg)
20–30	21	0 to 1.73	0 to 13
	40	2.4 to 3.5	18 to 26
	60	2.9 to 6.0	22 to 45
	100	2.9 to 5.9	22 to 44
40–50	21	0.5 to 2.3	4 to 17
	40	2.5 to 7.9	19 to 59
	60	3.3 to 10.4	25 to 78
	100	4.4 to 10.9	33 to 82
60 and over	21	1.2 to 3.5	9 to 26
	40	4.9 to 10.9	30 to 82
	60	5.2 to 15.0	39 to 113
	100	3.4 to 14.2	27 to 107

outside the body and this curve does not represent the true physiological behaviour of the body.

(v) *pH has immediate relevance to the assessment of respiratory failure.* The pH of the blood is the best measure we have of the acidity or alkalinity of the blood. Expressed in an alternative terminology, the pH is a measure of the hydrion concentration. The normal range at rest is 7.35–7.45 units. The pH of blood is related to the balance between acid and base and this relationship is given by an equation known as the Henderson–Hasselbalch equation.

$$pH = 6.1 + \log \frac{\text{(bicarbonate)}}{\text{(carbonic acid)}}$$

When some constants have been added to the above equation, a quantitative relationship is obtained. It is then possible to calculate one of the three variables if the remaining two variables are measured. In the blood–gas laboratory of the ICU, the PCO_2 and pH are measured and the bicarbonate can then be calculated. Some blood–gas machines perform the calculation automatically and display the result on the instrument. If this luxury facility is not available the bicarbonate can quickly be obtained by use of a chart (known as a nomogram) shown in Figure 6.5. To use this chart a straight edge or taut thread is placed across the chart so that the pH and PCO_2 are on the straight edge. The bicarbonate is then read off. The value for

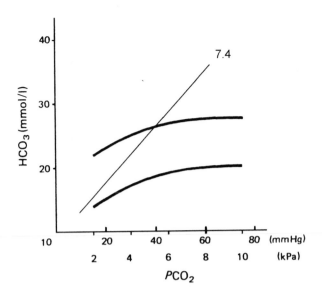

Figure 6.4 Carbon dioxide titration curves obtained *in vivo* on healthy subjects. Normal values lie within the two curves and pH 7.4 lies along the oblique straight line (From *Essential Intensive Care*, with permission)

bicarbonate obtained in this way is adequate in most cases, but in the remaining patients it is necessary to measure the bicarbonate, and for research this must always be done. To return to the experiments referred to earlier, during which the PCO_2 was varied within the range 2.5–9.0 kPa (19–68 mmHg). The pH was measured at the same time and the relationship of this variable to PCO_2 is shown in Figure 6.6. It will be seen that when the PCO_2 rises, pH falls and vice versa. The underlying physiology is straightforward. An increase in PCO_2 leads to an increase in carbonic acid and the concentration of hydrion increases, that is the pH falls. The defences of the body against such a pH change are minimal when the increase in acid occurs rapidly. Parallel changes occur when the PCO_2 falls due to over-ventilation of the alveoli. In this case the concentration of carbonic acid falls and the pH rises above normal. A fall in pH below 7.35 is termed acidosis (or acidaemia) and a rise above 7.45 an alkalosis. The pH limits compatible with survival are 6.8 and 7.8 units. When the pH is reduced by an excess of carbonic acid (hypercapnia) the term respiratory acidosis is used and a high pH due to a reduced concentration of carbonic acid (hypocapnia) is labelled a respiratory alkalosis. This and other aspects of acid-base balance are considered further in Chapter 5.

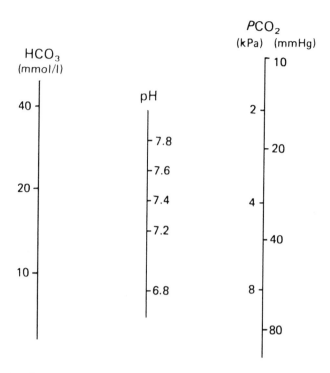

Figure 6.5 Nomogram relating pH, PCO$_2$ and HCO$_3$. A straight edge placed against any two variables will give the third variable (From *Essential Intensive Care*, with permission)

7. Circulation

Since pulmonary function consists of the exchange of gas between blood and air, examination of the circulation is an essential part of the assessment. A disorder of the circulation can be the primary cause of the respiratory failure, the lungs being previously normal; for example acute myocardial infarction. Alternatively, a specific disease of the lungs may have caused secondary changes in the circulation, as in severe asthma. The assessment of the circulation can vary in its depth from palpation of the pulse to measurement of the pulmonary artery pressure or cardiac output; a few examples are introduced at this stage.

(i) *The pulse and blood pressure.* The heart rate – assuming sinus rhythm – is of limited value in the assessment; this is because very varied and numerous pathological processes can cause a sinus tachycardia. Trends in

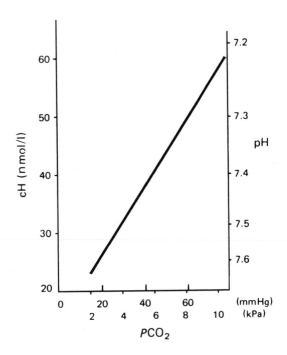

Figure 6.6 Relationship *in vivo* between cH, PCO_2 and pH in healthy subjects (From *Essential Intensive Care*, with permission)

the heart rate help to assess progress, good or bad. In severe asthma the pulse rate is very valuable in assessing the severity of the attack; a rate of 120 per min means severe respiratory failure and when the rate reaches 140 the disease is an immediate threat to life. Also in asthma the strength of the pulse can vary significantly during the respiratory cycle – *pulsus paradoxus*. This is an ominous sign because it means that the airways obstruction is so severe that the filling and emptying of the heart are impeded. When a major pulse cannot be felt then cardiac arrest is probable and respiratory arrest invariably follows. Hypotension is less dramatic but also important in the assessment. This is because most patients in severe hypotension have hypoxaemic respiratory failure even though lung structure is normal.

(ii) *Signs in the heart.* Examination of the heart can help in one of two ways. A cardiac diagnosis, e.g. mitral stenosis tells us the cause of the acute respiratory failure. A gallop rhythm would point to left ventricular failure and pulmonary oedema as the cause of the defective gas exchange. In contrast signs in the heart can be used to assess the severity of the respiratory failure when the heart is not primarily involved in three conditions, asthma, chronic lung disease and severe pulmonary embolism. Right heart strain due to pulmonary hypertension can be predicted when a rapid forceful heart beat is felt immediately below the xiphisternum.

(iii) *The pressure of blood in the vena cava is known as the central venous pressure (CVP).* Measurements of CVP are routine in the ICU and help to determine the cause of acute respiratory failure and assess the severity of the cardiovascular disturbances. Thus a raised CVP can help to determine the cause of pulmonary oedema. Conversely a low CVP in the shocked patient implies hypovolaemia.

(iv) ECG. Assessment of the circulation is incomplete without a standard 12-lead ECG. The ECG helps to place the cause of the acute respiratory failure into one of two pigeon holes; heart disease came first or it is secondary to lung disease. In the first instance the ECG can confirm a diagnosis of acute myocardial infarction, or show left ventricular strain in a patient with pulmonary oedema due to hypertension. In the second group of patients with cardio-respiratory failure, lung function failed first and led to secondary heart failure. Examples are the obstructed airway or depressed ventilation due to drugs. Initially, the ECG shows sinus tachycardia and only when the state of asphyxia is advanced will signs of injury appear. In two lung diseases the ECG helps to assess the stresses on the heart. In severe asthma the ECG can show certain danger signs, and in acute respiratory failure due to chronic lung disease the ECG signs of right ventricular hypertrophy or 'strain' point to the advanced stage of the disease. Finally, the obvious should be emphasized, namely that a normal ECG does not exclude acute respiratory failure.

8. Chest radiograph

Radiographs of the chest taken with a mobile machine are routine practice in the assessment of the severely ill or injured patient. This principle applies to all illnesses and not only to diseases of the lungs and heart. The technique requires brief consideration. For optimum interpretation of the film the patient should be upright (the erect film of the ambulatory), but in the critically ill we make do with the trunk elevated to about 30° to the horizontal. When there is severe hypotension, the patient is left supine. The posture is noted on the X-ray request form. A plate is positioned behind the thorax in direct contact with the skin. The X-ray tube is adjusted so that the beam is perpendicular to the plate and at a distance of about 2 metres. When

Table 6.9 Chest radiograph of the intensive care patient: radiological terminology (From *Essential Intensive Care*, with permission)

	Term	Signs
1.	Absorption collapse:	Homogeneous or irregular shadowing in part or the whole of the lung field without an air bronchogram. Wedge shaped shadow of segmental collapse.
2.	Consolidation:	Homogeneous or irregular shadowing in part or the whole of the lung field with an air bronchogram.
3.	Oedema:	Enlarged hila: increase in the hilar shadows. Woolly opacity: circular opacity of 2–3 cm in diameter. Prominent vascular pattern. Homogeneous opacity: uniform opacity in part or whole of a lung field.

possible, the exposure is made at the height of inspiration. The following radiographic data are recorded on a small blackboard adjoining the patient; milliamperes (mA), kilovolts (kVp), time in seconds. This arrangement facilitates a comparison of sequential radiographs of a patient. In the patient with a closed chest injury additional films may be required to recognize one of the following: fractured ribs, torn diaphragm or mediastinal emphysema.

A brief account on the interpretation of the X-ray is needed by the trainee. Experience in this unit has shown that many of the commonly used terms are frequently inaccurate and are certainly of no value to the therapeutic team. Examples are 'inflammatory shadowing bacterial infection or consolidation/collapse'. The ICU will need a standardized terminology of the acute changes in the lung fields leaving aside obvious lesions such as lung abscess or pneumothorax. Our interpretation is based on the use of simple descriptive terms which can be correlated with one or more of the following pathological processes in the lung: absorption collapse, consolidation or oedema. The diagnostic signs used are given in Table 6.9. A few further points require emphasis. The chest radiograph in sedative poisoning, paralysis of the respiratory muscles or severe asthma can be quite normal and cannot therefore be used to assess respiratory failure due to one of these causes. Secondly the radiographic signs of pulmonary oedema occur relatively late in the evolution of this condition. Unfortunately, this also applies to the Adult Respiratory Distress Syndrome.

7
Shock and heart failure

I   DEFINITION, CLASSIFICATION AND CAUSES
II ASSESSMENT OF THE CIRCULATION

I DEFINITION, CLASSIFICATION AND CAUSES

Shock is one of many patterns of circulatory failure. To be more precise there are several patterns of shock, hence the term 'shock syndromes'. There are two denominators common to each syndrome; hypotension and a general failure to distribute blood and therefore oxygen to the tissues. The consequences are functional or structural changes in the organs and tissues; at best they are temporary and reversible. The other end of the spectrum is death. The onset of shock is sudden or rapid and its duration is minutes or hours; the important exception is septic shock, shortly to be described. We believe that shock should be separated from transient hypotension. This presents as vasovagal syncope and the blood pressure usually returns to normal spontaneously. It may follow interventions such as physiotherapy, turning of the patient and administration of sedatives or anaesthetic agents. Shock can be classified into three types (Table 7.1) according to the principle disturbance in the circulation. In hypovolaemia shock the dominant patho- logical process is a reduced circulating volume. This is textbook shock. The acute hypovolaemia results from loss of either blood, plasma or saline from the circulation. The causes (Table 7.1) are therefore readily understood; external or internal haemorrhage, burns, fractures and saline depletion. Shock due to saline depletion (dehydration) represents severe losses of sodium and water (Chapter 4). The saline is most commonly lost from the gastrointestinal tract either as vomit, gastric aspirate or diarrhoea. Occa- sionally the kidney wastes saline and the resulting depletion causes shock. In the second type the primary fault is in the heart, a failure of the ventricular muscle. This type of shock is labelled cardiogenic but this term is sometimes restricted to the severe and persistent shock of acute myocardial infarction. A very different pathological process can also cause heart failure. Mechanical obstruction to the emptying and/or filling of the heart when both acute and severe leads to shock. This shock syndrome can be seen in one of four conditions: asthma, tension pneumothorax, severe valvular heart disease, or massive pulmonary embolus. A fifth cause, pericardial tamponade, is so

Table 7.1 Classification of shock, causes and pathophysiology (From *Essential Intensive Care*, with permission)

Type	Cause	Pathological process
Hypovolaemic	Haemorrhage, burns, saline depletion, soft tissue injury, fractures, anaphylaxis	Reduced circulating volume
Heart failure	Acute myocardial infarction Acute poisoning Bacteraemia, toxaemia	Muscle failure, dysrhythmia
	Asthma, tension pneumothorax	Impaired filling and emptying of the heart hypoxaemia
	Pulmonary embolism	Impaired emptying, hypoxaemia
Neurogenic	Head injury, subarachnoid haemorrhage, tetraplegia	Damage to the medullary control centre

rare in the general ICU that it can be safely omitted. In the third type of shock, neurogenic, the primary lesion is either in the brain or the spinal cord. Neurogenic shock is seen in the general ICU during the state of brain death. These various types of shock may co-exist in various combinations, particularly in the elderly. For example, the patient with cardiac impairment who has had inadequate peri-operative fluid replacement and then develops a chest infection will be seen by all trainees in hospital practice.

The next problem is to define the type of shock associated with systemic inflammation and microbial infection. Let us start with two familiar illnesses. A patient with a chronic urinary tract infection develops a bacteraemia, subsequently confirmed. There is shivering, fever, tachycardia, hypotension and cold skin. One or more other body systems may suffer damage to give delirium (Chapter 10), oliguria or coagulopathy (Chapter 13). This is shock caused by a bacteraemia. The second illness has a contrasting natural history, with or without clinical sepsis. Intra- abdominal abscesses indicate a microbial cause. In contrast, a patient with multiple injuries, properly resuscitated, develops signs of systemic inflammation and hypotension. Similarly, cases of severe haemorrhage, burns, acute pancreatitis or inflammatory bowel disease show the same clinical picture. The signs are: a 'toxic' looking patient; temperature commonly above 38°C, but may be below 36°C; warm, dry skin; tachycardia and hypotension but the cardiac output can be high; increased breathing; WBC count greater than 12 or less than 4 ($\times 10^9$/l). Even in the clinically septic patient the blood cultures are frequently sterile and unfortunately we still do not have a reliable test for bacterial toxaemia. This syndrome has found an acceptable label, the Systemic Inflammatory Reaction Syndrome (American College of Chest Physicians, 1992). When a microbial cause is proven the term septic shock is applied. Our definitions are complete.

II ASSESSMENT OF THE CIRCULATION

Assessment of the shock patient has to be fitted into the priority list for the individual. In nearly every case the priority list reads: upper airway, ventilation and circulation. The assessment of the circulation aims at obtaining information on the performance of the heart and on the blood flow to the tissues, especially those most susceptible to hypoxia. An ideal assessment would provide the following information: the cardiac output, peripheral vascular resistance, and distribution of blood flow to the brain, kidney and muscles. This is a tall order even for the most elaborately equipped shock units; in the poor district general hospital it is sheer fantasy. Fortunately simple methods of assessment will give enough information to treat patients and to obtain good results. The methods of assessing the circulation can be placed into one of three grades (Table 7.2) starting with the purely clinical and extending to haemodynamic data obtained by invasive methods. Our practice is to regularly use Grades I and II and to employ electronic pressure measurements when this is essential and then earlier rather than later. The performance of the heart is assessed by the pulse, blood pressure, CVP and measurement of the PAWP. The blood flow to the skin, brain and kidney is assessed by clinical examination, by measuring the skin temperature, by assessing cerebration and, lastly, by recording the urine output. Disturbances in pulmonary gas exchange or acid–base balance are assessed by measuring the pH, $PACO_2$ and PaO_2 of the arterial blood.

1. Pulse and blood pressure

From a forefinger on the radial pulse an experienced observer obtains valuable information on the circulation. The relevant observations are rate, rhythm and the volume of the pulse. A pulse which is excessively slow (less than 40) or very fast (greater than 160) suggests that a dysrhythmia is a contributing cause of the shock. Similar considerations apply to an irregular pulse. Changes in the pulse rate over minutes or hours, i.e. trends, can be recorded accurately by the intensive care nurse. A sinus tachycardia in the shocked patient which showed a downward trend would indicate improvement in the circulation. The volume of the pulse is the best clinical guide

Table 7.2 Assessment and monitoring during shock: the three grades of technology (From *Essential Intensive Care*, with permission)

Grade	Equipment
I Pulse, BP, cerebration, skin temperature, urine output	Trained observer
II I plus CVP plus measured skin temperature ECG Blood gases	Trained observer, CVP line, saline manometer, electrical thermometer ECG monitor Blood gas machine
III I plus II plus intravascular pressures, cardiac output Lactate	I plus II plus electronic equipment Biochemical laboratory

we have of the arterial flow. A reduced pulse volume is an important feature of both hypovolaemic shock and heart failure. Taking the blood pressure with a mercury sphygmomanometer is necessary for the diagnosis and invaluable for assessing the severity and response to treatment. The intensive care nurse can obtain reliable, i.e. reproducible results, and the trends are especially reliable. In severe shock when the systolic pressure is below 50.0 mmHg there is a significant discrepancy between the value obtained by the sphygmomanometer and the true intra-arterial pressure measured electronically. In this situation the sphygmomanometer reads low. When this limitation is recognized measurements of the blood pressure made by the intensive care nurse are of the utmost value, a fact substantiated by extensive investigations.

2. Skin

Clinical examination of the skin supplemented by measurement of its temperature can be used to assess the blood flow through the skin and in turn used as an indirect assessment of the circulation. The clinical observations are described first. A pale, cold and sweating skin is a characteristic feature of haemorrhage leading to hypovolaemic shock; excess circulating catecholamines are responsible. The observations are made on the skin of the dorsum of the hand and foot and over the shins. A low temperature and pallor are the more reliable signs and are found in both hypovolaemic shock and heart failure. These two signs indicate circulatory insufficiency and repeated observations are valuable in monitoring the course of the shock. Thus persistence of the signs is unfavourable but a rising skin temperature and return of colour indicate improvement. Blood flow through the capillaries is assessed by examination of the nailbed of a finger and toe. Pressure on the nail with the finger produces blanching of the nailbed. When the circulation is normal then the colour returns immediately after the release of pressure. A delay of several seconds indicates circulatory insufficiency, at least in the hand or foot. Clinical monitoring is invaluable and in some units is supplemented by measuring the skin temperature electronically. The electrical thermometer is robust, reliable and the technique is non-invasive, causing no discomfort. An electrode is attached to the skin with micropore tape. The recording sites are usually the big toe or the lower limb a few centimetres above the ankle. The electrical thermometer is switched on and the skin temperature read and then recorded along with the core temperature. Readings of 20–25°C are low and values of 23–35°C are high. Repeated observations will indicate a trend.

3. Brain

A precipitous fall in the blood flow to the brain causes immediate changes in function and these are easily recognized clinically. Depending on the degree of cerebral hypoxia the symptoms vary from impaired intellect to coma. Simple clinical observations will suffice to monitor cerebral function and the results provide indirect evidence of blood flow to the brain. The examination consists of determining the level of consciousness and recording the result on a scale; we use the Glasgow coma scale (Teasdale and Jennett, 1974; Chapter 10). The assessment of brain function in common with the other assessments must be modified according to the clinical situation. During severe shock more attention is paid to treatment than assessment. The assessment of brain function may be impossible or difficult when there is an associated head injury, general anaesthesia or when a potent analgesic has been given.

4. Kidney

During shock blood flow to the kidney is reflected in the urine flow. This didactic formula is very valuable but limitations on its interpretation will be emphasized. When shock is anything other than transient the bladder should be catheterized so that urine formation can be accurately measured. For this purpose the end of the catheter is connected to a urinometer. During the early and often hectic minutes of resuscitation the urine flow can be judged by the drip rate from the catheter into the urinometer and later the volume is recorded at hourly intervals. For the present purposes anuria is defined as no detectable urine and oliguria as a flow of urine of less than 50 ml/h. Before and during the treatment of shock oliguria implies defective blood flow and an increase in the flow points to an improvement in the overall state of the circulation. This interpretation is incorrect if the oliguria could be the result of a nephrotoxic drug or bacterial toxin. In this instance the oliguria is due to intrinsic renal failure. When, following treatment, the urine flow exceeds 50 ml/h the circulation is adequate to maintain vital functions; the results of the other assessments will decide whether the circulation is now normal. In contrast oliguria may persist although the blood pressure brain function, skin temperature and CVP are either normal or lie within 'safe' limits. Oliguria can be due to one or more pathological processes and it is important to investigate this systematically. To help speed the investigation and to avoid omissions we have constructed a flow chart (Figure 7.1)

5. The central venous pressure (CVP)

In the general ICU the central venous pressure is measured in the majority of patients whether or not they are shocked. CVP measurements are required in shock unless this is known to be of the hypovolaemic type and also responds quickly to treatment. The significance of the CVP in shock was described in 1943 by the Nobel prizewinner André Cournand and his colleagues. Its invaluable use in therapy was established by McGowan and Walters (1963) and by Sykes (1963) . The trainee must appreciate that the CVP together with the other assessments cannot tell him the cardiac output, contractility or peripheral vascular resistance. Nevertheless this simple measurement will certainly help to determine the kind of shock and also guide the treatment. This measurement has undoubtedly saved thousands of lives and for once a controlled trial is unnecessary.

(a) Technique

To measure the CVP it is necessary to pass a cannula into the venous system so that its tip lies within the thorax, and in the subclavian vein or the superior or inferior vena cava. The cannula is introduced in one of the following sites: the cephalic vein, subclavian vein, femoral vein or internal jugular. To facilitate training and the supply of equipment it is important to standardize on the technique. We use the subclavian vein approached from above or below the clavicle and the other routes are detailed in the monograph by

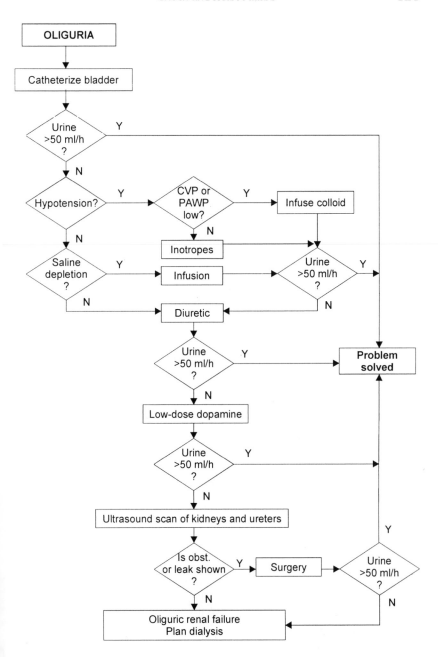

Figure 7.1 Algorithm to facilitate the management of oliguria

Peters (1983). Fortunately most of the equipment is readily available in kits pre-packed and ready for instant use. This is a convenient place to describe the essential equipment, since the techniques encompass circulatory monitoring and i.v. fluid therapy. There are two variations on a common theme, and, like other medical techniques, one or other tends to go in and out of fashion. The newcomer should have examples available for hands-on inspection.

(i) Seldinger technique.   This was invented by a Swedish radiologist in 1953 and greatly facilitated the cannulation of arteries or veins. The new item is called the guide wire but in reality is a finely wound coil of wire (that is, a spring) which has flexibility and elasticity. The leading end of the wire is made floppy for extra safety. The cannula is made to a sliding fit over the Seldinger guide wire. The sequence of operation is readily understood. A needle with stilette the same diameter as the wire is placed in the vessel. The wire is substituted for the stilette and threaded a short distance. The needle is withdrawn leaving the wire in place. The cannula is threaded over the wire through the wound and vessel wall and directed until the distal end is where it is intended to be.

(ii)   The introducer/cannula.   The introducer/cannula is a short plastic tube fitted with a hub and tapers at the distal end. A steel needle slides into the introducer/cannula and the bevelled tip protrudes slightly beyond the plastic. The sequence for placing the cannula is summarized in Figure 7.3.

Before starting the patient is reassured and the procedure is briefly explained. The procedure is carried out under conditions resembling those of an operating theatre, with the operator wearing sterile gown, surgical gloves and so forth. The patient lies flat with a pillow or the bed is tilted 10° head down. Either the right or left vein can be used and the following description applies to cannulation of the right subclavian vein from above the clavicle. The patient's head is rotated about 10° towards the left. The skin is cleaned with alcoholic hibitane and three surface markings are identified and marked with gentian violet or iodine. These are the centre of the sternal angle, the sterno-clavicular joint and the posterior border of the clavicular head of the right sterno-mastoid muscle (Figure 7.2). If this muscle cannot be identified because of obesity, oedema, haematomas or surgical emphysema, an alternative point on the upper surface of the clavicle is chosen at the junction of the inner third and outer two-thirds. For the remainder of the procedure, the operator kneels at the head of the bed. At the apex of the angle formed by the clavicle and clavicular muscle-head, the skin and subcutaneous tissues are infiltrated with 1% lignocaine, and a stab wound made with a scalpel blade. It will be appreciated that the point of

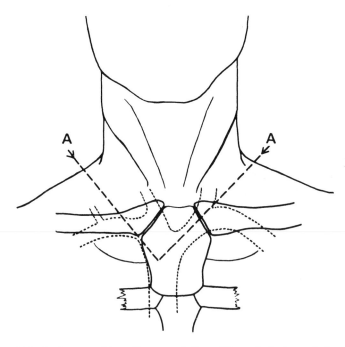

Figures 7.2 Surface markings for cannulation of the subclavian vein from above the clavicle. A, direction of the needle. (From *Essential Intensive Care*, with permission)

entry lies in the supraclavicular fossa. The introducer is placed over the needle which is attached to a 5 ml syringe containing about 2 ml of heparinized saline. The needle plus introducer is passed through the wound and advanced horizontally with the point directed towards the imaginary perpendicular line which passes through the surface marking (A). The needle has been passed behind both the clavicle and the sterno-clavicular joint. The operator can usually feel that the needle has traversed the wall of the subclavian vein. When correctly positioned, blood will flow into the syringe of its own accord or with gentle suction. Following the venepuncture the CVP catheter is placed in the vena cava in a sequence shown in Figure 7.3. Cannulation of the subclavian vein or jugular vein can cause serious, even life-threatening complications which are described on page 131. At this point we would emphasize that most of the complications are avoidable if cannulation is carried out by the right doctor (this is not a job for cowboys) and the system then cared for by the right nurses. Before the CVP line is

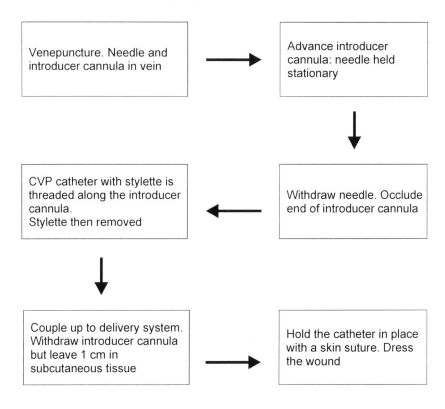

Figure 7.3 Sequence for placing a central venous catheter

used for measurements or infusions the position of the cannula is checked by X-ray.

We like the distal end of the cannula to lie in the superior vena cava. The central venous line is kept patent by a flow infusion of heparinized dextrose (10 000 units of heparin in 500 ml of 5% dextrose). The proximal end is connected both to the dextrose–heparin and to a disposable manometer (Figure 7.4) The manometer is fitted to a vertical scale reading in centimetres. When the cannula has been introduced and is connected to the measuring equipment, it is then necessary to set the zero point of the manometer scale at the same horizontal level as the sternal angle (angle of Loewi), or some other fixed point of reference. This adjustment is made with the aid of a levelling device, of which there is a choice. A spirit level attached to a length of tubing is fitted to the manometer stand so that the tubing

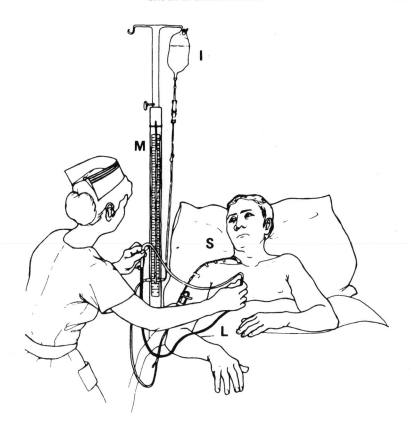

Figure 7.4 Arrangement for measuring the central venous pressure. 1, infusion apparatus; S, central venous line; M, manometer; L, level (From *Essential Intensive Care*, with permission)

corresponds with the zero of the scale. The spirit level is used to fix the tube in a horizontal position. The next step is to place the eye adjacent to the tube as if it were a telescope. The tube is kept horizontal but is raised or lowered until the sternal angle is sighted; the zero of the manometer scale will now be at the same level as the sternum angle.

The alternative apparatus (D.M. Morrison) is simpler, easier to obtain and decidedly cheaper. The principle has been used by builders for 4000 years! Flexible transparent tubing 6.0 mm bore and 2.0 m in length is half- filled with coloured fluid and the open ends jointed together. Figure 7.4 shows how the liquid column within the plastic tube is used to adjust the levels. The three-way tap on the measuring equipment is adjusted so that the CVP can be read. The reading is invalid unless the level can be seen to fluctuate with respiration. The level rises and falls during expiration and inspiration respectively. The converse occurs during IPPV. The proximal end of the CVP line may also be connected directly to a transducer and both pressure and wave-form are displayed on a monitor. It is still important to site the transducer at the correct height with respect to the patient, as already described. The reading of the CVP, correct to 1.0 cmH$_2$O or 1.0 mmHg is entered in the patient's notes.

(b) Interpretation

The CVP is affected by changes in intrathoracic pressure. Such changes may be physiological, the CVP falling during inspiration and then returning to the former value during expiration. Alternatively during IPPV in healthy subjects the CVP is higher than during spontaneous breathing. The actual increase in CVP will depend on the rise in intrathoracic pressure which in turn is related to the intratracheal pressure measured on the ventilator (Chapter 19). To obtain the CVP during IPPV it usually suffices to subtract 5.0 cm from the reading. When more precision is required then alternative methods can be used. It may be possible to disconnect the patient from the ventilator for long enough to take a reading during spontaneous breathing. Alternatively intrathoracic pressure may be measured by passing a Ryle's tube into the oesophagus so that the tip lies mid-distance down the oesophagus. The tube is filled with water and the intraoesophageal pressure measured. This reading is an accurate value of the intra-thoracic pressure. A high in-trathoracic pressure and therefore a raised CVP occurs in tension pneumo-thorax, a fact to be remembered in the patient with both shock and thoracic injuries. To return to the interpretation of CVP in the shocked patient. For general intensive care measurements are commonly made in mmHg pres-sure and the sternal angle taken as a zero point on the scale. We cannot interpret readings made on patients without knowing control values and as so often happens there are too few observations on healthy controlled subjects. Results from the literature gave a range of −1.0 to +1.0 mmHg for subjects breathing spontaneously.

At this stage in learning, the beginner should recall that most of the blood volume is contained in the veins and capillaries rather than the heart and arteries; it follows that the CVP reflects the circulating volume. Here are some didactic guides to interpretation. (i) A low CVP means hypovolaemia. (ii) Hypovolaemia can exist with a normal CVP. (iii) A high CVP is much more complex, but can usually be unravelled by following the flow chart (Figure 7.5) Having excluded valvular heart disease and hypervolaemia due to intravenous infusions or transfusions then a raised CVP means heart failure.

This rule-of-thumb will occasionally need indirect measurements of pressure in the left side of the heart.

6. Haemodynamics

Pressure and flow in the circulation can be measured electronically rather than assessed clinically by sphygmomanometer, saline manometer or skin temperature. Given the money and maintenance engineers it is a simple exercise to substitute electronic measurements for the clinical and to display or record the arterial blood pressure, CVP, cardiac output and so on. The facilities are useless and dangerous without trained medical and nursing staff and competence means regular usage; invasive haemodynamics are not for cowboys. To illustrate the subject the measurement of the pulmonary artery wedge pressure (PAWP) has been chosen because this is essential in the diagnosis and treatment of some cases of shock.

(a) Background physiology

We use the PAWP to give us an indication of the pressure in the left atrium. How this is achieved can be understood by referring to Figure 7.6. A catheter is placed into the right atrium just like a CVP line, but then steered through the right ventricle into the pulmonary artery; the resulting pressure trace is shown in Figure 7.7. The systolic, diastolic and mean PAWP are thus obtained. But the value we seek can only be obtained when the catheter occludes (becomes wedged) in a branch of the pulmonary artery, the arterial pulse disappears, but the lumen of the catheter is open to the capillary bed. Figure 7.6 shows how the vessel was readily occluded by inflating a small balloon placed near the tip, rather like an ET tube; this is the Swann–Ganz catheter invented in 1970. The blood pressure recorded (Figure 7.7) is no longer arterial, but is that transmitted from the left atrium through the capillary bed and for our purpose is a reliable indicator of the left atrial pressure. These pressure readings are in mmHg, referred to the sternal angle and atmospheric pressure; the normal value is 8.8mmHg, but there is considerable variation between the control patients.

(b) Equipment and technique

An essential of intensive care is that the equipment is always 'at the ready'. This comprises an electronic pressure system and the essential software – the Swann–Ganz catheter. The latter is a double lumen tube, one channel for measuring the pressure at the distal open tip and the second for inflating

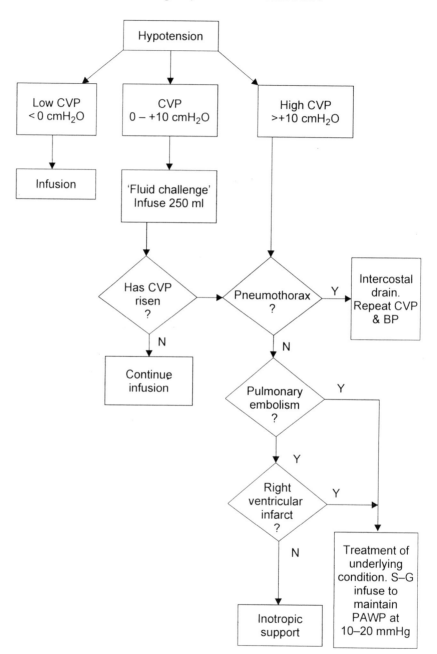

Figure 7.5 Flow chart to aid interpretation of the central venous pressure

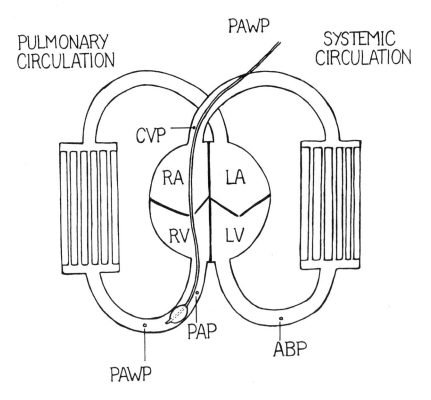

Figure 7.6 Anatomy of the pulmonary artery wedge pressure (PAWP)

or deflating the balloon sited proximal to the tip; 1.25 to 2.0 ml of gas is required to inflate sufficiently to occlude a pulmonary artery without causing damage. The method of placing the Swann–Ganz catheter in the pulmonary artery used at the RPA hospital can be broken down into the sequence shown in Figure 7.8. The Seldinger method is used to place an introducer/cannula into the subclavian vein. This permits the Swann–Ganz catheter to be advanced along the superior vena cava into the right atrium. Inflation of the balloon with 1.25–2.0 ml of air will 'flow-direct' the catheter into the pulmonary artery (Figure 7.6). The catheter is advanced until the wedge trace (Figure 7.7) is seen. The goal is nearly achieved. The balloon is next deflated and slowly re-inflated, noting the volume of air, until the wedge trace is again obtained. The volume of air required must exceed 1.0 ml to ensure that the occluded artery is not too small; adjustments may be necessary. Three further points. The system must be flushed continuously, the trace moni-

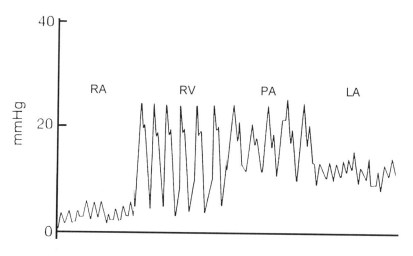

Figure 7.7 Waveforms in health using the Swann–Ganz catheter. RA, right atrium; RV, right ventricle; PA, pulmonary artery; LA, left atrium. (After Branthwaite and Morgan, from Miller, 1989, with permission)

tored continuously and a sterile sheath retained around the exposed part of the Swann–Ganz catheter.

The Swann–Ganz method is done at the bedside and X-ray screening is not essential but some units like to observe the pathway of the catheter by means of a portable image-intensifier.

(c) Interpretation

For the present purpose we use the PAWP to tell us the left atrial pressure (normal 8.0 mmHg) and to diagnose left ventricular failure. We jump to the conclusion, which would not satisfy the purist, that a PAWP above 15 mmHg means left ventricular failure. When the PAWP reaches 25 mmHg the pulmonary capillaries will leak plasma and blood cells, that is, pulmonary oedema has developed. The PAWP at which pulmonary oedema develops depends on the strength of those forces which oppose the PAWP. The opposing forces are osmotic and the chief one to remember is the plasma albumen; the lower the plasma albumen, the lower the PAWP needed to cause capillary leak.

(d) Indications

We are very selective about the Swann–Ganz catheter and only make this measurement when there is a good chance of rescuing a patient from life-threatening shock. Certainly the technique is never used because the doctor thinks it's a party trick or has no other clinical task awaiting him! We measure the PAWT in patients following surgery, bacterial shock and in obstetric emergencies. The one and only indication is a combination of shock and pulmonary oedema and the question which needs a quick answer is, will an intravenous infusion increase the cardiac output?

(e) Complications of CVP and Swann–Ganz catheters

A chapter would be required to deal thoroughly with these, so we will confine ourselves to the fundamentals. Negligence can perforate or thrombose a vessel or introduce infection during insertion; the remedy is obvious! Infection can be reduced to a minimum by reducing colonization as described in Chapter 27. The CVP line used for resuscitation is polyethylene which can abrade the vascular endothelium sometimes leading to right-sided endocarditis. A softer tube made from silicone rubber is substituted when the line is used for prolonged intravenous therapy. The Swann–Ganz catheter has also caused life-threatening complications, especially rupture or thrombosis of the pulmonary artery. Prevention depends on correct technique and a time limit of 48 hours for removal.

Having inserted a Swann–Ganz catheter it is logical to obtain the maximum amount of information, and this includes the cardiac output (CO). The essentials of a commonly used technique are next described. A Swann–Ganz catheter has two additional features; a port opening into the right atrium (RA) and a 'thermometer' at the distal end which lines in the pulmonary artery (PA). The 'thermometer' is a semi-conductor adapted to measure temperature and called a thermistor. This device is very small, will measure very small changes in temperature and responds very quickly. The reader should now visualize the 'anatomy' of the technique from Figure 7.6. The cuff of the Swann–Ganz catheter is deflated. A measured volume of ice-cold water is injected into the RA and mixes with the blood in the RA and RV before reaching the thermistor in the PA. The thermistor, already recording the blood temperature, shows a small and transient drop due to the bolus of cold water. From this recording and the physical properties of the water and blood, the CO is calculated by a computer. The measurement can be repeated as often as indicated, since the injectate is harmless. The CO can be expressed in relation to the surface area of the patient to give the cardiac index. This result, together with other physiological measurements, can be

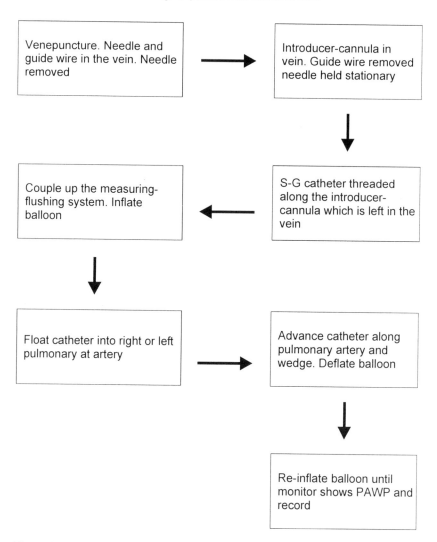

Figure 7.8 Sequence for placing a Swann–Ganz catheter (RPA hospital)

Table 7.3 Physiological measurements and derived information

Measurements	Derived variables
	Surface area
Haemoglobin	Cardiac index
Heart rate	Left atrial pressure
Pressure:	Left ventricular stroke work index
CVP	Right ventricular stroke work index
arterial	
pulmonary artery	
PAWP	
Flow:	
cardiac output	Oxygen consumption
	Oxygen delivery
Arterial blood:	
oxygen content	
Mixed venous (*PA*) blood:	
oxygen content	
Respiratory gases:	
inspired and expired oxygen	
concentrations	

used to calculate valuable assessments of the circulation and the delivery of oxygen to the tissues (Table 7.3). A word of caution; the beginner must avoid the pitfall of treating physiological data rather than the patient!

7. Blood gases

The blood gases should be measured when shock is either severe or prolonged or both. Examples would be the patient with multiple injuries, crushed chest, diabetic acidosis or severe self poisoning. The blood gases are of limited value in the assessment of the circulation. This is because the four variable pH, $PaCO_2$, HCO_3, PaO_2 are also influenced by the functioning of the lung, kidney, liver, nervous system and by disturbances of intermediary metabolism. To the extensive list must be added the effects of blood transfusions, intravenous infusions and drugs! (Chapter 5). Nevertheless some deductions are of value. Hypoxaemia is commonly found and low PaO_2 probably indicates more severe shock than a normal value. A metabolic acidosis again implies severe shock and is due to an increase in lactic acid due to tissue hypoxia.

8

Cardiac arrest

    I   **DEFINITIONS AND CAUSES**

   II   **DIAGNOSIS**

We apply the term cardiac arrest when a patient collapses due to cessation of the heart beat, rather than to the arrest which inevitably ends the process of dying. Recognition is simplicity itself and its management is an easily performed task for the staff of any ICU. Cardiac arrest will be a rare event in a general ICU unless the unit also admits cases of acute myocardial infarction. The general ICU may or may not participate in the cardiac arrest team serving the whole of a general hospital. The staff of a general ICU certainly have an important educational role; in teaching the prevention of arrest,, the criteria for treatment and regular training in the techniques of resuscitation (Chapter 21).

I DEFINITION AND CAUSES

The condition of cardiac arrest was only recognized during the development of general anaesthesia, in particular chloroform. In medicine a simple definition is usually the best. 'Cardiac arrest is best defined as the abrupt failure of the heart to pump sufficient blood to keep the brain alive' (Gilston and Resnekow, 1971). It is evident that the heart has failed to beat, what of the electrical activity? By far the commonest disturbance of rhythm is ventricular fibrillation (VF) but alternatives also occur; ventricular tachycardia, very rarely ventricular asystole and extreme bradycardia (including block). More than one dysrhythmia can occur in rapid succession. The beginner should be prepared for a surprise electrical finding; the ECG trace is normal but there is no output, a state given the grand label of electromechnical dissociation.

Only a few of the causes are common. Heart disease, especially coronary heart disease, tops the list (Table 8.1) and all the remaining causes are infrequently seen in the district general hospital. Although heart disease is the most frequent cause it is important to recognize that there are conditions which can cause the normal heart to arrest. These conditions consist of severe and usually rapidly developing changes in the composition of the extracellular fluid (ECF). The deviations are given in Table 8.2 Two or even

135

Table 8.1 Pathophysiology of cardiac arrest (From *Essential Intensive Care*, with permission)

Coronary heart disease acute myocardial infarction	Ischaemic or infarcted heart muscle, hypoxaemia
Asthma, tension pneumothorax	Impaired filling and emptying of the heart, hypoxaemia
Pulmonary embolism	Acute pulmonary hypertension, shock, hypoxaemia
Brain damage	Obstructed upper airway - hypoxia
Brain death	Destruction of medullary centre
Acute poisoning	Obstructed upper airway, shock, dysrhythmia induced by drug
Bacteraemia, bacterial toxaemia	Bacterial toxin on the heart, hypoxaemia
Iatrogenic Drugs Surgery Diagnostic procedures, e.g. cardiac catheterization, bronchoscopy	Direct action of drug Vagal reflexes ?

three such changes can be found in the same patient and it is probable that the effects are additive. The real importance of these biochemical abnormalities is that some can be prevented or at the worst detected early and promptly corrected. In this way the cardiac arrest is prevented. The knowledge required to achieve this is described in other chapters. To return briefly to the pathological processes in the heart which can cause cardiac arrest omitting the primary biochemical disturbances already referred to. Common things are commonest. Coronary heart disease can arrest the heart by causing ischaemia or infarction of the muscles; in turn this leads to VF or less commonly one of the other three dysrhythmias. In contrast a healthy heart can arrest due to one or more pathological processes operating singly or in combination (Table 8.1) Drugs taken as self-poisoning arrest by the direct toxic action on the heart or by hypoxic arrest, a sequel to an obstructed upper airway. Drugs used in therapy are not blameless! Again the normal heart can arrest due to the combined action of hypoxia and mechanical impedance. Such is the state of affairs in severe asthma or tension pneumothorax. Both lead to severe hypoxaemia and impair the filling and emptying of the heart.

Table 8.2 Causes of cardiac arrest according to biochemical abnormalities (From *Essential Intensive Care*, with permission)

Acidosis, metabolic or respiratory; pH less than 7.0

Hyperkalaemia; Kp greater than 7.0 mmol/l

K depletion and hypokalaemia; Kp less than 2.0 mmol/l

Acute hypoxaemia; PaO_2 less than 50 mmHg

Hypothermia; core temperature less than 26°C

Table 8.3 Signs of cardiac arrest (From *Essential Intensive Care*, with permission)

Arrest highly probable	abrupt unconsciousness absent major pulses
Additional signs	dilating pupils apnoea or gasping cyanosis VF asystole heart block extreme bradycardia

Cardiac arrest is rapidly followed by widespread tissue hypoxia. In man the most susceptible organs are the brain, liver and kidney. The brain dies in about 4 minutes and the liver and renal damage are irreversible after 15 minutes and 1 hour respectively. The widespread hypoxia of muscle and liver results in the accumulation of lactate in turn causing a metabolic acidosis (Chapter 7). This acidosis disturbs cell and organ function; defibrillation is less likely to succeed. Other important metabolic changes quickly follow cardiac arrest. In the blood there is a striking increase in the concentrations of adrenaline and noradrenaline. This finding should be remembered when using one or more of these substances in treatment.

The management of cardiac arrest is given in the chapter on resuscitation (Chapter 21) which includes an account of the sequelae and their treatment.

II DIAGNOSIS

Two signs, and only two signs, are required to recognize cardiac arrest – abrupt unconsciousness, and absent major pulses. Either the carotid or femoral pulse should be sought, depending on whether the neck or groin is the more accessible. Valuable time is often lost looking for additional signs, relating to the pupils or respiration (Table 8. 3). As a generalization, the size of the pupils is an unreliable sign both of arrest and the response to resuscitation. The ECG in cardiac arrest can show one of four rhythms but more than one dysrhythmia can also occur in rapid succession. When resuscitation fails, bizarre and often widened QRS complexes appear on the monitor, often referred to as an agonal ECG. External cardiac compression produces a synchronous QRS complex, which a beginner may mistake for a return of spontaneous heart actions. A display or record of the ECG is required as part of the treatment of cardiac arrest, never for the diagnosis.

9

Renal failure

What is man, when you come to think upon him, but a minutely set,
ingenious machine for turning, with infinite artfulness, the red wine of
Shiraz into urine.   Isak Dinesen, in Seven Gothic Tales

I   DEFINITION AND CLASSIFICATION
II   ACUTE RENAL FAILURE
III   CHRONIC RENAL FAILURE

In the District General Hospital the epidemiology and natural histories of
renal failure show similarities to those of respiratory failure (Chapter 6). The
inexperienced doctor or nurse must appreciate that like respiratory failure,
renal failure is ubiquitous and the more it is sought the more often will it be
found. Depending on its severity and duration, renal failure may or may not
require any special treatment; the same is true of respiratory failure; only a
small percentage of patients either require or are likely to benefit from
intensive care. In this field the functions of the ICU are twofold; (i) to
investigate and treat patients with either acute or chronic renal failure. The
investigatory aspect is important because some patients will need intensive
therapy pending an accurate diagnosis. Experience throughout the world
has shown that acute renal failure is best treated in an ICU because the
special treatments are readily available and because other body systems
may fail and such failure must be promptly recognized and energetically
treated. (ii) Educational; to teach the prevention and early recognition of
renal failure to junior doctors and qualified nurses.

I DEFINITION AND CLASSIFICATION

The kidney has many functions. Which of these diverse functions should be
used to define renal failure? Various definitions have been used during the
past 30 years and these have confused rather than helped the trainee doctor
and nurse, The writers like to keep things simple and therefore adopt a
straightforward definition which depends on a single measurement, itself
readily available in all hospitals or clinics; 'Renal failure is a high blood urea,
irrespective of the cause' (Robson, 1975), Obviously, the definition is based
on the failure of the kidney to excrete nitrogenous waste rather than a failure
to maintain a balance of electrolyte or acid–base balance, The term uraemia

Table 9.1 Signs and symptoms of uraemia (From *Essential Intensive Care*, with permission)

Neurological	Lethargy, drowsiness, confusion, fits, coma
Gastrointestinal	Thirst, anorexia, nausea, vomiting, constipation, diarrhoea, coated tongue, haematemesis
Respiratory	Increased breathing ('air-hunger') hiccough, pulmonary oedema
Urinary	Oliguria, polyuria, nocturia
Haematological	Uraemic coagulopathy, anaemia, leucocytosis

remains a confusing one, because it is used in two contexts – a clinical picture, or a state of the blood, namely a raised urea, Clinical uraemia is a syndrome of symptoms and signs attributed to severe renal failure and the textbook picture (Table 9,1) is most often seen in chronic renal disease, In such a case the blood urea is markedly raised (50–100 mmol/l, 300–600 mg/ml) and the serum creatinine is also very high, Despite prolonged research many of the symptoms and signs have defied a biochemical explanation, Another term which includes the word uraemia and which is of value in clinical practice is 'the uraemic emergency' (taken from Wrong, 1972), which implies that one or more biochemical changes are an immediate threat to life, and call for prompt action,

The classification of renal failure into acute or chronic is of equal importance to the patient and to the unit staff; the separation is not always an easy one. Acute renal failure means that the blood urea has risen from normal during the preceding few hours or days and this will not have escaped notice when the patient is in hospital.

Acute failure is readily diagnosed before the patient shows any of the clinical features of uraemia. Chronic renal failure means that the blood urea has been elevated for months or years and this is often accompanied by other biochemical changes. Another classification is of value, both in relation to treatment and prevention; this is to classify the failure according to the anatomical site of the primary disease or pathological process (Table 9.2) Pre-renal – often due to a saline depletion – means that the kidney is capable of functioning normally and will do so when the pre-renal process is corrected. Intrinsic means that the pathological process is in the kidney and this may be reversible over days or weeks, provided metabolic balance is maintained by artificial means; in the less fortunate, the pathological process is irreversible. In the third group of causes the site is post-renal and

Table 9.2 Classification of renal failure (From *Essential Intensive Care*, with permission)

A.	Pre-renal	
B.	Intrinsic renal	acute reversible acute irreversible chronic irreversible
C.	Post-renal	obstructive nephropathy

Table 9.3 Some causes of acute renal failure (From *Essential Intensive Care*, with permission)

Department	
Casualty/accident	Shock, cardiac arrest, multiple injuries, self-poisoning, accidental poisoning
Surgical unit	Shock, dehydration, potassium depletion, jaundice, cholangitis, pancreatitis, abscesses, obstructive nephropathy, transfusion reactions Following cardiac surgery Following renal transplantation
Aortic aneurysm	Shock, ischaemia, infarction
Burns	Shock, muscle damage
Medical unit	Acute mycoardial infarction Glomerulonephritis Nephrotic syndrome Hypertension Drug sensitivity Acute auto-immune disease Viruses Acute hepatic failure, (viral, drugs, cholangitis) Terminal cirrhosis Following anti-cancer therapy
Obstetric unit	Severe toxaemia, (eclampsia, antepartum haemorrhage, intrauterine death)
Gynaecology	Septic abortion
Intensive care	Shock, cardiac arrest, secondary Gram-negative infection
Common to all units	Bacteraemia, endotoxaemia, drugs

this invariably means obstruction at some site in the urinary tract, from the renal tubules to the urethra.

II ACUTE RENAL FAILURE

It required the medical experiences of two world wars to obtain the natural history of acute renal failure. Trauma, shock and sepsis were the first causes to be recognized and acute tubular necrosis was a corresponding histological pattern. These three conditions remain important causes of acute renal failure, although it is now appreciated that there are hundreds more! Many of these are relatively rare and can only be seen in a specialized renal unit. For the purpose of general intensive care a useful classification is based on the diseases of the DGH; this is done in Table 9.3. Bear in mind that this list applies to adult practice and excludes tropical diseases. Even a brief description of acute renal failure would occupy this book and therefore only a few of the natural histories will be described. It is imperative that specialized diagnostic help be available to the staff of a general ICU together with an adequate reference library on this topic. In common with all 'disease' the possibility of renal failure being due to drugs used therapeutically should never be forgotten; the briefest shortlist is given in Table 9.4.

Acute renal failure, like acute respiratory failure, can follow one of several natural histories and some of these are next described. It is appropriate to intensive care that the reversible forms should take priority over the irreversible types.

Table 9.4 Drugs and poisons which can cause acute renal failure (From *Essential Intensive Care*, with permission)

Drugs	Antileukaemic and anti-neoplastic drugs
	Penicillins
	Thiazides
	Frusemide
	Aminoglycosides
	Cyclosporin A
	Non-steroidal anti-inflammatory drugs
	Paracetamol
Poisons	Aniline
	Arsine
	Carbon tetrachloride
	Ethylene glycol
	Mushroom poisons
	Paraquat
	Venoms

1. Acute oliguric renal failure

This natural history is textbook acute renal failure; oliguria and uraemia follow shock, bacteraemia, multiple injuries, peritonitis, ulcerative colitis, etc. The corresponding renal histology is acute tubular necrosis and as far as is known this is usually reversible. Hypovolaemic shock is now a rare cause, because resuscitation is better organized and more efficient. In our experience the commonest causes are bacterial infections and toxaemias. The cardinal features are oliguria and a rising blood urea. In the early stages the symptoms are those of the cause or due to disturbances in the balance for water, sodium or potassium (Table 9.5). Unless dialysis is used, the symptoms of uraemia will develop (Table 9.1). Oliguria always commands investigation and the beginner should have a clear programme of the investigation of this sign which will also enable him to recognize acute renal failure at an early stage, even before the blood urea is significantly raised. The clinical situation is a familiar one. A patient is seriously ill due to injury, bacteraemia, haemorrhage, keto-acidosis, poisoning, emergency surgery, peritonitis, ulcerative colitis and so on. Despite apparently adequate resuscitation, there is oliguria. Investigation of the patient proceeds in a logical manner, outlined in Figure 9.1. Except for emergency pyelography details of the methods were given in previous chapters.

An IVP should be included in the scheme when the patient has a fractured pelvis or closed abdominal injury which could involve the kidney; haematuria is likely. One purpose of the IVP (and cystogram) is the detection of a torn

Table 9.5. Clinical findings in acute renal failure
(From *Essential Intensive Care*, with permission)

---

1. The cause; multiple injuries, sepsis
2. Water and sodium imbalance
       oliguria
       overhydration (saline excess)
       oedema
       hypertension
       increased breathing, dyspnoea, crackles
    Water intoxication
       headache
       fits
3. Potassium intoxication
       usually none (cardiac arrest when Kp
       is greater than 7.0 mmol/l)
4. Potassium depletion
       apathy, confusion, weakness
       hypotension, dysrhythmias
       paralytic ileus

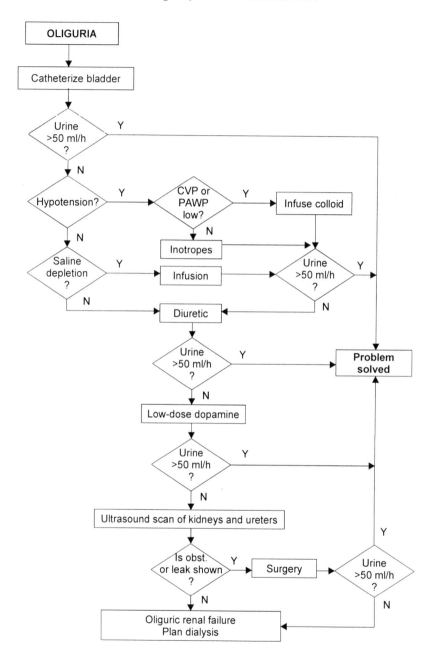

Figure 9.1 Algorithm to facilitate the management of oliguria

Table 9.6 Composition of the urine and the urine/plasma values in saline depletion and acute intrinsic renal failure (U = urine, P = plasma) (From *Essential Intensive Care*, with permission)

	Saline depletion	*Acute renal failure*
Urea (mg/100 ml)	>2000	<1100
(mmol/l)	333	183
Urea U/P	20	14 decreasing to 5
Sodium (mmol/l)	<15	10–100
Osmolarity U/P	>20	1.7 decreasing to 1.0 incipient >1.05 established <1.05

bladder or rupture of the renal pelvis. At the completion of the programme there are alternative outcomes; the urine output improves to a value in excess of 50 ml/h or oliguria persists. The latter outcome strongly suggests acute renal failure is incipient. The next step is to make additional measurements which help to confirm or refute the diagnosis. Samples of blood and urine are collected and the following measurements made on both; sodium, potassium, osmolarity, urea. Ratios for each component – urine/plasma – are calculated; a sort of instant clearance. The laboratory results are compared with those given in Table 9.6 which shows values for saline depletion and incipient or established renal failure. When the results support a diagnosis of acute renal failure a diuretic test is next performed. This test has two values; firstly diagnostic and secondly therapeutic. The test consists of giving one or more diuretics intravenously and observing the urine output over the ensuing minutes or few hours. We use frusemide in a dose of 80–125 mg. A brisk diuresis, that is one within 15 min, and a subsequent output of over 50 ml/h means that the diagnosis of acute renal failure is again in doubt. Following the frusemide, an infusion of dopamine is given as a 'low dose' of 1–5 µg/kg/min. It may be that this drug has already been started as a prophylactic measure (Chapter 20). Low dosage dopamine greatly increases renal blood flow and this in turn may re-start the urine flowing. A feeble response to either or both treatments means that acute renal failure is now a certainty; in this case a therapeutic plan is drawn up. To return to the natural history of acute oliguric renal failure. The oliguria lasts for days or weeks, the average duration being 11 days; the urine is usually cloudy, brown in colour and contains protein, red cells and casts. Even when the intake is severely restricted, there is retention (positive balance) of water, sodium, potassium and a progressive rise in the blood urea. The rate at which the blood urea rises depends on two factors, the degree of catabolism and the nutrition given, especially on the intake of energy. In the special example of extensive burns, other treatments can influence the catabolic rate. When, despite good nutrition, the blood urea shows a daily rise of 10 mmol/l (60 mg/100 ml) or more, the label of hypercatabolic renal failure is applied. Highly skilled intensive therapy may carry the patient through to the diuretic phase, when, over a period of a week or so, the urine output increases progressively from values of 50–500 ml per day to 2.0 litres or more. This can mean that the state of balance for water, sodium and potassium changes for the good, but the urine is a poor imitation of normal, containing little urea. In consequence, the blood urea continues to be elevated, modified by dialysis. Survival now depends on resolution of a causative disease and on the patient escaping the dreaded complications of bacterial infection, bacterial toxaemia or gastrointestinal haemorrhage. Indeed, the natural history is beset by 'ifs'. If the renal lesion heals, and a stage is reached when dialysis or filtration is no longer required to maintain metabolic balance, then one can speak of cure. The less fortunate patient has impaired function but can remain healthy for more than 30 days, then an irreversible lesion is probable. The diagnosis is best resolved by means of renal biopsy. The possible results are irreversible tubular necrosis (cortical necrosis), irreversible acute inter-stitial nephritis or unsuspected acute glomerulonephritis. At any time during the oliguric or diuretic phase the natural history can change dramatically for the worse. Any one of the following can cause a fresh assault on the kidney, and renal function returns, as it were, back to square one; laparotomy (perhaps a second), intra-abdominal abscess, bacteraemia, bacterial toxae-mia, haemorrhage, recrudescence of acute pancreatitis. Obviously in such patients the chances of survival are further reduced.

2. Acute polyuric* renal failure

Instead of oliguria, the same causes can result in renal failure with a normal output of urine or polyuria; the reasons for such striking differences are unknown. Another important cause of acute polyuric renal failure is potas-sium depletion. The ICU has an important role to play in the prevention, early recognition and treatment of potassium depletion of which acute renal failure is one of the many pathological processes (Chapters 4 and 16). In our experience the acute renal failure of potassium depletion is due to loss from the gastrointestinal tract; chronic benign pyloric stenosis or paralytic

---

*   This label is preferred to non-oliguric.

ileus treated by 'drip and suction' without adequate potassium. Whatever the cause of the acute polyuric failure, the renal lesion is tubular and the treatment is based on the assumption that the pathological process is reversible; time will show whether this is correct. Recognition of this type of renal failure depends on clinical vigilance and routine measurements of the blood urea. Unlike the oliguric type, the condition can pass unrecognized. Symptoms and signs are attributed to the cause or to saline depletion, potassium depletion, metabolic alkalosis or hyperosmolarity of the ECF, or to a combination of these states. The recovery of the patient depends on resolution of the primary pathology, e.g. pyloric obstruction, peritonitis, acute pancreatitis; the resolution of the tubular lesion; restoring and then maintaining a state of metabolic balance.

3. Obstructive nephropathy

Some causes of obstruction which can cause acute renal failure are shown in Table 9.7. Taken together they account for only a few cases in the general ICU. In this unit papillary necrosis is the commonest of the obstructive causes. Obviously in this group there is oliguria or anuria. The role of the unit is to help a physician or surgeon to find the cause, e.g. myeloma, papillary sloughing, and secondly, to main metabolic balance. Specific treatment is planned, assuming there is any.

4. Bacterial infection

Acute renal failure caused by a bacteraemia or by circulating bacterial toxin follows one of two natural histories. The first pattern has a dramatic onset. The patient is undergoing cystoscopy or exploration of the bile ducts, a 'D & C', or, unknown to the hospital staff, is receiving an infusion fluid contaminated with bacteria. Quite unexpectedly the patient 'collapses'. There is shock cyanosis, a rigor and a precipitous rise in temperature. Blood cultures will show retrospectively that a bacteraemia occurred. Acute renal failure quickly becomes evident. If recognition and resuscitation are both performed promptly, the patient may show only transient oliguria. The alternative natural history is quite different. The patient is seriously ill (ulcerative colitis, peritonitis, burns, acute pancreatitis) or has multiple injuries and is therefore in a surgical ward, accident unit, or intensive care unit. The circulation is stable and metabolic balance is maintained. Oliguria develops 'out of the blue' and is accompanied by other signs; the secondary illness is attributed to bacterial toxin, often the endotoxin of Gram negative bacteria. Blood cultures are usually sterile and, unfortunately, the assay of

Table 9.7 Acute renal failure due to obstruction (obstructive nephropathy) (From *Essential Intensive Care*, with permission)

1. In the renal pelvis
    Sloughed papillae
        Chronic analgesic nephropathy
        Pyelonephritis
        Diabetes
2. In the ureters
        Cancer of bladder or uterus
        Calculus anuria
        Retroperitoneal fibrosis
        Surgical ligation of ureters (pelvic operations)
3. In the renal tubules
        Bence-Jones protein (myelomatosis)
        Casts
            Muscle damage
            A pathological process in ATN
        Crystals
        Acute and severe hyperuricaemia

endotoxin is of no diagnostic value. Within 12 h the blood urea has doubled and the urine osmolarity and urea are low. The renal lesion runs the course of acute tubular necrosis, but all too often the patient dies from the effects of bacterial toxin on the brain, heart, gut or liver.

III CHRONIC RENAL FAILURE

It is a sad fact that each year thousands die from chronic renal failure and many more suffer disabling uraemia. At any one time 4000 patients in the UK await renal transplantation and in Australia the figure is 1200. The condition therefore involves the general practitioner, urological department, regional renal unit, etc. Patients with chronic renal disease fall into one of two groups. In the first group the disease has been diagnosed so that the patient and his general practitioner are aware of the problem, even if treatment is not yet required. On the other hand, indifferent health can steal up on the patient unnoticed, or he may adopt a stoical attitude and dismiss the symptoms. In this group, neither the patient nor his general practitioner are aware of the diagnosis. Patients in either group may at any time take a turn for the worse and this can occur quite rapidly. This acute episode can either be quickly and correctly diagnosed as uraemia or be mistaken for anaemia, intestinal obstruction, confusional state, left ventricular failure, etc. Such a patient can be admitted to a surgical ward, psychiatric unit or medical ward. The important point is that the patient is seriously ill, even

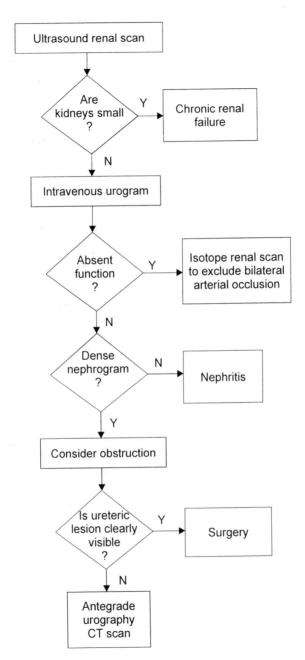

Figure 9.2 Diagnostic imaging for obstruction

Table 9.8 Some causes of chronic renal failure which may present as a uraemic emergency (From *Essential Intensive Care*, with permission)

Disease	Clues to diagnosis
Glomerulonephritis	History of AGN. May be none
Auto-immune disease	Lupus, polyarteritis
Pyelonephritis	Urinary infections, bacteriuria
Interstitial nephritis	Abuse of paracetamol. Non-steroidal anti-inflammatory drugs. Gout
Tuberculosis	Lesion in lung, bladder or bone
Amyloid	Rheumatoid, chronic sepsis, tubercle, myeloma
Myelona kidney	Bence-Jones proteinuria
Diabetes mellitus	Long history, other complication
Malignant disease	Lymphoma, leukaemia
Obstructive nephropathy	Nocturia, dysuria, enlarged prostate, malignant disease, renal colic/calculi
Polycystic disease	Family history, palpable kidneys
Sarcoid Involvement of other organs; skin,	lymph nodes, eye, liver, spleen
Drug-induced	Non-steroidal anti-inflammatory drugs

critically ill, so that immediate investigation is impossible or severely restricted. Indeed a useful label for this case is 'the uraemic emergency'. The situation is such that treatment of the uraemia must precede diagnosis; traditional medicine back to front. An important exception is the rapid relief of obstruction in the bladder or urethra; a catheter is passed and left in place. The clinical situation now calls for a quick decision; intensive care or not? The patient himself is too ill to make any rational contribution; 'Don't listen Doc, it's the uraemia talking', said Professor Merrill's patient. The decision is based on information obtained from the relatives and GP; the age and personality of the patient; the attitude of the relatives; the existence of other chronic disease. When it is decided to employ intensive care, then a priority list for treatment is quickly drawn up. The patient is examined for the following disturbances, which are then arranged in a list according to their priority; saline depletion or excess; potassium depletion or hyperkalaemia; metabolic acidosis; hypertension/hypotension; respiratory failure;

left ventricular failure. A blood sample is taken for the following; full blood count, urea, creatinine, uric acid, sodium, potassium, calcium, phosphate, serum proteins and phosphatases. The urine is examined for protein (including Bence–Jones), red cells, casts, pus cells, and is also cultured. In the group of patients with 'renal failure cause unknown' many other tests may be required to determine the nature of the renal disease; they can often be postponed until intensive care has tided the patient over the life-threatening emergency. The treatment is based on fluid therapy and nutrition, together with the control of the uraemia by dialysis. Other treatments, such as oxygen therapy or antibiotics, may be part of the therapeutic plan. Details of these treatments are given in other chapters.

By the 3rd or 4th day of intensive care there should be a dramatic improvement in the condition of the patient. Treatment now depends on whether the renal disease is 'known' or 'unknown'. In the case of the former, investigation is unnecessary and management will be by diet, with or without further dialysis. The second group of patients need further investigation, in an attempt to determine the renal lesion, with special emphasis on a search for something treatable. The primary diseases causing renal failure are legion and only a few of these are to be seen in the general ICU; a sample is found in Table 9.8. The second assessment should proceed according to a pre-determined plan. A new history is taken from the patient, who is now able to remember symptoms more accurately. The results of the tests carried out on admission are also reviewed; hypercalcaemia, pyuria, bacteriuria, raised muscle enzymes, positive antinuclear antibodies* can help to recognize the cause. The ECG may point to long-standing hypertension. During this re-think on the problem, the radiologist is enlisted to draw up a programme of diagnostic imaging. There are two aims, to check and re-check for obstruction and to measure the size of the kidneys and determine their anatomy. The programme will depend on whether the department has a CT scanner or gamma camera. A plan is shown in Figure 9.2. A note on retrograde or antegrade urography; both have a morbidity, and are used only when imaging results confirm obstruction. Routine renal biopsy is out, because in these patients it is both difficult and dangerous. The chief indication is 'suspicion of a potentially reversible cause other than ATN' (Kerr, 1985).

---

* Anti-neutrophil cytoplasmic antibody (ANCA), anti-glomerular basement membrane antibody (AGBMA)

10
Brain failure

Or emptied some dull opiate to the drains.
One minute past, and Lethe-wards had sunk.

John Keats, 1820

I	COMA AND IMPAIRED CONSCIOUSNESS
II	BRAIN DEATH
III	DELIRIUM
IV	STATUS EPILEPTICUS

A few minutes' reflection will demonstrate to yourself that one definition will not fit brain failure. Impaired intellect, coma, madness, and epilepsy are all types of failure. So we are forced to a negative definition, the brain not doing what it should be able to do. Our classification of brain failure will not please Professor Know-all, but it worked for intensive care, so here it is: impaired consciousness, brain death, delirium and status epilepticus.

I COMA AND IMPAIRED CONSCIOUSNESS

1. Diagnosis

Three clinical findings lead to a diagnosis of coma, and all three are negative, that is something is absent from the normal; compare this with jaundice. The signs are: the eyes do not open spontaneously; there is no response to the command 'put out your tongue'; thirdly, intelligible speech is absent, but the patient may grunt or moan. The third sign cannot be sought when the patient is intubated!

2. Causes

The reader should already be familiar with the causes shown in Table 10.1 and information relevant to intensive care is in the chapters quoted. With one exception cerebrovascular disease will not be considered because intensive care cannot benefit these patients. The exception – an important one – is Spontaneous Subarachnoid Haemorrhage. When this terrible condition is due to rupture of an intracranial aneurysm or arterio-venous anomaly, then the patient is transferred to intensive care. Following the initial assessment the 'well' patient is quickly referred to a neurosurgical unit

153

Table10.1 Some causes of coma or impaired consciousness

		Chapter reference
Hypoxia	Respiratory failure	6
	Shock	7
	Cardiac arrest	8
Cerebrovascular accident	Thrombosis Embolus Haemorrhage	
Poisoning	Accidental Self	
Trauma	Head injury	4
Metabolic	Hyperglycaemia	4
	Hypoglycaemia	4
	Hypercalcaemia	4
	Hepatic failure	11
Microbial	Bacteraemia	15
	Bacterial toxaemia	15

in the hope that a second bleed can be prevented by an operation. The moribund patient remains in the ICU and receives all necessary supportive therapy. When brain death ensues, then organ donation may be possible – 'a gift of life'. The preventive role of the intensive care unit should not be forgotten. The reader might try to recall disasters which could have been prevented; these can be recalled from Table 10.1.

3. Monitoring of impaired consciousness

You would not get very far recording the temperature of the body with the back of your hand, but this was the type of recording applied to coma until 1974. Our clinical notes contain some amazing rubbish – 'a little lighter today', 'showing spontaneous movement'. As with temperature we now have a scale for charting impaired consciousness and, like the degree Celsius, this is used internationally*. The Glasgow coma scale (Teasedale and Jennett, 1974) measures three aspects of behaviour, referred to as the Best Motor Response, the Best Verbal Response, and Eye Opening. Each measurement is made independently of the others according to the methods

---

*   One of Professor Bryan Jennett's treasured possessions is the Glasgow coma scale in Japanese

Table 10.2 The Glasgow Coma Scale 'Order Out of Chaos' (From Teasdale and Jennett, *Lancet* **1974; 2: 81–83, with permission)**

I   BEST MOTOR RESPONSE
      The scale is from 6 to 1 as follows:

6.   Obey commands
      Command the patient to move an arm, protrude the tongue or open the eyes. If no response, apply a painful stimulus to the hand. If flexion is observed, apply a painful stimulus to the head and trunk to test for localization.

5.   Localized pain
      A localizing response indicates that a stimulus at one or more sites causes a limb to move so as to attempt to remove it.

4.   Withdraws
      Rapid withdrawal associated with abduction of shoulder.

3.   Abnormal flexion
      Associated with extension movement in either arm or leg at the time of examination.

2.   Extension to pain
      Extensor posturing is obviously abnormal and is usually associated with adduction, internal rotation of the shoulder and pronation of the forearm.

1.   No response
      No response is usually associated with hypotonia.
      When recording motor response as an indication of the functional state of the brain as a whole, the best or highest response from any limb is recorded.

II   BEST VERBAL RESPONSE
      The scale is from 5 to 1 as follows:

5.   Orientated
      Orientation implies awareness of the self and the environment.
      The patient should know who he is, where he is, and why he is there; know the year, the season and the month.

4.   Confused conversation
      Confused conversation is recorded and attention can be held and the patient responds to questions in a conversational manner but indicates varying degrees of disorientation and confusion. It is here that verbatim reporting of the individual patient's responses can be useful.

Table 10.2 (Glasgow Coma Scale) continued

3. Inappropriate words

Inappropriate speech describes intelligible articulation but implies that speech is used only in an exclamatory or random way, usually by shouting and swearing. No sustained conversational exchange is possible.

2. Incomprehensible speech

Incomprehensible speech refers to moaning and groaning without any recognizable words.

1. None.

III   EYE OPENING

Eye opening is tested as follows, and the results recorded on a 4 to 1 scale:

4. Spontaneous eye-opening with sleep/wake rhythms is most highly scored on this part of the scale and it indicates that the arousal mechanisms in the brain stem are active.

3. Eye-opening in response to speech is a response to any verbal approach, whether spoken or shouted, not necessarily the command to open the eyes.

2. Eye-opening in response to pain should be tested by a stimulus in the limbs, because the grimacing associated with supraorbital or jaw-angle pressure may cause eye closure.

1. None

summarized in Table 10.2. Each examination is repeated according to the natural history of the disease and the trends are recorded in a chart.

Finally in this section, a word on management dealt with again in Chapter 26. The management is simple enough but so important to avoid the misuse of intensive care. When coma is due to cerebrovascular disease then large trials have shown that the outcome is awful with or without intensive therapy including IPPV. The burdens far exceed the benefits.

11 BRAIN DEATH

This is easily diagnosed and the care of the patient standardized. The difficult problem is the care of the bereaved and of those who care for the brain dead. Brain death means that you are dead and despite all the life support systems of intensive care, the heart will arrest for good in a few hours or days. When gas exchange is maintained mechanically, then the heart, kidneys and liver continue to function for hours or days. The beginner should know that there are no 'ifs' or 'buts' about brain death. Brain death occurs when there is irreversible damage to the cortex and brain stem and is recognized when all activity above the foramen magnum is shown to be absent by a series of simple bedside tests. It is agreed throughout the UK that brain death can be diagnosed by recognizing death of the brain stem alone; the tests were designed accordingly. In Australia the legislation refers to whole brain death and additional tests for cortical death may be performed, but these are not mandatory. The next thing to learn is when the diagnosis must not be attempted and the beginner will need a check list. Starting with the antecedent conditions, poisoning of any kind or severe hypoglycaemia; accidental hypothermia – the core temperature must be 35°C. Next, treatment given before or following admission; the diagnosis of brain death is not attempted if a sedative drug or muscle relaxant is still acting. What is the brain dead patient doing in an intensive care unit, a place for treating those deemed recoverable? The answer is that some brain dead patients are potential organ donors; those with head injury or spontaneous subarachnoid haemorrhage. This is a convenient point to hammer home the fact that your ICU won't contribute to the transplant programme unless the administration ensures that all these patients are admitted to the ICU before brain death develops, if this tragedy ensues. Contraindications to donation comprise infection, extra-cerebral malignancy, hypertension, chronic pyelonephritis, diabetes, and widespread atheroma.

Tests

These tests assess the vital centres and pathways of the brain stem. The equipment is really very basic. An electrical thermometer to measure oesophageal temperature; bright light to test the pupils, ice-cold water to inject into the ear.

In the absence of poisoning and hypothermia brain death is diagnosed as follows:

(1) There must be no response when the pupils are examined with a bright light in a darkened room. The size of the pupils is irrelevant but they will commonly be dilated.

(2) There must be no response to corneal stimulation with cotton-wool.

(3) There must be no response to the presence of the endotracheal tube nor any evidence of cough when suction is applied to the trachea.

(4) There must be no eye movements when 20 ml of ice-cold water is injected into each ear, clear access to the drums having been established.

(5) There must be no response to painful stimuli to the head and neck – for example, supraorbital pressure and firm pinching of the ear lobes.

(6) Spontaneous breathing must be absent during hypercapnia – this may be tested in either of two ways:

(a) The ventilator is disconnected and a 2-litre reservoir bag filled with oxygen substituted. Oxygen is stopped and the pressure valve closed. The bag is then squeezed about four times a minute for three minutes. Assisted ventilation is then stopped. The bag is observed for respiratory movements, which must be absent for 5 minutes. Cardiac contractions cause movement of the bag synchronous with the heart beat and should not be confused with respiratory movements.

(b) Arterial carbon dioxide pressure is measured. If this is below 4.8 kPa (36 mmHg) alveolar ventilation is reduced to attain normocapnia. This is achieved by lowering the minute volume by reducing the frequency and either tidal volume or pressure. The concentration of inspired oxygen is increased to prevent hypoxaemia. Table 10.3 gives the predicted ventilator settings required to achieve normocapnia. After 15 minutes the patient is disconnected from the ventilator and oxygen delivered at 2 lites/min through a fine cannula introduced into the trachea. The patient's chest is observed for 5 minutes, during which there must be no spontaneous respiratory movements. An additional extra is to then measure the blood gases to ensure that the $PaCO_2$ is above 50 mmHg (6.7 kPa). These tests should be performed by two doctors independent of the transplant team on two occasions. If any test gives an equivocal result, however, treatment should be continued and testing repeated at 4-hour intervals. In the UK electroencephalography is not required to diagnose brain death and may even be misleading. In contrast, the EEG is used in some Australian units to diagnose cortical death, along with test for diabetes insipidus. In a few patients severe facial injuries make it impossible to examine the pupils

Table 10.3 A guide to setting a ventilator to achieve normocapnoea (From Luksza, *Br Med J* 1979; 1: 1316–1319, with permission)

Body weight (kg)	Minute volume (l)
20	2.4
40	4.2
60	5.4
70	6.0
80	6.9
100	8.4

and eye movements or the reflex response to pinching the ear lobe. We then demonstrate the greatly reduced blood flow throughout the cerebral hemisphere by means of angiography or isotope scanning.

III DELIRIUM

The first thing to learn about delirium is that in intensive care it is often missed! The word is derived from delira, a furrow; the mind is in a furrow. The formal definition is really jargon – delirium is global impairment of cognitive processes. For us, this needs translating! Here is a sketch of acute delirium occurring in a patient who may require intensive care or who is already on the receiving end. The patient is awake and can hold a conversation, but the memory, perception and comprehension are impaired. You can work out for yourself how to diagnose these signs. The patient is restless and sleep is disturbed. Hallucinations may be experienced. Remember that the signs fluctuate over hours and are usually worse in the late evening or night; this is called sundowning. Time is not properly comprehended – disorientation.

In the acute medical or surgical patient we must search diligently for delirium, but what does it mean? Delirium might be expected as a manifestation of brain failure in some patients, especially those in the older age group. Thus it might accompany head injury, follow hypoxia, or hypoglycaemia, or bacteraemia. When the cause is not clear-cut, urgent survey is made to ensure that we do not miss the treatable. When you even suspect that the breathing pattern is abnormal (Chapter 6) measure the minute volume ventilation and analyse the arterial blood gases. The plasma concentrations of glucose, potassium, calcium and inorganic phosphate may give a quick answer to the problem. Consider deficiencies of folate and vitamins B and if either is likely, then treat right away. If this important survey, carried out within an hour, does not provide an explanation, the problem still requires urgent solution. To start with 'bugs and drugs'. Bacteraemia or bacterial toxaemia (Chapter 15) may first manifest as delirium and time is vital if the patient is to recover. The WBC is examined and three blood cultures taken. Delirium can be caused by many drugs, taken accidentally or given by the ICU staff. Poisoning of the brain by heavy metals or metabolites such as porphyrins may be the cause. Finally, to enhance the diagnostic challenge the patient may have two or three causes of delirium! Table 10.1 may help. However, you cannot look for a cause if you fail to recognize the condition!

IV   STATUS EPILEPTICUS

Remember a patient in casualty, fitting continuously, cyanosed, and with clenched teeth; secretions or even vomit running out of the mouth. Your ears tell you that the airway is partly obstructed. Five seconds is all the time required to assess the problem, but what would you do? Would you hope that someone else will act quickly or make futile efforts with a mouth gag, suction catheter, or oxygen mask? The intensive care doctor or accident and emergency consultant will act reflexly, as in cardiac arrest. This introduces status epilepticus, a killing state, and one which demands a right patient in the right place at the right time. The organizational problem is that an average district general hospital will only see a few patients a year. Status epilepticus is usually a variant of idiopathic grand mal epilepsy; inadequate drug treatment or alcohol can set off the condition. Hypoglycaemia is a cause not to be forgotten and, more rarely, encephalitis or brain tumour.

11

Gastrointestinal tract failure: acute upper gastrointestinal haemorrhage: liver failure

I	GASTROINTESTINAL FAILURE
II	ACUTE UPPER GASTROINTESTINAL HAEMORRHAGE
III	LIVER FAILURE

I GASTROINTESTINAL FAILURE

1. Definition

Our declared aim is to keep things simple, so why invent the label 'gastrointestinal failure'? The justification will become apparent if you reflect on the patients at present in the unit where you are a learner. In how many is the gastrointestinal tract (GIT) functioning to provide the fluid and nutrition appropriate to the disease? It would be surprising if the answer is more than half the patients. The absorption of fluid and nutrient was selected from the many other processes to provide a simple definition of GIT failure. Thus defined, GIT failure is very common, and of relevance both to diagnosis and therapy.

It is helpful to compare GIT failure with respiratory and renal failures. When nutrients do not reach the stomach, then a normal GIT cannot perform the tasks described; when the thoracic cage and diaphragm fail to move air (drug overdose, Guillain-Barré syndrome) then normal lungs cannot exchange healthy gases. When the blood flow fails to supply the glomerulus (shock); then a healthy kidney cannot excrete water and electrolytes.

GIT failure is present in two groups of patients. Firstly, as the presenting problem, ileus, ulcerative colitis, and can then rarely escape notice. But failure to digest and absorb is also common in such diverse conditions as fractured pelvis, bacteraemia, or acute self poisoning. In this group GIT failure, like respiratory and renal failure, must be sought out and supportive therapy planned. We conclude this introduction with a caution on patient selection in gastrointestinal disease. For each disease, consensus management will formulate the criteria for admission (Chapter 3) – the which and when of intensive care. These rules (yes, they are rules) largely avoid the need to carry out a rescue. Also, patients with incurable disease will not be admitted as part of a medical cover-up. Remember that the supportive therapies of intensive care cannot mend holes in the gut!

2. Pathophysiology

Three pathological processes dominate: obstruction, diarrhoea and inflammation. The first can occur without the last, but the diarrhoeas are accompanied by inflammation; the consequences of the pathophysiology are serious or life threatening. The worst examples of saline depletion and potassium depletion are caused by obstruction or diarrhoea. It is important to remember that during ileus huge volumes of ECF can accumulate in the bowel – up to 30 litres; this fluid is lost (outside) to the body. When the ileus resolves then mobility and absorption are restored and there is a large, and potentially dangerous intake of water and electrolyte. The deficits or excesses also affect acid–base balance as previously described. Rather than repeat the information here the reader should try and work out for themselves the acid–base consequences of 'drip and suck' or diarrhoea. The deficits are water and electrolyte can cause shock, renal and brain failure. Hand-in-hand with these deficits' there is acute malnutrition with all the physiological consequences as already described (Chapter 4). For the patient morbidity and mortality are increased. It is hoped that the trainee in intensive care will quickly learn that such disastrous changes in the body fluids can be prevented.

Turning next to the third component, inflammation. There may be a clear bacterial origin such as peritonitis or cholangitis, but equally serious inflammation can occur from unknown causes and inflammatory bowel disease is especially important. Fever and leucocytosis are easily remembered, but the toxaemia can readily cause failure of one or more of the distant organs such as the heart, brain, or lung.

When there has been either trauma, infection, or toxaemia then the destructive process of hypercatabolism invariably develops, getting into top gear, as were, in a few days. The reader will recall that the whole of metabolism is deranged: increased urea production, loss of lean muscle and body fat, accelerated glucose synthesis and hypoproteinaemia.

Much easier to understand are the mechanical consequences of abdominal distension. This reduces the vital capacity of the lungs, and, more seriously, leads to basal collapse; consolidation may then follow.

In most acutely ill patients the normal flora of the gut changes, and such changes are accelerated by antibiotics. In particular, the aerobic Gram negative bacteria take over from the anaerobes which predominate in health. The Gram negatives colonize the small bowel and can spread to the stomach. Indeed, this process was first described in patients with paralytic ileus. The next migration of pathogens is not surprising; to the pharynx and mouth, from which the trachea is quickly reached. Thus pulmonary infection is a common and potentially lethal sequence of gastrointestinal failure. It is easy to understand how endotoxaemia can follow peritonitis or cholangitis, but this lethal process is also seen without overt infection. An increased production in the gut of endotoxin, together with impaired neutralization in the liver is an attractive hypothesis to explain these clinical events, but remains hypothesis and not fact. The stomach may again be involved even when not the primary site of disease. Stress ulceration is common (how common is unknown) and occasionally (how frequently is also unknown) causes serious haemorrhage. This brief survey of the pathophysiology ends by mentioning the haematological changes. These are normochromic anaemia, and the hypercoaguable state of the blood. Leucocytosis accompanies inflammation.

3. Causes and assessment

One of the fascinations of general intensive care for both nurse and doctor is the variety of diseases or conditions treated. This variety challenges the knowledge of the service doctor who should be familiar with the natural histories of the diseases listed in Table 11.1. The patient selection is paramount to success, and depends on the right patient being admitted at the right time. All too often in gastrointestinal disease the wrong patient is admitted; those who cannot benefit or are unlikely to benefit.

Having achieved the difficult objective then the assessment and monitoring follow the essentials already described. Remember the first two principles in any illness: pain and sleep! To the assessment of the whole patient two additional diagnostic processes are added. Firstly, the use of scales for specific diseases and which are based on accurate studies on large numbers of patients. We have chosen three of these to illustrate the point, and they are shown in Tables 11.2 and 11.3. Such scales are like the admission criteria agreed by each hospital (consensus management) and then enforced. The second essential is endoscopy, at any time of the day or night 365 days of the year. Oesophagoscopy, gastroscopy, sigmoidoscopy and colonoscopy have to be made available at the drop of a hat.

Table 11.1 Disease or conditions causing gastrointestinal failure (failure to absorb)

Mouth, oesophagus	Strictures or tumours
Stomach	Pyloric stenosis, tumours
Biliary tract	Obstructive jaundice
Bowel	Peritonitis, abscesses, trauma, bands strictures Inflammatory bowel disease, ulcerative colitis, Crohn's disease, pseudomembraneous colitis Infective diarrhoeas: Salmonella, bacillary dysentery Intestinal fistula
Pancreas	Acute pancreatitis
Central nervous system	Head injury, spinal cord injury, Guillain-Barré syndrome
Systemic	Bacteraemia, bacterial toxaemia Hypoxia Poisoning

Table 11.2 Assessing the severity of Crohn's disease (From de Dombal, 1988)

Score one for each feature present.

Pain present
Bowel action; more than six a day or
    blood and mucus in the stools
Perianal complications
Fistula
Mass present
Wasting
Temperature above 38°C
Abdominal tenderness
Haemoglobin below 10 g/dl
Other complication

Table 11.3 Assessing the severity ('risk factors') of ulcerative colitis (From Truelove and Witts, 1954)

Pulse
Temperature
Bowels
Haemoglobin
Erythrocyte sedimentation rate

II ACUTE UPPER GASTROINTESTINAL HAEMORRHAGE

Two aspects are relevant to general intensive care. A minority of patients are best admitted to reduce the morbidity and mortality, so we must treat the right patient in the right place at the right time. Have you read this before? Secondly, and again a minority, gastrointestinal bleeding complicates the initial illness and can then load the dice against recovery.

1. Causes and pathophysiology

The apprentice is now on familiar ground and should try self-assessment: list the causes of haematemesis and melaena in the frequency of their occurrence. Now add coagulopathy (Chapter 13) to your list. The haemorrhage from the oesophagus, stomach, or duodenum arises from a capillary ooze, an eroded artery, or a ruptured vein. Acute haemorrhage leads to hypovolaemic shock and if this is not quickly treated, then failure of one or more vital organs is inevitable (Chapter 7). The acute upper gastrointestinal haemorrhage secondary to multiple injuries, burns, acute renal failure, is due to stress ulcers in the stomach or lower oesophagus or to a coagulopathy.

2. Assessment

The priority list is very simple: the circulation and endoscopy to describe the lesion or lesions. Assessing the circulation in hypovolaemic shock can be done quickly and effectively by the staff of intensive care, A & E, or the recovery room; the methods were described in Chapter 7. At the same time the reactions of the patient to haematemesis are weighed up; would you feel anxiety or sheer terror? We now need to determine the natural history of the bleeding: previous peptic ulcer? diagnosis of cirrhosis? The assessment extends to disability due to chronic lung and heart disease – the CHE of the APACHE system. This information will influence the plan of action. The patient's blood is cross-matched and a blood count and clotting screen

Table 11.4 Assessing the patient with acute upper gastrointestinal haemorrhage; factors which influence morbidity and mortality

Age: over 60

Pre-existing disease. Examples are: cirrhosis, hypertension, chronic bronchitis

The blood loss. Assessing the circulatory changes as described in Chapter 7

A second or third acute haemorrhage

The endoscopic findings; varices or multiple erosions are worse than a single ulcer

carried out along with analysis of plasma chemistry. Anaemia usually means acute-on-chronic haemorrhage. Endoscopy of the oesophagus, stomach, and duodenum will be available at the drop of a hat. In three-quarters of cases the lesion, ulcer, ruptured varix, will be visualized and the anatomical site carefully noted.

The criteria for admission to intensive care will be taught to the trainee; those used at the Whiston Hospital were given in Chapter 3. Similarly, the indications for surgical treatment of the haemorrhage would have been formulated by consensus. No experience is required to know that continuing haemorrhage is nearly always preventable.

III LIVER FAILURE

1. Patterns and pathophysiology

Impaired functioning of the liver is common in the critically ill, irrespective of the primary disease; fortunately this is slight and rarely threatens life. In sharp contrast, acute life-threatening liver failure can be the central problem. Whichever pattern of liver failure, the beginner should appreciate that there is no nice simple test of failure as exists in renal failure. For didactic teaching the problems can be broken down as follows:

(a) Hypoxic damage

Can you remember the quote from J.S. Haldane 'anoxaemia not only stops the machine, but wrecks the machinery'. Which organs are most susceptible to hypoxia? The novice should list the organs in their susceptibility. Hypoxia due to shock or respiratory failure damages the liver and histologically the centre of the hepatic lobule suffers most. Clinically we will not be able to

Table 11.5 The body systems in acute liver failure

Body fluids	Potassium depletion, hypoglycaemia, respiratory alkalosis, metabolic alkalosis, lactic acidosis
Lung	Increased ventilation, pulmonary oedema, respiratory failure.
Circulation	Hypotension (septic shock), dysrhymias
Kidney	Renal failure
Brain	Delirium, impaired consciousness, coma, tremor, decerebrate states
Liver	Jaundice, foetor, blood shows raised unconjugated bilirubin and high amino-transferases
Blood	Consumptive coagulopathy

recognize this dysfunction, and diagnosis is suspected when the plasma transaminases are high.

(b) Jaundice

This can develop following trauma or sepsis. The serum bilirubin varies widely, from 30–600 μmol/l (normal 5–13). The commonest histological finding is stasis in the bile ducts within the parenchyma, but the pathophysiology still awaits solution. Both hypoxic damage and 'ICU' jaundice probably influence the chances of recovery, but the proof of this would require a large trial.

(c) Acute or subacute liver failure

This is a much more tangible subject. Firstly, it is the primary problem; secondly, the cause can be found; and lastly we have a clinical definition of its more severe form: fulminant hepatic failure is diagnosed when encephalopathy occurs within 8 weeks of the first symptoms. The causes are easily dealt with: the accidental or suicidal ingestion of chemicals or drugs. Carbon tetrachloride and paracetamol are examples. Very rarely a drug taken therapeutically in the correct dose causes acute liver failure, and the reaction is labelled idiosyncratic, but the label tells us little. One or more of the many viruses of hepatitis can cause acute failure. Irrespective of the cause the damage is widespread so that the numerous functions of the organ are deranged. But, as in so many acute illnesses, the pathology is widely disseminated as summarized in Table 11.5. But do not expect to find them all in one patient or at the same time! The changes in brain function require emphasis because of their clinical implications. Brain oedema causes the expected rise in intracranial pressure, and a general intoxication caused perhaps by an excess of normal metabolites.

2. Assessment

This follows the standardized methods of intensive care. The clinical and laboratory methods must prevent the spread of hepatitis viruses! The clinician should bear in mind that it is so easy to miss delirium (Chapter 10). When there is delirium or impaired consciousness, this means that the patient has developed hepatic encephalopathy.

12

Metabolic failure

The most destructive processes seen in the study of body composition are those that combine severe injury with starvation and invasive sepsis. The body cell mass quickly melts away into a hypotonic ocean of extra-cellular fluid.

Francis Moore, 1963

    I   **THE METABOLIC RESPONSE TO INJURY**
    II   **DIABETIC KETO-ACIDOSIS**

This chapter summarizes the metabolic response to injury and diabetic ketoacidosis. The first is an inevitable sequence to injury, major surgery, and many other conditions; it requires intensive monitoring and appropriate supportive therapy. Diabetic ketoacidosis is included for two reasons. Firstly because selected patients need the ICU to survive, and secondly it illustrates perfectly all the principles of general intensive care. The other causes of metabolic failure require emphasis – hypoxia, for example. To requote J.S. Haldane 'Anoxaemia not only stops the machine, but wrecks the machinery'.

I THE METABOLIC RESPONSE TO INJURY (MRI)

This pattern of disturbed metabolism was first identified in 1924 by the late Sir David Cuthbertson, and the serious student is advised to read the review written by the discoverer some 56 years later! (Cuthbertson, 1980) We must emphasize that the MRI is completely different to the semi-starvation of healthy subjects, by accident, by malice, or simply slimming. The term physiological response to injury is sometimes used, but is incorrect; MRI is unphysiological and can prolong illness or itself kill the patient. A vital factor influencing the signs and outcome is nutrition. For the patients in this group appropriate nutrition (Chapter 17) can make the difference between life and death.

1. The patient

During the 'ebb phase' the signs are those of hypotension, pale skin, and maybe oliguria. After a few days things hot up, as it were. Fever is the rule, the skin is warm and flushed; the pulse rapid, and of large volume. Body weight falls – unless too much fluid is infused – and the loss of subcutaneous fat and widespread muscle wasting become evident with associated weakness; the extent is often masked because of interstitial oedema. There is apathy and depression. Wound healing is impaired as is the whole immunological system. Anaemia is variable. The recovery phase occupies weeks or months. Further symptoms can develop due to errors or omissions; hyperglycaemia or folate deficiency for example.

2. Metabolic findings

(a) Prior to resuscitation, metabolism is deranged due to shock, energy expenditure may be reduced and tissue hypoxia can lead to an anaerobic type of cell metabolism. The production of catecholamines is increased. The plasma free fatty acids are often high but the blood sugar may fall. Acute deficits of salt and water can follow diarrhoea, ileus, obstruction or extensive burns. The core temperature can either fall below the normal due to heat loss during anaesthesia and surgery or the temperature may be raised due to extensive inflammation or infection. An imbalance of electrolyte and water following injury can be directly attributed to a metabolic response rather than the obvious causes previously described. The imbalance takes the form of a reduced renal excretion of sodium and water and it follows that when normal basal intakes of water (2.5 litres) and sodium (100–150 mmol/l) are given a positive balance of one or both is likely to occur and thus cause saline excess (overhydration) and oedema. In the critically ill patient it is rarely possible to disentangle this cause of a positive balance from the other causes, namely preceding dehydration and renal failure. The imbalance is probably mediated through excessive secretions of aldosterone and antidiuretic hormone; a balance can be restored by means of a diuretic.

(b) A few days after the injury or established infection, energy expenditure increases and thus energy requirements rise. Some of the causes are obvious; fever, tissue healing, increased cardiac work or respiratory work (muscles of respiration). Extensive burns lead to enormous loss of energy from the body because of the evaporation of water from the raw areas. But the energy expenditure can rise to levels for which we cannot account. This increased expenditure of energy persists for 1 or 2 weeks after major surgical operations or multiple injuries, but in the circumstances like burns, or continuing infection, the imbalance persists for many weeks. An increased metabolic rate can readily be worked out by the reader. The body weight falls but not as much as might be thought because of the 'ocean of hypnotic fluid'. By using isotopes it was possible to show how the four body compartments undergo striking change. The ICF volume is commonly reduced and that of the ECF increased. The physiological balance between synthesis and catabolism is deeply disturbed. Synthesis of protein (don't forget this includes all enzymes) is depressed so that there is anaemia, low plasma proteins, depleted immunoglobulins, and many more deficits. Catabolism is accelerated hence the label hypercatabolic state. All protein is degraded resulting in increased gluconeogenesis and the production of huge amounts of nitrogenous waste. The latter is chiefly urea but also creatinine and urate. The huge increase in urinary nitrogen leads to a severe negative balance (Chapter 4) which defies correction by treatment but is reduced by appropriate nutrition. You must understand that the negative nitrogen balance is not some interesting laboratory finding, but mirrors the muscle wasting – 'endogenous cannibalism' as our colleague M.J.T. Peaston called it; a negative nitrogen balance kills patients. When 70% of the body nitrogen has been consumed the outcome is certain. To date no treatment can switch off this devastating metabolic failure. The intracellular compartment is also depleted of other components, phosphate and zinc for example. The beginner must get to grips with the nitrogen balance in quantitative values on individual patients. To refresh the memory, the information given in Chapter 4 is repeated here. Figure 12.1 shows the external balance for saline, potassium and nitrogen following a 'routine' cholecystectomy for gall stones and that following multiple injuries. The first produces a moderate metabolic response and the latter causes severe alterations to the body structure and function. In each case the balance shown is for the fifth day following the 'injury' and both patients were given dextrose and saline. By way of self-assessment, the reader should be able to describe and then interpret the balance for saline and potassium then write down the clinical consequences. The nitrogen balance is easy. In both cases the output of nitrogen is increased despite an intake of almost none. For the injured patient, the negative balance was 20 g of nitrogen per day, mostly urea. What was the source of this urea? Day after day of this accelerated protein catabolism would kill in 2 weeks. Later in the book we will learn that this destructive state is modified by the nutrition denied this patient.

(c) Glucose intolerance.   Some 60 years ago the 'diabetes of injury' was recognized but the mechanisms are very different from those of insulin dependent diabetes mellitus. In the glucose tolerance following trauma or accompanying invasive sepsis, the plasma concentration of endogenous insulin and cortisol are elevated. Hyperglycaemia can occur in the patient who has – wrongly – been starved or only becomes evident when appropriate carbohydrate is given, usually i.v. glucose. It is important to recall that the

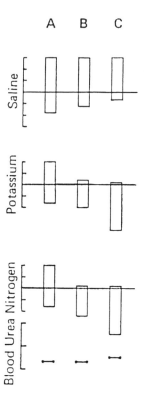

Figure 12.1 Balance data for saline, potassium, nitrogen and blood urea. A, control; B, following cholecystectomy; C, following multiple injuries. Details are given in the text (From *Essential Intensive Care*, with permission)

more glucose oxidized the greater the carbon dioxide production, which means increased alveolar ventilation.

(d) Recovery.   Nature heals, doctor takes the credit! When the patient and supportive therapy win through, the metabolic madness gradually subsides. Insulin therapy is no longer required, the nitrogen balance starts to swing from negative to positive, muscle is therefore restored and enhanced synthesis means that anaemia, hypo-albuminaemia are reversed. If interesting facts interest you, then transferin is one of the last proteins to be restored. The pathophysiology of the MRI is complex; here is an aid to memory. Changes occur in the following ten parameters: oxygen consumption, cardiac output, body temperature, plasma glucose, plasma lactate, plasma free fatty acids, catecholamines, glucagon, cortisol, insulin. In the flow phase, all are increased. In the ebb phase the first three and the last are decreased, and the remainder increased.

II DIABETIC KETOACIDOSIS

1. Principles of general intensive care

Diabetic ketoacidosis can be used to illustrate the essentials of intensive care. The right patient in the right bed at the right time. The management of the patient in a general ICU is a piece of cake and there will be no errors or omissions; in a general ward the exercise may be a struggle and horrific complications occur – inhalation of vomit, undiagnosed bacteraemia for example. The staffing levels at night or on Christmas Eve may mean that the other patients get second-rate care. Intensive care can guarantee effective management, but cannot prove that it saves money, but then high standards of anything in life costs more! Another principle is that the centralization of the care will facilitate the teaching of this emergency by standardized methods – yet another essential of intensive care. When recovery is underway then the factors leading to this preventable state are analysed and steps taken to avoid it. Education of the patient, general practitioner, community nurse are obviously considered. Finally, a psychological aspect – no, not the patient, the service doctor. If a general ICU resists the admission of the diabetic, asthmatic, or epileptic, then the whole service must be critically examined. For example, if a patient is turned away because of medical ignorance or resentful personality traits, then a new service doctor is required.

2. Pathophysiology

The post-basic nurse or house officer will already be familiar with those changes in physiology characteristic of diabetic keto-acidosis; this section is therefore a brief one. The disturbances in the metabolism of carbohydrate fats and body proteins lead to changes in the body fluids which in turn lead to failure of one or more systems. Indeed the changes in the physics and chemistry of the ECF can reach extremes, for example an arterial pH of 6.8 or a blood sugar of 30.0 mmol/l. Cell function is consequently severely affected or there is cellular death, depending on the severity of the disturbance and the duration. So far we have described changes in concentrations (hydrion, sugar) but equally disastrous changes occur in the whole body but these may be less obvious to the beginner. Deficits dominate and are readily revealed by means of the external balance method described in Chapter 4. The results obtained during treatment have shown that the total deficits may

Table 12.1 The body fluids in diabetic keto-acidosis; common findings

The compartments	
ECF	volume decreased
Blood volume	reduced, haematocrit raised
ICF	volume decreased, depleted in K, P, Ca, Mg
Blood chemistry	
Nap	normal or low '
Kp	normal or high despite depletion
Clp	low
Cap	normal
Mgp	normal
Inorganic P	normal or high despite depletion
pH	low or very low
$PaCO_2$	low or very low
HCO_3	low or very low
Osmolarity	high
Acetone	100–400 times normal
Aceto-acetic acid	high
3-hydroxybutyric acid	high
Insulin	low
Cortisol	high
Catecholamines	high

be 6–8 litres of water; 500–600 mmol sodium, and 300–400 mmol potassium. When sodium and water deficits are extreme (say 900 mmol sodium and 8 litres of water) shock develops with hypotension, low central venous pressure, oliguria, and hypoxaemia. The reader should pause and explain to themselves the apparent contradiction of a huge potassium deficit with hyperkalaemia. The increase in the production of aceto-acetic and 3-hydroxybutyric acids causes a metabolic acidosis. These acids diffuse from the cell and are, at first, buffered by the plasma bicarbonate, proteins and inorganic phosphates. The concentration of bicarbonate in the plasma falls. The rising concentration of acids increases alveolar ventilation and the $PaCO_2$ falls. This compensates for the fall in bicarbonate and helps to keep the pH nearer to normal. As the acidosis progresses the buffering capacity of the blood and other fluids is overwhelmed and the pH falls progressively,

Table 12.2 The body systems in severe diabetic keto-acidosis

The lung	Hyperventilation: increased frequency and $\dot{V_E}$
Heart and circulation	Hypovolaemia, heart failure, shock
Kidney	Oliguric renal failure (pre-renal, intrinsic, obstructive), proteinuria, increased white cells
Gastrointestinal tract	Vomiting, stomach distended and emptying delayed. Increased risk of acute pancreatitis
Liver	Increased gluconeogenesis, uptake of precursors, triglyceride deposits and ketogenesis. Absent glycogen
Brain	Failure: delirium

despite minute volumes of 28–30 litres and $PaCO_2$ values of 1.3–2.7 kPa (10–20 mmHg). A quick revision; the pathophysiology is summarized in Tables 12.1 and 12.2.

3. The patient

Diabetic acidosis develops over 8–72 h. The dominant symptoms are thirst and polyuria; nausea and vomiting are common. Abdominal pain is a frequent symptom, particularly in children; the pain is usually generalized, may be severe and associated with dilatation of the stomach. The pathological processes causing the pain are unknown. The patient is found to be drowsy or unconscious. The tongue and mouth are dry and the elasticity of the skin and muscles greatly reduced. The respirations are deep and rapid, the breath smells strongly of acetone. The skin is pale except for that of the face which is flushed. The pulse is rapid and weak and the systolic, diastolic and pulse pressures lowered. The abdomen may be tender to palpation and occasionally shows rigidity. A precipitating cause may be found from the relatives or during the clinical examination or by examination of the urine or chest radiograph.

The general ICU will have to deal with other, much rarer, metabolic emergencies, acute porphyria for example. Also, other endocrine emergencies are relevant; Addison's crisis, myxoedema, coma, extreme hyperthyroidism or tetany. The problems of diagnosis and therapy are outside the scope of this book, but information is readily to hand in the ICU library – that's the justification for a library which never closes! We are grateful to Professor GKAW Alberti for help with Tables 12.1 and 12.2.

13
Disorders of coagulation

I	THE HYPERCOAGUABLE STATE
II	DISSEMINATED INTRAVASCULAR COAGULATION (DIC)
	OF INJURY AND INFECTION
III	DIC OF OBSTETRICS

The first and second disorders are exceedingly common and fortunately the coagulopathy of obstetrics is rare and, unlike the others, largely preventable. From your student days it will be recalled that blood clotting is complex and it should be no surprise that the coagulopathies relevant to intensive care are also complex. This chapter is an over-simplification of the problems and therefore didactic; it is not intended for clot doctors. Let us take heart by starting with the easy one!

I THE HYPERCOAGUABLE STATE

Quickly following a fracture or any surgical operation, the blood becomes more coaguable and clots form, chiefly in the veins of the feet and calves. Although these events are nearly ubiquitous, your experience may have misled you to conclude that they rarely cause harm. This is not so, because the postmortem has shown that thromboembolism is a common cause of morbidity and mortality in the hospitalized person. Haemorrhage renders the circulating blood hypercoaguable. Ponder for a moment at the genius of a William Hewson who demonstrated this fact in 1772. He observed that when sheep were exsanguinated or patients were subjected to blood letting 'the blood which issued last coagulated first'. The hypercoaguable state can be demonstrated in a blood sample by comparing tests on your own blood with those from a patient. It is a good practical exercise to see the tests of Table 13.1 performed and to remember the results. When the one or more processes causing the blood to clot have ceased then a repair process comes into operation, thrombolysis or fibrinolysis. This occurs as a physiological process in healthy subjects, so that in the hypercoaguable state we are really talking about accelerated or enhanced fibrinolysis. Increased fibrinolysis can be demonstrated by laboratory tests directly or by measuring the increase in the breakdown products – fibrin degradation products (FDP) which are excreted in the urine. In some intensive care patients, for example,

13.1 Basic laboratory tests for diagnosis of coagulopathy (From Bain, 1982, with permission)

Test	Function tested
Platelet count	
Bleeding time	platelet number and function
Prothrombin time (PT)	extrinsic and common pathways
Activated partial thromboplastin time (aPTT)	intrinsic and common pathways
Thrombin clotting time (TCT)	the conversion of fibrinogen to fibrin, and therefore the level and function of fibrinogen, the presence of heparin and the presence of other antithrombins such as fibrin/fibrinogen degradation products
Fibrinogen level	
Fibrin/fibrinogen degradation products (FDPS)	lysis of either fibrin or fibrinogen
Clot observation	excessive fibrinolysis

ARDS, the early acceleration of fibrinolysis is followed by depression which means that the repair process stops or is slowed down. The reader is already familiar with the clinical manifestations of hyper-coagulopathy; deep venous thrombosis and pulmonary embolus. Although out of context, a word on prevention is important. Early ambulation and physiotherapy are beneficial but do not influence the incidence of thromboembolism. Only heparin, started before the anaesthesia is induced will reduce mortality and morbidity. More information on this is given in Chapter 28.

II DIC OF INJURY AND INFECTION

Although intravascular clotting is a cardinal feature this must be separated from thromboembolism. The striking difference is the site of the clotting. In DIC the intravascular coagulation takes place in the capillaries. The blood is often hypercoaguable and the clotting is triggered by activators. In turn the activators are triggered by catecholamines or corticosteroids – and these familiar hormones increase during stress states. Alternatively, the DIC is triggered off by thromboplastin which reaches the circulation from damaged tissue, for example crushed muscle; circulating endotoxin is also a very powerful initiating agent. From this information we can deduce the clinical causes – trauma or bacterial toxaemia. When DIC is severe, which probably means widespread, then the clot formation uses up clotting factors and is labelled consumptive coagulopathy. It is necessary to digress for a moment to refresh your knowledge on the balance between production and destruction or consumption. In your own blood the platelet count is steady because the two opposing processes are nicely balanced. A reduced platelet count means defective production (e.g. folate deficiency) or increased consumption – DIC. The catch is that in the ICU patient a normal count or concentration of clotting factors may be due to increased production with increased consumption – potentially harmful. The body continues to produce these elements but the consumption can outstrip production. Hence there is thrombocytopenia, a reduced concentration of clotting factors and less commonly hypofibrinogenaemia. When consumptive coagulopathy goes far enough, then haemorrhage will result. To return to the intravascular coagulation. This could lead to failure of any organ – the liver, kidney, brain etc. But it is difficult to know whether organ failure is due to the DIC or to the cause of the DIC, especially in bacterial toxaemias.

This is an appropriate place to define the three facets of this coagulopathy. DIC is strictly a histological diagnosis made on a sample of tissue at autopsy or biopsy; the blocked capillaries causing organ failure. The next facet is the consumptive coagulopathy diagnosed by blood test. It is a pity that there is no clear-cut pattern to the blood tests; several tests are required and the overall picture interpreted. Neither are there agreed criteria for consumption. The usual laboratory findings in DIC are: a reduction in the platelet count to less than 100×10^9/l; prolongation of the PT, aPTT and usually the TCT; a reduction in the fibrinogen level to 0.5–1.5 g/l or less; and elevation of the FDP level, usually to 20–80 mg/l or higher. Low levels of plasminogen and antithrombin III are usual. A rapid deterioration of the platelet count or fibrinogen level suggests DIC, since normally both have long half lives. Since no single laboratory test is always abnormal, strict criteria cannot be laid down and tests must be interpreted in the light of the usual findings in the underlying disease.

Lastly, the patient! DIC can lead to haemorrhage from puncture sites, wounds or cause gastrointestinal haemorrhage; alternatively or concurrently we attribute respiratory, renal or brain failure to DIC. The incidence of DIC in the intensive care patient is not known with accuracy because the laboratory findings are so variable and internationally agreed criteria are not yet formulated. As with other system failure we must search out the conditions in all patients following major injury, during bacterial or viral infections, inflammatory bowel disease, pancreatitis – it would be easier to list the conditions when DIC is improbable!

This section concludes by mentioning an iatrogenic coagulopathy, heparin-induced thrombotic thrombocytopenia. This develops in a few percent of patients on heparin and is an immune response to this agent. The condition is easily missed. The hallmarks are progressive thrombocytopenia with or without thrombotic effects. A suspicion is confirmed or refuted by demonstrating that the heparin given will cause platelet aggregation. For once the treatment is simple; stop all heparin.

III DIC OF OBSTETRICS

This is separated off from the DIC of intensive care, not for the obvious reason of childbirth but because the clinical and laboratory findings are clearer, which makes life easier. DIC of pregnancy is extremely rare and like all rare conditions is likely to be missed. When recognised early, and treatment is correct, then intensive care of organ failure can be avoided. The missed case treated incorrectly will die. The occasional patient who does need intensive care provides an exciting challenge to the staff because complete recovery is the aim but this will only be achieved by meticulous attention to every organ of the body, including the psyche; a single error or omission can rarely be corrected. The causes are given in Table 13.2.

1. Pathophysiology

The pathology is straightforward even if the mechanisms are obscure as summarized in Table 13.3. You will need to be a generalist to cope with this lot! The consumptive coagulopathy follows a uniform pattern at least when compared to that of trauma or sepsis. There is thrombocytopenia, low clotting factors, and a low fibrinogen. Is this triggered off by the foetus, placenta or amniotic fluid? The answer is don't know. The shock is routine to the ICU and here is a real justification for measuring the pulmonary artery wedge pressure to sort out the mechanisms and to transfuse correctly (Chapter 20). Turning briefly to the renal physiology. This illustrates the problem of acute renal failure in the ICU, commonly there are several possible mechanisms, and in this case shock or the DIC. One or both, take your pick. In the study of acute renal failure this obstetric disaster became a well-defined natural history. The oliguria was both diagnostic and pre-dialysis – impossible to treat. Today, the oliguria is nearly always preventable by correct management of intravenous fluids and the early use of low-dose dopamine: dialysis has become a simple technical exercise (Chapters 22–25). The lung failure follows the pattern of ARDS but there are three possible mechanisms; intravascular coagulation in the capillary bed which

Table 13.2 Causes of DIC in the obstetric patient

Acute

    Abruptio placentae

    Amniotic fluid embolism

    Saline termination

    Septic abortion

Subacute

    Retained dead foetus

    Hydatidiform mole

    Pre-eclampsia and eclampsia

    Syndrome of haemolysis, elevated
      liver enzymes and low platelets

    Degenerating leiomyoma

Table 13.3 Pathophysiology of obstetric DIC

Site	Pathology	Mechanism
Uterus	Table 13.2 plus inflammation and infection	Trauma, opportunistic infection, decreased immunity
Blood	Consumptive coagulopathy, anaemia, leucocytosis	?
Circulation	Shock, microvascular thrombosis	Hypovolaemia, heart failure. Activated coagulation
Kidney	Acute tubular necrosis, renal cortical necrosis	Shock, ?DIC
Lung	Adult respiratory distress syndrome	Intravascular thrombosis, massive blood transfusions
Liver	Centrilobular necrosis	Hypoxia
Metabolic	Citrate poisoning	Citrated whole blood

we know is a histological feature of ARDS, massive transfusions of bank blood which contain aggregates capable of blocking the same capillaries, lastly bacterial toxaemia. You will know already that ARDS of itself has a death rate of 50%, no matter how skilled the therapy. Uterine pathology (Table 13.3) needs no expansion. Finally, an important metabolic disorder. Shock, heart failure and bacterial toxaemia all damage the liver – a syndrome of centrilobular necrosis. Impaired function means that the liver cannot metabolize the citrate present in some banked blood. This results in high blood levels of citrate (1000 μmol/l) and hypocalcaemia. Nothing could be worse for blood clotting!

2. The patient

For an early diagnosis all that is necessary is to consider the diagnosis every time one of the causes of Table 13.2 is encountered! A few simple blood tests (the jargon is clotting screen) will confirm or refute and early treatment is then possible. When this practice is neglected (medical negligence) then the diagnosis will depend on bleeding from puncture sites, respiratory distress (increased breathing especially important) or oliguria or shock. At this late state the patient is transferred to the ICU when a priority list is drawn up (10 minutes the maximum) and the therapeutic plan put into operation. The latter embraces the contents of this book as can be appreciated from Table 13.3.

14

Trauma

I   PATHOPHYSIOLOGY
II   HEAD INJURIES
III   CHEST INJURIES
IV   ABDOMINAL INJURIES

Trauma is a 'morbid condition of the body produced by wound or external violence' (*OED*). Trauma is a continuing plague of human activity and, tragically, major trauma is a significant cause of civilian deaths, particularly in younger age groups. Quite logically, the media keep the fearful statistics before us and the message is repeated yet again in Table 14.1 as related to two countries. The reader will know that only prevention can reduce this slaughter. This chapter concentrates on the knowledge essential to understand the intensive care of the injured. We assume that the reader has an elementary knowledge of fractures and dislocations.

I   PATHOPHYSIOLOGY

The causes of trauma as seen in a general ICU are forces which crush tissues or penetrate the tissues or cavities of the body. A proportion of patients sustain injuries that the beginner is unlikely to see, because they kill in the first few minutes or hours. Examples are transaction of a major blood vessel or the trachea; brain penetration. Of those who survive trauma, the main features can be grouped as early (minutes) and late (hours, days or weeks).

1. Early manifestations

These will depend on the site or sites of trauma as described in the sections to follow. But irrespective of the site there are two features of cardinal importance, chiefly because early recognition and prompt treatment are essential. These pathological processes are respiratory failure and continuing haemorrhage. Both subjects have already been described but a brief recapitulation may help. The essential pathophysiology of respiratory failure is shown in Table 14.2. The upper airway and impaired consciousness were dealt with in Chapters 6 and 10, and chest injury will follow. A few supplementary facts on failure due to spinal injury are given because this is too

Table 14.1 Civilian casualties due to trauma

	United Kingdom		Australia	
	Major injuries	Deaths	Major injuries	Deaths
Roads	45 000	3700	*	3000
In the home	130 000	5000	*	*
At work	16 000	400	*	*

*Data not available

Table 14.2 Pathophysiology of respiratory failure and the implications for treatment

1.	Obstructed upper airway due to impaired consciousness or foreign material	Restore and protect the airway (Chapter 18)
2.	Injured chest wall	
3.	Lung pathology, pneumothorax, bruises, gastric aspiration, early pneumonia.	Section III
4.	Spinal injuries	

often missed. In the multiple injured a search for paraplegia or tetraplegia must be part of a systematic examination. The essentials in diagnosis are paralysis, sensory loss, and the autonomic effects such as retention of urine and priapism. In the conscious the diagnosis is straightforward and the effects on pulmonary gas exchange can be assessed – paralysed intercostal muscles cannot move air! The recognition of paralytic respiratory failure is difficult or missed when there is either impaired consciousness, chest injury, or both. In these patients there are two or three processes which can cause respiratory failure.

Continuing haemorrhage. The trainee will now be familiar with the pathophysiology and signs of hypovolaemic shock; the tissue hypoxia and hypoxaemia 'stops the machine and wrecks the machinery'. Continuing haemorrhage is easily recognised even before the arterial blood pressure falls, so why the problem? In penetrating wounds the haemorrhage will continue until the surgeon can stop it. In the crushed patient, finding the site can be all too easy or all too slow. The essentials can be learned by starting at the patient's head and moving down the body. Severe haemorrhage from the scalp can hardly be missed but continuing haemorrhage concealed by bandages can kill; the implications are obvious. Haemorrhage in the thorax is recognised by radiograph and chest drains; more than 500 ml of blood per hour requires thoracotomy. Continuing haemorrhage into the abdomen is Catch 22. Abdominal pain and distension make the diagnosis probable. Peritoneal lavage and computerised tomography are valuable aids. An essential principle is that when intra-abdominal haemorrhage is a suspected cause of persistent shock then laparotomy is urgently needed.

Severe trauma induces endocrine, metabolic, and haematological changes and the metabolic rate is depressed; this was called the 'ebb phase', to be quickly followed by the 'flow phase' (Chapter 12). The circulating blood becomes hypercoaguable (Chapter 13).

2. The late features

From the mass media or the experiences of relatives or friends you will be familiar with the late death or disabilities which can follow trauma. Prompt first aid, expert resuscitation lead at first to a 'stable condition', as the hospital spokesman would have it, but during the next week or so progress changes for the worse. Indeed a great deal of the intensive care of the injured centres on the prevention or treatment of the late pathophysiology. This is summarized in Table 14.3 and the features are described below or in other chapters. Should the newcomer to intensive care find these complications both bewildering and depressing then try to imagine the feelings of the patient and relatives. Examples are all too with numerous: following a head injury with short-lived unconsciousness the patient talks only to lapse into deepening coma and apnoea. A case of fractured pelvis is 'doing well', until increased breathing is observed and ARDS is diagnosed.

II HEAD INJURIES

It is convenient to start by revising your knowledge of the anatomical lesions. In a general ICU the trauma is nearly always due to deceleration/acceleration forces and rarely due to penetrating wounds. Here is a brief list to jog your memory: contusions, haematoma (intra- or extradural) and shearing of the white matter; the latter can be appreciated by shaking a trifle: a blow to the containing dish will cause the sweet to oscillate but one layer will also shear from the next. Quickly following the initial impact, one or more secondary lesions can develop; these invariably threaten life. Congestion and oedema lead to swelling of the brain and an increase in the intracranial pressure (ICP). In health ICP is below 15 cm; 15–30 cm is high, and over 30 cm is

Table 14.3 Pathophysiology of trauma: late features

Organ or system	Pathophysiology
Brain	Expanding intracranial haematoma Generalized brain swelling Brain ischaemia Brain death Meningitis
Chest	Absorption collapse Microbial infection Pulmonary oedema ARDS
Abdomen, pelvis	Ileus Continuing haemorrhage
Kidney	Renal failure (Chapter 9)
Cardiovascular	Heart failure (Chapter 7) Septic shock (Chapter 7) Fat embolism. Thrombo-embolism
Aorta	Rupture of pseudo-aneurysm
Blood	Coagulopathy (Chapter 13)
Metabolic	Metabolic response to injury (Chapter 12)
Immune	Impaired resistance to microbial infection

probably lethal. Should haemorrhage continue, either resulting haematomas will cause focal ischaemia by pressure, but also cause a rise in ICP. No matter what the cause of the intracranial hypertension, the result is potentially lethal, ischaemia of the whole brain leading to brain hypoxia and cell death. The hypoxia will occur more readily when the arterial blood pressure or cardiac output are low and may be compounded by hypoxaemia. This can be due to an obstructed upper airway, and this tragedy, like untreated shock, has been called the 'second injury'.

The pathological disturbances form the basis of the clinical picture, but may not correlate with the anatomical lesions. In general intensive care the dominant physiological disturbance is altered consciousness; the spectrum of slight impairment to brain death was described in Chapter 10. Less common, but just as important are focal deficits such as monoplegia and excitatory phenomena, convulsions or delirium. Two natural histories will help to understand the pathophysiology. The initial trauma results in persistent coma with extensor limb responses; there is no skull fracture and no haematoma on CT scan. The pathophysiology is diffuse brain damage;

indeed macroscopically the brain may look normal. This natural history is comparable to non-traumatic hypoxic damage following cardiac arrest. The second natural history illustrates the consequences of the primary and secondary pathophysiology. A fall results in loss of consciousness for 10 minutes; there is a skull fracture. The patient recovers consciousness and talks during a 'lucid' interval. But this only lasts an hour. Coma follows and persists. Four hours later there is decreased breathing, then apnoea and brain death. You are dismayed that an intracranial haematoma was not diagnosed and removed! In about three-quarters of such patients a haematoma would be the fatal secondary event. In the remainder there is no discrete haematoma but diffuse damage has caused brain swelling. We have deliberately omitted the natural history of lucid interval coma with one dilated pupil and a contralateral hemiplegia. This natural history should now be relegated to the history books because, when due to a haematoma, severe secondary damage has occurred by the time the clot is removed.

III   CHEST INJURIES

Injuries to the thorax fall into one of two classes. Open injuries are produced by a knife stabbed into the chest, or by a bullet wound. In contrast, the second class are closed injuries and caused by a blunt impact which exerts a crushing force on the thorax. The latter are caused by traffic accidents either when a pedestrian or cyclist is in collision with a motor vehicle or the occupants of a motor vehicle when this is in violent collision. Closed injuries also occur in the building trade, coal mining and at the dock-side. A summary of the primary pathophysiology is given in Table 14.4 and a few of the problems are now described.

1. Shock

Shock is caused by tissue damage and loss of blood into the pleural cavity, lung substance or tissues of the chest wall. In addition to blood loss, other lesions can reduce the cardiac output; tension pneumothorax or pericardial tamponade either of which interferes with the filling or emptying of the heart.

2. Haemorrhage

Massive haemorrhage can be caused by a penetrating wound of the heart or a large vessel but similar haemorrhage can also follow a closed injury which tears the aorta or a pulmonary artery. Less dramatic but still life-threatening haemorrhage can take place in the lung parenchyma (haema-

Table 14.4 Crushing injuries of the chest: primary pathophysiology

Anatomical site	Results
Thoracic cage	
ribs, sternum	fractures
	flail chest
intercostal vessels	tears, haemothorax
intercostal muscles	contusions
Main bronchus	tears
Mediastinum	
major blood vessels	tears
lung	mediastinal emphysema
heart	contusions, tamponade
Lung	pneumothorax
	haemothorax
	contusions
Diaphragm	rupture
	hernia of stomach or bowel
Circulation	shock
	heart failure

tomas, lacerations) or the pleural space (haemothorax); in the last example the bleeding can originate from the lung or an intercostal vessel.

3. Pneumothorax

Unilateral or bilateral pneumothorax means that air has leaked into the pleural space, commonly from a punctured lung or rarely from a tear of a bronchus. When the puncture is valvular, allowing the air to flow in one direction only, that is into the pleural space, the pneumothorax becomes a tension one; this causes alveolar hypoventilation, also the resulting increase in the intrathoracic pressure impedes the filling and emptying of the heart, resulting in fatal shock.

4. Chest wall

The pathology depends to a large extent on whether the injury is penetrating or crushing in nature. A penetrating injury consists of one or more holes with a variable amount of surrounding muscle destruction – more with a high velocity bullet than with the knife. A large penetrating wound is obvious, but when bomb fragments are the cause, it may be impossible to decide which of the many skin wounds is penetrating. The pathology of a crushing injury is very different. The skin may show only minor abrasions; the muscles may be pulverized over one or more areas the size of the hand; many ribs or costal cartilages can be fractured; the sternum can break. Within a short time of the injury the tissues of the chest wall swell due to oedema or surgical emphysema. A distinct lesion of the chest wall is known as a flail segment, which can lead to paradoxical movement of the segment, the hemi-thorax or even the entire thoracic cage. The pathology is as follows: fractures of adjoining ribs, or fractures of ribs in two places causes a flail segment or area. During inspiration the thorax expands normally but the flail segment is drawn inwards; the underlying lung cannot inflate normally. A flail segment is more commonly seen anteriorly or laterally than posteriorly because the rib cage has the additional protection of the scapula and scapular muscles. Multiple and bilateral fractures of the costal cartilage cause the sternum to become flail. At one time it was thought that some inspired air would be drawn into the healthy lung from the lung underlying the flail segment. Physiological studies showed that this to-and-fro rebreathing (called pendelluft) did not occur.

5. Lung

Both penetrating and crushing (closed) injuries can cause bruising (haematomas), lacerations or localized oedema. Generalized pulmonary oedema can be due to a blast from an explosion or alternatively caused by fat embolism of the lungs. It is important to appreciate that the oedema may not become apparent on X-ray or may not influence gas exchange for hours or days.

6. Main bronchi

A rare development following a closed injury is rupture of a bronchus. The main bronchi are usually involved and the majority of bronchial tears occur within 2.5 cm of the carina. Unilateral and bilateral pneumothorax may result and air is present in the mediastinum. The diagnosis is likely when large volumes of air are seen escaping through the intercostal drains. X-rays of the chest shows mediastinal emphysema and air is also present in the deep cervical tissues. Pneumothoraces are present despite drainage and the lung or lungs remain collapsed.

7. Rupture of the diaphragm

This can be due to either a penetrating wound or a blunt injury to the thorax. A rupture is found more commonly on the left than on the right side and takes the form of a tear in the diaphragm through which may herniate the stomach or bowel. In turn this can cause gastric bleeding or intestinal obstruction.

A crushing force to the chest produces quite different trauma depending on the resilience of the thoracic cage, which is greatly reduced in the elderly. Thus a child of twelve may have no rib fracture but severe pulmonary contusions; a senior citizen may have eight rib fractures but no detectable lung damage.

IV ABDOMINAL INJURIES

A little imagination will enable the reader to envisage the pathology of intra-abdominal injury which may follow stabbing or shooting; just anything can result, although haemorrhage is the immediate threat to life. The anatomy of crushing injuries to the abdomen is more predictable. Tears of the spleen or liver top the list. Contusions of the large retro-peritoneal spaces can cause huge haematomas. Occasionally the gut is torn. A kidney can be contused or the renal pelvis torn.

Fractures or dislocations of the pelvic bones can be graded as minor or major. A unilateral fracture of the pubic ramus is minor. In contrast, when one or more of the pelvic bones are broken, the resulting haemorrhage is life-threatening. When this trauma is caused by a crushing force, then the haemorrhage can be self-arresting by the process of tamponade, already familiar in the pericardium. It follows that blood losses of ten litres or more will occur when there is an open wound in the perineum. The most catastrophic pathology is that associated with compound fractures of the pelvis. In addition to haemorrhage, the injured bowel is devitalized and sepsis follows. Those who survive the early phase of pelvic injury may look well for several hours or days following vigorous resuscitation. This can be misleading because the consequences of bowel devitalization and myoglobin injury to the kidneys may still endanger life for several weeks ahead. Despite early surgery and repeated debridements, late death remains common. The pathophysiology of the late disease is given in Table 14.3

15

Microbial infections

Microbial infections are a central theme of intensive care, and cast a long dark shadow over every activity. The result is as familiar to the lay relative as to those who work full time in units – infection too often kills the patient who should have walked out.

The accumulation of huge amounts of information on these problems has unfortunately not yet lifted the threat to the injured or surgical patient, and the intensive care of conditions like primary pneumonia leave room for improvement. Nevertheless, the benefits for selected patients outweigh the burdens. It is important to stress again the teaching role of the ICU, in particular to critically analyse the errors and omissions, and to help enforce the antibiotic policies of the hospital.

I CLASSIFICATION

We use simple classifications as an aid to teaching. The anatomical classification is given in Table 15.1 and needs no explanation. Infection at any one site can be grouped as primary or secondary, that is complicating a disease or therapy; for example, multiple injuries are complicated by respiratory infection. It is important to recognise those puzzling cases with a proven bacteraemia or all the signs of toxaemia but with sterile blood in which we cannot prove the origin of the infection.

II SOURCES AND MODES OF SPREAD

It may help to commence with the familiar. Recall for example the origins of the following: cholangitis, primary pneumonia due to *Legionella pneumophila*, meningococcal meningitis. These occur sporadically or in epidemics, but for each disease the sources remain the same. Hospital

Table 15.1 Infections and toxaemias related to intensive care

Lung	Primary pneumonia Complicating chronic bronchitis Complicating intubation or IPPV
Gastrointestinal tract	Peritonitis Gastroenteritis, dysentery Complicating inflammatory bowel disease Cholangitis
Urinary tract	Primary pyelonephritis Complicating obstructive uropathy Complicating catheterization
Obstetrics and gynaecology	Septic abortion Puerperal sepsis Complicating obstetric DIC
Brain and spinal cord	Meningitis Encephalitis Guillain-Barré (?infective) Tetanus Botulism
Blood and blood vessels	Bacteraemia and endotoxaemia of unknown origin Complicating intravascular cannulation or catheterization Complicating i.v. therapy

acquired infection has plagued our hospitals for centuries; knowledge has replaced ignorance, but the problems remain. Each year in the UK 100 000 patients acquire infection in hospital and this costs £100m. The beginner in intensive care will quickly recognise how the problem can change success into failure. There are literally hundreds of sources of infection in the intensive care unit. Indeed from its inception intensive care has made an important contribution to knowledge, but sadly the elimination of secondary infection is yet to be realised; the progress so far is given in Chapter 27. Some of the sources are given in Table 15.2 and this is next briefly expanded. A useful starting point is to group the sources as is done in Table 15.3 and to detail some examples. A patient develops pulmonary infection with *Pseudomonas aeruginosa* and laboratory tests showed that this originated in the faeces of another long-stay patient. How did the transmission occur? (i) The skin or bedlinen became contaminated with faeces and the *Pseudomonas aeruginosa* was transmitted to another patient on the fingers of a member of staff. Having colonized the pharynx or trachea the bacteria

Table 15.2 Sources of infection

Disease	Pathogen	Source
Primary pneumonia	*S. pneumonia* *M. pneumoniae* Influenza A *S. aureus*	Human carrier
	L. pneumophila	Lakes, reservoirs, air conditioning
Secondary pneumonia Complicating intubation or IPPV	Enterobacteriae *S. aureus*	Staff, equipment, solutions, patient's stomach, nutrients
Via the diaphragm	As for peritonitis	The peritoneum
Peritonitis		Patient's bowel
Cholangitis		
Wound infection, abscesses, bacteraemia	Staphylococci	Self-infection, other patient, staff environment

reached the bronchi by its own mobility or during suction. (ii) Nurse*. The nurses' fingers can be contaminated from one of many sources; own skin or nostril, contaminated handcream, saliva, faeces, wound fluid, infected urine, or gastric aspirate, and many more. Hand washing, although essential, will not ensure safe hands. Hence it is so easy to contaminate a suction catheter or the patient's mouth with *S. aureus*, or *Klebsiella* spp. (iii) A CVP line provides a wound for colonization by Gram positive skin bacteria, not forgetting Gram negative and fungi. The microbes reach the wound by droplet infection or carried on fingers when dressing. The colonists cause inflammation of the wound but unfortunately there is a high risk of a bacteraemia. (iv) The mechanical ventilator, was, in the early days of intensive care, a potential source of infection because of contamination from previous use and the difficulty of sterilization. Autoclaving of the patient's circuit has largely solved this one, but remember the casing can readily be contaminated, especially when wet.

---

*   Nurse gets the blame, but does most of the work; doctor is the real sinner (Chapter 27)

Table 15.3 Sources and transmission of hospital-acquired infection

Patient	Nostrils, mouth, pharynx, Skin Sputum, gastric aspirate, faeces Wounds, drains, burns
Staff	Nostrils, expired air (talking, coughing) Skin, fingers, hand cream, clothing
Immediate environment	Air, dust Walls, floors, trolleys Bed linen Handbasins, taps, lotions, soaps Shaving equipment, toothbrushes, Thermometers
Equipment	Suction apparatus Ventilators, anaesthetic machines Dialysers, filters Catheters
Nutrition	Beverages, ice-cubes, food Intragastric feeds I.V. infusions

III PATHOPHYSIOLOGY

We briefly digress into the physiology to ensure that the reader is familiar with the bacterial flora. In healthy adults, two sites of the body are colonized by bacteria which are labelled normal flora; these sites are the oropharynx and the large gut. The distribution of the various types of bacteria is fairly uniform. In the colon the anaerobes compose 99.9% of the population, and 0.1% are Gram negative (GN) aerobes. This balance is partly maintained by a process of bacterial interference; thus the anaerobes prevent expansion of the GN aerobes. Healthy subjects regularly inhale bacteria from the oropharynx, but these are quickly dealt with by the defence mechanisms. In a few healthy subjects with achlorhydria, the stomach is colonized by bacteria.

During very varied illness (and in addition to the neoplastic diseases), following surgery or trauma, changes occur in the defence system and in the bacterial colonists. Within a few days the oropharynx is colonized by GN aerobes and the latter increase in the colon. In addition, these bacteria colonize the small gut and stomach, the latter then becomes a bacterial

Table 15.4 Some effects of infection of toxaemia

Site	Result
Lung	Consolidation Adult respiratory distress syndrome
Heart and circulation	Syndrome of warm hypotension Heart failure, shock
Brain	Delirium, impaired consciousness
Kidney	Renal failure with or without oliguria
Liver	Impaired function, jaundice
Blood	Anaemia, rarely acute lysis Leucocytosis or leucopenia Coagulopathy
Metabolism	Glucose intolerance Accelerated metabolism Impaired protein synthesis
Any site	Inflammation, sepsis

reservoir. These changes occur with or without antibiotic therapy. The same patients are also likely to be colonized by bacteria from other long-stay patients which can be transmitted, for example, on the hands of the hospital staff or by equipment. The same sites, oropharynx, stomach or gut are colonized as well as the skin or bladder. These facts help us to better understand the mechanisms of bacterial infection in the 'intensive care patient', even when the environmental sources have been largely eliminated. Infection is particularly common in those with an intubated airway, catheterized bladder, intravascular devices or naso-gastric tube. We now move from facts to hypothesis. In the naso-pharynx, either the normal flora including *H. influenzae* and *S. pneumoniae*, or the new colonist like *Klebsiella* spp. can readily reach the lung and colonize the tracheal/bronchial tree or cause infection. It is also probable that the GN aerobes reach the lung from the gastric reservoir. Infection of the lung by *S. pneumoniae* or *Haemophilus influenzae* tend to develop early during intensive care, and the GN ones later on.

We assume the reader to have an elementary knowledge of clinical bacteriology, so try a self-assessment: name the enterobacteriae: what is the armoury of the hospital staphylococcus? By what means do strains of *E. coli* damage the organs of the body? The effects of infection or toxaemia are brought together in Table 15.4. We must emphasize again that bacterial toxaemia often occurs without a bacteraemia. For example, a patient can show warm hypotension and delirium or oliguria, but the blood is sterile. These signs, with or without other system failure, call for prompt action to provide any chance of survival. A few additional words on immunology are necessary, but what follows is a mixture of theory and fact. Let us start with the familiar. The defences are impaired by anything which damages the skin or mucous membranes; intravascular lines, nasogastric tubes, an endotracheal tube or a tracheostomy; urethral catheters, surgical or accidental wounds; pressure due to immobility; absence of the normal blinking of the eyelids. Body defences also depend on normal gut mechanics and are impaired when motility is decreased due to disease or therapeutic drugs. But to these dangers must be added impairment of the immune system of the body. Many of the following factors acting singly can be shown to impair defence against bacterial invasion: increasing age, trauma or surgery, malnutrition, renal failure, prolonged anaesthesia. A useful hypothesis is that when a few of these factors are present together, then the scene is set for life-threatening bacterial infection – the colonists become the invaders. Unfortunately, most of the factors are beyond influence but we can concentrate on malnutrition and the prevention of colonization. Thus the intensive care patient can start off with the dice loaded against survival. And yet another unfavourable factor must be mentioned. Should a broad spectrum antibiotic be given – quite logically – to treat an infection, when a few days later another life-threatening infection can develop. The pathophysiology is as follows. The antibiotic inhibits and diminishes the normal bacterial inhabitants of the body. A resistant micro-organism initially present as a small minority can then multiply and become dominant. The same mechanism allows resistant micro-organisms – which reach the patient by the methods described in Section II – to colonize and maybe cause infection. The end result is that the normal flora composed mainly of antibiotic sensitive organisms is replaced by secondary flora of resistant organisms. Examples are *Klebsiella, Serratia* spp. and *Candida* spp. This is not the end of the depressing story. Broad spectrum antibiotics commonly cause diarrhoea and rarely contribute to a life-threatening condition labelled pseudomembraneous colitis; the pathogen is *C. difficile*.

IV DIAGNOSIS AND MONITORING

1. Diagnosis

The diagnosis of any infection whether primary, like meningococcal meningitis, or secondary like that complicating prolonged IPPV will require a thorough knowledge of the natural history of the conditions, including the probable pathogens; relevant radiographs and lastly tests on blood and other body fluids. The latter fall into three categories: haematological to determine the bone marrow response, microbiological to isolate the pathogens, and immunological to obtain direct evidence of the causative organism. The natural history of the primary infections is beyond our brief and the reader will be familiar with some of the secondary infections; like those associated with diabetic keto-acidosis, peritonitis, pyelonephritis, or chronic bronchitis. These problems are straightforward but not so those infections which are secondary to occult conditions; for example, undiagnosed infection with HIV or any one of the viruses of hepatitis. Recognition of the infections complicating IPPV was given in Chapter 19. If the reader feels that they should revise their medical microbiology, we have recommended a reading list at the end of the chapter. We would urge the beginner not to lose heart at a bewildering number of micro-organisms isolated during intensive care; a few weeks charting them as described later will result in some familiarity. A provisional diagnosis, good enough to start therapy may be obtained in a few minutes by microscopy of a sample of sputum, cerebrospinal fluid, or urine. Isolation of the pathogen by culture will take hours or days; for Gram-negative organisms 18 h but for Gram-positive bugs or yeasts, 48 h. Hence in some cases, having taken the appropriate samples, therapy is started blind (Chapter 27). A recurring problem in a variety of acute illnesses is to decide whether or not severe inflammation is due to microbial infection. Examples are acute pancreatitis, inflammatory bowel disease, closed injuries to the chest or abdomen. In both instances, there is fever, leucocytosis, and often other signs of toxaemia; tachycardia, warm hypotension, and the pattern of increased breathing. Differential diagnosis can be made more accurate by definitions and we use those published by an impressive group of American Chest and intensive care physicians (1992). The inflammatory illness just described then becomes the Systemic Inflammatory Response Syndrome (SIRS). If SIRS is proved to be due to infection, then the label becomes sepsis (Appendix 2 to Chapter 15).

2. Monitoring

Believe it or not, the aim of monitoring is to contribute to recovery rather than to collect data for a PhD! Charting the course of an infection is part of the monitoring of the patient as a whole; not forgetting to ask how the patient feels! The simplest observations on body temperature and white cell count are of cardinal importance. Depending on the primary site of the infection, imaging techniques will help monitor progress. Thus in the lung the daily chest radiograph is invaluable. In contrast, in monitoring peritonitis

Table 15.5 Bacterial monitoring of the patient during IPPV

Non-selective daily routines	Swabs or specimens from the following sites: nose pharynx trachea stomach wounds drains
Selective routines	
High risk or suspicion of bacteraemia	Blood cultures
Cross infection	Search for the source as shown in Table 15.3

or meningitis imaging techniques contribute little. The metabolic trends would certainly help: less insulin for the same food intake is a favourable sign.

The strictly bacterial monitoring is carried out by methods which are standardized but tailored to the disease. The aims are two-fold. Firstly to determine whether one or more pathogens are eliminated; examples would be the disappearance of *Kl. aerogenes* in the tracheal aspirate or sterile blood which previously grew *S. pneumoniae*. Our second aim is to detect as early as possible the development of secondary infection which is itself secondary to colonization. This is a large undertaking for the bacteriological laboratory, but is a must in the surgical or trauma patient and during IPPV or dialysis. An example of a standardized method is given in Table 15.5. Also part of the fabric of intensive care is the bacterial monitoring of staff, environment and equipment. We will leave this preventive monitoring to Chapter 27.

Dr HKF van Saene assisted with this chapter.

APPENDIX 1

Abbreviations

Genus	Abbreviation, with individual species
Acinetobacter	*A. calcoaceticus*
Aspergillus	*A. fumigatus*
Bacteroides	*B. fragilis*
Moxarella	*M. catarrhalis*
Citrobacter	*C. freundii*
Clostridium	*C. perfringens*
Enterobacter	*E. cloacae*
Escherichia	*E. coli*
Haemophilus	*H. influenzae*
Klebsiella	*K. pneumoniae*
Legionella	*L. pneumophila*
Morganella	*M. morganii*
Proteus	*P. mirabilis*
Pseudomonas	*P. aeruginosa*
Serratia	*S. marcesens*
Staphylococcus	*S. aureus*
Streptococcus	*S. pneumoniae*

APPENDIX 2

Definitions (1 to 10 HKF van Saene, personal communication; 11 to 13 modified from American College of Chest Physicians/Critical Care Medicine Consensus Conference, 1992)

1. Infection. A diagnosis needs symptoms together with a sample from a given site which yields $>10^5$ colony forming units from 1 ml.
2. Superinfection. A new infection caused by a new organism or the primary organism which has become resistant while the patient was on i.v. antibiotics, or within a week of stopping treatment.
3. Exogenous infection. An infection caused by micro-organisms introduced into the patient from the environment by staff or equipment. The micro-organisms are introduced to the site where colonization and infection then occur, e.g. *Pseudomonas pneumoniae* following the use of a contaminated bronchoscope.
4. Primary endogenous infection. An infection caused by micro-organisms acquired either in the community or the hospital, and which are already carried at the start of the illness; examples are, *H. influenzae* pneumonia, *P. mirabilis* infection following intra-abdominal surgery.
5. Secondary endogenous infection. An infection caused by micro-organisms acquired after admission to the ICU and which are invariably 'hospital' bacteria, e.g. *Acinetobacter* pneumonia caused by a strain originating in another long-stay patient and transferred via the hands of the staff. After acquisition, carriage develops, followed by colonization and infection.
6. Colonization. The microbial presence at a body site which is normally sterile. The diagnostic sample must yield $<10^5$ colony forming units from 1 ml
7. Carriage. The isolation of identical micro-organisms from two consecutive surveillance samples (saliva, gastric fluid, faeces, vaginal fluid) in any concentration over a minimum period of one week.
8. Surveillance samples. Samples from the throat and rectum are obtained on admission and afterwards twice weekly, e.g. Monday and Thursday. These specimens are needed (i) to detect the carriage of potential pathogens, (ii) to evaluate their eradication by non-absorbable anti-microbials and (iii) to detect the carriage of resistant strains.
9. Diagnostic samples. These are sent to the laboratory when clinically indicated, (i) to diagnose infection and (ii) to evaluate the results of antimicrobial therapy.
10. Outbreak. An event wherein two or more patients develop a superinfection by an identical and multi-resistant bacterium.

11. Systemic Inflammatory Response Syndrome (SIRS). This follows a variety of severe insults, some microbial, some not; for example multiple injuries, pancreatitis, inflammatory bowel disease. The signs are: temperature >38° or <36°, tachycardia, increased breathing, leucocytosis or leucopenia.
12. Sepsis. This is SIRS due to infection.
13. Septic shock. This is sepsis with hypotension despite adequate fluid resuscitation. There may be oliguria, delirium or acidosis.

SECTION THREE
PRINCIPLES OF THERAPY

16
Fluid therapy

... the pure syndromes, like Platonic universals, scarcely deign to show
themselves in this workaday world.   D.A.K. Black, 1967

There must be an orderly process in treatment ... they should be nudged,
not kicked. in the right direction.   Francis Moore, 1959

  I   **INTRODUCTION**
  II   **FLUID THERAPY**
  III   **ACID–BASE THERAPY**

I INTRODUCTION

When healthy, we enjoy the eating and drinking essential to maintain a state
of metabolic balance. Drinks other than water contain electrolyte, energy and
protein; conventional food contains water and electrolyte. Consequently, in
health our fluid therapy and nutrition are inseparable. The same may be true
for the intensive care patient but in other cases, or at some stage of an illness,
the fluid therapy and nutrition require separate plans. It is important to
remember that fluid therapy can readily be given without giving nutrition, but
nutrition always includes fluid therapy. The newcomer to intensive care
should appreciate that the treatment of each patient admitted to a general
ICU has to be arranged in a priority list which includes therapy and nutrition,
but these are often third or fourth on the list. Since nutrition tends to be
forgotten, we have made a rule that all patients requiring intensive care for
more than 48 h must be given appropriate nutrition. The requirements for
fluid therapy must depend on the disturbances caused by the disease and
these were described in Chapter 4. Nevertheless the requirements of most
ICU patients can be predicted from published observations. This means that
standardized schemes can be drawn up; such policies form one of the
essentials of intensive care as was described in Chapter 2. To practice fluid
therapy and nutrition the trainee requires knowledge of the disturbances
described in Chapters 4 and 5. To facilitate description the therapy of
acid-base disorders is given in a separate section. Aseptic methods and the
techniques of tube feeding and central venous cannulation are skills that are
readily acquired. The appropriate attitudes were described in Chapter 2.

II FLUID THERAPY

For the great majority of intensive care problems, fluid therapy can be simplified to the three components, water, sodium and potassium. The fluid therapy for a particular disease or the individual patient has to be fitted into the general priority list of treatment. The planning is then taken one step further (Table 16.1). The deficits or excesses of water, sodium and potassium are arranged in the order of their importance so that each can be dealt with in turn, or several disturbances can be treated at the same time. When major deficits or excesses – the former are more commonly found – have been corrected then the maintenance fluid therapy can be planned. A general principle is that maintenance fluid therapy should be incorporated in a scheme for nutrition. The fluid therapy of the four common disturbances are next briefly described but it should be borne in mind that the patient often requires more than one therapy, given consecutively or concurrently.

1. Saline depletion (dehydration and hypernatraemia)

The treatment of saline depletion depends on three principles: the size of the deficits of sodium and water; whether the continuing losses of sodium and water exceed the normal; whether the sodium and water can be given by the gastrointestinal tract or can only be given intravenously. Moderate saline depletion implies a deficit of 250–500 mmol of sodium and 2–4 litres of water. The deficit can be corrected by giving frequent beverages or by giving a standard tube feed, providing that the gastro- intestinal tract is functioning normally and the continuing losses of sodium and water are normal. In other cases the deficit is corrected by intravenous fluid therapy. In most examples the Nap is normal or low and the salt and water are then given as normal saline (sodium chloride injection BP 0.9% w/v. (Table 16.2). A provisional plan would be to infuse normal saline at 250 ml/h for 12 h and then re-assess. Progress is monitored by the mental state, the elasticity of the tissues. the urine output and the blood urea. The Nap cannot be used to control the therapy for the reason given in Chapter 4. When the Nap exceeds 155 mmol/l, either on admission or during treatment,, then weaker salt solutions (31 or 77 mmol/l, Table 16.2) or 5% glucose (glucose injection BP 5%) are included in the scheme.

Severe saline depletion corresponds to a deficit of 500–1000 mmol of sodium and 5–7 litres of water and should always be treated by intravenous infusions of saline. When the saline depletion has resulted in hypovolaemic shock then there is a strong argument for using a colloid in saline rather than normal saline.

Table 16.1 Overall plan for fluid therapy and nutrition (From *Essential Intensive Care*, with permission)

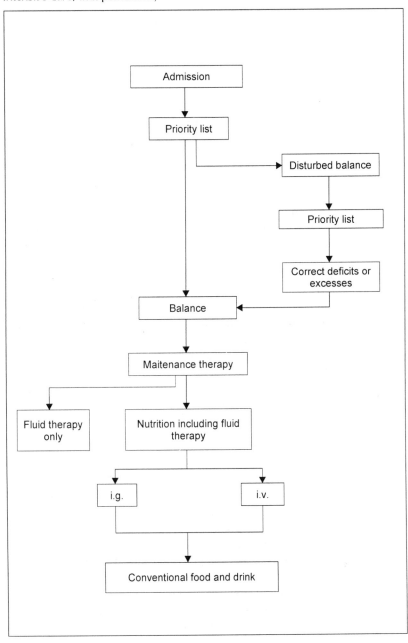

Table 16.2 Commercial intravenous solutions of sodium chloride (From *Essential Intensive Care*, with permission)

	Per cent (g/100 ml)	mmol/l
Sodium chloride injection BP	5.0	855
	1.8	308
	0.9	154
	0.45	77
	0.18	31

A colloid of gelatine in saline is infused at a rate of 500–1000 ml over 20 min and the circulation monitored (Chapter 7). If this treatment results in both restoring the circulation and a urine output of greater than 50 ml/h then the fluid therapy is continued with normal saline. Should the colloid fail to restore the circulation then the further investigation is necessary as described in Chapter 7. On the other hand oliguria with a satisfactory circulation needs investigation according to a well-defined plan (Chapter 9).

Severe hypernatraemia merits a direct therapeutic attack in addition to the treatment of the cause (Chapter 4). The hypernatraemia is treated by infusion 5% glucose or 1/5 normal saline (31.0 mmol/l) at a rate of 250 ml/h until the Nap, measured 2-hourly, falls to 150 mmol/l. When the hyperna-traemia is accompanied by hyperglycaemia, then hypotonic saline is used and 5% glucose is not given. When the Nap is down to 150 mmol/l, the emergency has passed and fluid therapy and other treatment are revised to prevent a recurrence. If not already in progress, balance data for sodium, potassium and water are collected.

2. Saline excess (over-hydration)

This means a positive balance for sodium and water occurring over hours or days; the positive balance is both inappropriate and harmful. Saline excess must be clearly distinguished from acute circulatory overload. (Chapter 4). The treatment of saline excess depends on whether it is due to the metabolic response to injury or infection, or caused by renal failure. The management of saline excess due to the former mechanism is quite straightforward. The intake is not restricted because these patients invariably have high nutritional requirements. The inappropriate retention of sodium and water is rectified by a diuretic. We give frusemide or bumetanide intravenously; a modest dose of either will cause a brisk diuresis and natriuresis. The saline excess often recurs after a day or so and the diuretic is repeated. Saline excess is so dangerous to the intensive care patient that early recognition is imperative and this can only be obtained by an external balance (Chapter 4). Saline excess is then recognized before the patient shows either oedema of the soft tissues or the lungs. Saline excess caused by renal failure requires a different approach. In acute renal failure, daily intake of water is reduced to 2 litres and that of sodium to 50 mmol. Saline excess is treated by haemodialysis or haemofiltration. In chronic renal failure, the intake is also reduced and the balance restored by one of two methods, used alone or together; these are larger doses of a potent diuretic and dialysis. These treatments will be detailed in Chapters 4, 23 and 24.

Hyponatraemia. This is a common finding in the ICU patient which sometimes needs a change in therapy. The treatment depends on the pathophysiology; (a) an excessive secretion of antidiuretic hormone, itself part of the metabolic response to trauma (Chapter 12). When the hyponatraemia is moderate (Nap 120–130 mmol/l) the feeding scheme is left alone or the volume decreased. On the other hand, severe hyponatraemia calls for direct treatment. The formula is to restrict the water intake and infuse hypertonic saline. The aim is to raise the Nap at a rate of 1.0 mmol/h because rapid correction can damage the brain stem (hence the Francis Moore quote at the start of this chapter). Hypertonic saline (5%, 855 mmol/l) is infused in small amounts (50–100 ml/h) until the clinical manifestations of hyponatraemia are alleviated and the Nap reaches 120 mmol/l. (b) When severe hyponatraemia complicates the course of acute renal failure the correct treatment is to increase the Nap by dialysis against a fluid having a sodium concentration of 140 mmol/l and to remove water at the same time. We prefer haemodialysis or haemofiltration to peritoneal dialysis and use a dialysate or replacement fluid containing 140 mmol/l. If peritoneal dialysis is used the dialysate contains the same concentration of sodium but water is removed by the osmotic action of 6.3% dextrose.

3. Potassium depletion and hypokalaemia

Serious potassium depletion can often be prevented by maintaining a normal intake (80 mmol/day) during acute illness or following surgery or trauma. When potassium loss exceeds the normal the balance method (Chapter 4) is used to keep up with these losses. The treatment of moderate potassium depletion is to increase the intake. This can be done by giving a 'good' diet, puréed ward food, a standard intragastric liquid diet (Chapter 17) or by means of intravenous potassium chloride. A tube feed provides about 100 mmol of potassium a day. The intake of potassium is increased by adding 50 mmol (2.0 g) of potassium chloride to one of the 3 litres of liquid diet. The standard intravenous diet (Chapter 17) also gives a normal potassium intake which can be increased by adding 25, 50 or 100 mmol potassium chloride to the amino acid solutions. The treatment of severe potassium depletion depends on three principles: (i) Whether potassium depletion is causing serious effects on the circulation, the bowel, brain, kidney or acid–base balance (Chapter 4). (ii) The degree of hypokalaemia; severe hypokalaemia is defined as Kp values in the range 1.5–2.5 mmol/l. (iii) Whether large potassium losses are continuing. If the clinical signs, ECG, balance data and Kp indicate the need for intensive replacement we invariably give potassium intravenously rather than by intragastric tube, even in the absence of gastrointestinal failure. The reason for this policy is that intensive replacement by mouth is too slow, uncertain and may cause intestinal ulceration. The replacement solution is made up from ampoules containing 10 or 20 mmol of KCl and from 5% glucose. This mixture can be delivered through a central venous line by one of two methods; (i) That used at the Whiston Hospital for 15 years is simple and cheap. A litre bag of 5% glucose is connected to 100 ml burette which is then half-filled with the glucose. The KCl, either 10 or 20 mol is next added from a syringe and the burette then filled to the mark and the contents shaken. The solution is infused into the superior vena cava usually at a rate of 10–20 mmol per hour. (ii) A KCl–glucose mixture is infused by means of an electronically-controlled pump. The aim of the therapy is to convert hypokalaemia from severe to moderate. This usually takes 12 h during which time the Kp is measured two to three times. During intravenous potassium therapy it is usually possible to start a diet of normal potassium content.

4. Hyperkalaemia

Following cardiac arrest (Chapter 8), during diabetic acidosis, or during starvation no treatment is required to correct the hyperkalaemia. in these states the total body potassium is normal or even reduced. Hyperkalaemia during large and rapid blood transfusions may require intravenous calcium to prevent cardiotoxicity. Hyperkalaemia requires specific treatment only when it complicates the natural history of acute renal failure or terminal (end-stage) renal failure. When hyperkalaemia is severe (Kp 6.5– 10.0 mmol/l) and especially when developing rapidly (that is over a few days), or when accompanied by a metabolic acidosis, then there is a serious risk of cardiac arrest. Let us consider acute renal failure first. In the main, hyperkalaemia can be avoided by a combination of an appropriate diet with early and intensive dialysis. Should the patient be able to take conventional food, then items rich in potassium are omitted. If, on the other hand nutrition is intravenous, then supplements of KCl are omitted. Potassium is removed from the body by using a dialysate containing about 2.0 mmol/l of potassium. When on rare occasions the diagnosis of acute renal failure has been delayed the patient can have severe hyperkalaemia. In this instance the treatment of choice is immediately dialysis. Should there be delay in arranging for this, then the Kp can often be lowered to a safe level and cardiac arrest thus avoided by an intravenous infusion of dextrose–insulin–calcium gluconate. A single injection is made of the following: 100 ml of 50% glucose, 50 units of insulin and 20 ml of 10% calcium gluconate. The correction of hyperkalaemia in chronic renal failure is also largely dependent on diet and dialysis. When the patient is known to have chronic renal failure then a climbing Kp will be one of several indications to start a programme of maintenance dialysis with a view to transplantation. If such methods are not available then the hyperkalaemia is partially controlled by a low protein, low potassium diet (modified Giovanetti). To hasten the falling Kp an ion exchange resin is given for the first few days – calcium polystyrene sulphonate, 15 g, 8-hourly by mouth. Hyperkalaemia presents a more difficult problem in the 'uraemic emergency' of the patient with previously unrecognized chronic renal failure. Clearly severe hyperkalaemia, especially when accompanied by a metabolic acidosis, requires urgent correction. The treatment now depends on the presence or absence of oedema. The oedematous patient should be started on dialysis or filtration right away as this will correct both acidosis and hyperkalaemia simultaneously. In the saline-depleted or normally hydrated patient with hyperkalaemia and acidosis the latter is ameliorated by giving intravenous sodium bicarbonate in a dose dictated by the arterial pH (Table 16.3). The hyperkalaemia is next treated by dialysis or by infusing the glucose–insulin–calcium gluconate solution referred to. The third priority in all such cases of chronic renal failure is to start adequate nutrition. by intravenous infusions if there is nausea, vomiting or diarrhoea.

III ACID–BASE THERAPY

1. Prevention

The ICU should devote considerable thought and effort to the prevention of acid–base disturbances, or failing this, to contain the disorder. This aspect of treatment is far more important than the occasional specific acid–base therapy, which means giving base (alkali) or, exceptionally, acid. This principle is of such importance that it will be illustrated by clinical situations. Respiratory acidosis; an acute respiratory acidosis can often be prevented altogether by (i) adequate care of the unconscious, (ii) prompt IPPV in sedative poisoning or polyneuropathy (iii) the early and correct treatment of

Table 16.3 Alkali therapy in metabolic acidosis. Initial dose of intravenous sodium bicarbonate to partially correct a metabolic acidosis (From *Essential Intensive Care*, with permission)

Arterial pH	Sodium bicarbonate, mmol
7.10–7.20	100
7.00–7.10	150
6.80–7.00	200

asthma. Metabolic acidosis; can be prevented or mitigated by (i) immediate defibrillation of the heart when the coronary patient develops primary ventricular fibrillation, (ii) prompt and efficient treatment of shock, (iii) appropriate nutrition of the surgical or trauma case, (iv) early admission and detailed management of diabetic acidosis, (v) early and intensive dialysis for hypercatabolic renal failure. All these aspects of intensive therapy are dealt with in the ensuing chapters.

Most disturbances of acid–base balance should call attention to the metabolic or respiratory care of the patient as a whole, but they do not require specific treatment. A severe change, especially when it occurs acutely, can maim or kill the patient and calls for immediate treatment to oppose the change. It must be stressed that the treatment – alkali therapy, dialysis or acid therapy – can only restore the internal medium for a limited time; they buy time to enable the causes to be investigated and treated.

2. Intravenous alkali

Alkali therapy means giving base, as a soluble salt, to replace or partly replace the deficit of bicarbonate in the ECF. Alkali therapy is given only in severe metabolic acidosis. Does one treat the pH or the bicarbonate? The answer is the former, since it is the low pH which can kill. During intensive care, the base is given intravenously as a single dose or intermittently. The first recorded successes were in the treatment of cholera; a case record in 1832 and a series of patients in 1910. The choice of alkali is important. It is logical to replace by bicarbonate, and all the evidence favours sodium bicarbonate rather than the potential alkalis sodium lactate or sodium acetate. Lactate is inferior to bicarbonate during critical illness because, with a notable exception of diabetes, the acidosis is often caused by an excess of lactic acid. Sodium acetate is rapidly converted to bicarbonate except in diabetic acidosis and is a satisfactory substitute for sodium bicarbonate, but commercial preparations are not readily available. For intravenous use we recommend only sodium bicarbonate. In the treatment of the dire emergency, such as cardiac arrest or the pulseless state, we use the 8.4% solution, since 100 ml (100 mmol) can be given quickly. When the pathological process allows a little more time, as in diabetic acidosis or renal failure, we use an isotonic solution (1.26%, 150 mmol/l); the reason for this is to reduce the risk of hypernatraemia. The dose required to convert a severe acidosis to a moderate is given in Table 16.3. It is quite safe to give the infusion quickly over a few minutes. Ten minutes later the pH and $PaCO_2$ are measured. and further alkali given according to the results. Alkali therapy has three important complications: alkalosis, saline excess (fluid overload, over-hydration) and hypernatraemia. Alkalosis means incorrect treatment. The usual cause is oversight during resuscitation. An 8.4% or 4.2% infusion is started, but not supervised and an excess is given. This error can be avoided by giving the bicarbonate with a syringe or by using an infusion set fitted with a burette. Another iatrogenic alkalosis occurs when a forced alkaline diuresis is used incorrectly. A moderate alkalosis (pH = 7.5–7.6) is probably harmless; a severe alkalosis will cause tetany. Saline excess cannot occur when bicarbonate is given to the dehydrated diabetic, but it is a real hazard when hydration is normal, but the kidney is unable to excrete the sodium load. This is likely to be the case in the following: cardiac arrest due to acute myocardial infarction; severe shock due to haemorrhage; acute oliguric renal failure; during the metabolic response to injury seen in the surgical patient or case of multiple injuries. In all these patients, the amount of sodium bicarbonate is kept to the minimum required to convert a severe acidosis into a moderate one. As soon as the emergency is over, oliguria is investigated and treated. A severe metabolic acidosis complicating acute oliguric renal failure should be corrected by dialysis rather than by intravenous sodium bicarbonate.

Hypernatraemia, when severe (160–170 mmol/l), leads to hyperosmolar brain damage. Infusions of sodium bicarbonate, especially the hyperosmolar ones, can cause hypernatraemia and the following patients are particularly at risk; diabetic acidosis with hyperglycaemia; the surgical patient with intestinal obstruction or paralytic ileus. To minimize the risk of hypernatraemia. the patient is given isotonic sodium bicarbonate (1.26%, 150 mmol/l) rather than the hyperosmolar solutions.

3. Oral alkali

This is required by a few intensive care patients. These have chronic renal failure and are admitted to the unit because of a rapid worsening of the uraemia, or because of concomitant hypertension. In those patients who survive the uraemic emergency, a metabolic acidosis may persist due to wasting of bicarbonate by the diseased kidney. The acid–base balance can lie maintained by giving alkali by mouth and sodium bicarbonate tablets BP (600 mg, 7.1 mmol or 300 mg, 3.6 mmol), adjusting the dose to compensate the dose for acidosis.

4. Dialysis

This is a powerful method for both restoring and then maintaining the acid–base balance of the blood and ICF. This is not however used for this purpose alone, but as part of the metabolic care of the patient with acute or chronic renal failure. Dialysis can correct a metabolic acidosis or alkalosis by the exchange of acid and base between the blood and dialysate. In the case of a metabolic acidosis, the excess of acid (lactic, phosphoric) diffuses into the dialysate and bicarbonate or potential alkali (acetate, lactate) diffuses into the blood. It will be immediately evident that when the acidosis is due to a high concentration of lactic acid (5.0 mmol/l), then a peritoneal dialysate containing lactate will aggravate the acidosis rather than correct it. It follows that in the case of a lactate acidosis, if found by laboratory measurement or suspected through the natural history, the dialysate must contain bicarbonate or acetate as the base. A severe metabolic acidosis is seen in hypercatabolic acute renal failure and intensive dialysis will usually control both the acidosis and the uraemia, and at the same time maintain fluid balance. Similarly, in chronic renal failure a metabolic acidosis is an important facet of the uraemic emergency. If such a patient has oliguria and oedema, then dialysis is used and alkali is not given. A distinct type of acute renal failure is seen in the general ICU with the following characteristics: potassium depletion with hypokalaemia, and a metabolic alkalosis together with polyuria and uraemia. Intensive dialysis or filtration (or both) is required to control the uraemia and the dialysis will also correct the metabolic alkalosis.

17
Nutrition

'Every careful observer of the sick will agree in this, that thousands of patients are annually starved in the midst of plenty.'

Florence Nightingale., 1859

I   INTRODUCTION
II   ENTERAL NUTRITION
III PARENTERAL NUTRITION
APPENDIX: EXTERNAL BALANCE FOLLOWING SEVERE
           TRAUMA

I INTRODUCTION

Food is essential to maintain the metabolism which in turn maintains the body. No matter how new to hospital practice you will be familiar with starving patients! Starvation increases morbidity and mortality – we don't need any more trials to prove this, but not all starving patients need appropriate nutrition. The very old with severe disabilities or those with terminal cancer must never experience thirst but heroic nutritional support is inappropriate. In contrast, if the aim is to get a patient better in the shortest time, then food is essential. Why this class of patient suffers malnutrition is a sad reflection on medical training in particular and on the attitudes of doctors to nutrition. The good news is that all patients in the ICU receive the appropriate nutrition, and the unit can give continuous training – rather preaching – on the consequences of malnutrition and on prevention; a process of educational feed-back. Fortunately, nutrition is an easy treatment and requires only minutes of medical time; 90% of the work is for the nurses!

The materials and equipment required were manufactured from 1960 onwards. The essentials were: glucose polymers to replace glucose, amino acid solutions and fat emulsions. In the early days a few essentials were forgotten: folic acid, fat soluble vitamins, zinc, and trace elements, such as manganese and copper. The CVP line (Chapter 7) transformed i.v. nutrition and prepacked kits with a silicone rubber catheter made for safety and efficiency.

II ENTERAL NUTRITION

Roughly half of the patients in the general ICU need either i.v. nutrition or tube feeding, but the remaining half should not be neglected; patients with acute myocardial infarction, heart failure, asthma, and the injured also need food.

1. Ward food

British hospitals do not have an enviable reputation for the food served to ward patients. Despite much criticism, the food, when analysed for its nutritional value will usually satisfy the basic requirements of physiological man at rest. This statement is as valid today as it was in early hospital records (Table 17.1). The various reasons why most severely ill patients cannot eat enough of hospital food to avoid semi-starvation were given in Chapter 4. It suffices to emphasize here that half-eaten meals or 'light diet' have no place in the intensive care unit. When it is obvious that a patient will be unable to eat sufficient conventional food, it may be that the food could be swallowed if made into a purée. For such cases the hospital kitchen is requested to supply lean meat, liver, etc. A portion is put into a household blender, a small quantity of vegetable and nutritious gravy added and the mixture then puréed and fed to the patient.

Table 17.1 Food at St. Bartholomew's hospital in 1687(From Drummond and Wilbraham, 1939)

10 ounces of Bread	
4 ounces of Cheese	
2 ounces of Butter	
1 pint of Milk Pottage	
3 pints of Beere	
Calories	2600
Proteins	80 g
Fat	110 g
Calcium	1.9 g
Phosphorus	1.85 g

2. Supplements

Tasty snacks of high nutritional value can help the patient with multiple injuries, burns or severe infection. Examples are listed in Table 17.2. The

Table 17.2 Nutritious snacks to supplement nutrition (From Grant and Todd, 1987, with permission)

	Protein (g)	Energy (kcal)	Volume (ml)
Peachy milk shake 150 g tinned peaches 50 g skimmed milk powder 200 ml milk	25	435	375
Cheap chocolate shake 50 g Complan 10 g drinking chocolate 250 ml milk	19	420	300
Ambrosia shake 150 g tinned rice pudding 100 ml milk 50 g Polycal	9	390	300
Orange juice 400 ml natural orange juice 100 g Polycose	3	532	450
Tomato soup + Caloreen 300 ml tinned tomato soup 50 g Caloreen	2.5	365	330
High protein soup 200 ml tinned strained soup 50 ml milk 10 g Caloreen 15 g Maxipro	18	250	275

Suppliers: Caloreen, Clintec; Complan, H J Heinz; Maxipro, Scientific Hospital Supplies; Polycal, Cow and Gate; Polycose, Abbott.

supplements must not be used as a substitute for an adequate diet, given by nasogastric tube or intravenously. Glucose polymers (Caloreen, Clintec) or Poly Joule (Sharpe) are preferred to glucose because they are much less likely to cause nausea, vomiting, or diarrhoea. Chocolate, spirits, fresh fruit and cream are other examples of food supplements. All help to match the increased requirements for energy and nitrogen, to maintain oral hygiene and by no means least, to maintain morale. Caloreen is a mixture of polysaccharides. It is highly soluble in water and much less sweet than glucose, only 3% of which is present. Caloreen can readily be served as an ice cream, pudding or high energy coffee. A solution made by adding an equal weight of water can be added to fruit, puddings, gravies, soups and beverages. This solution provides 2500 kcal/l.

3. Liquid diet

When a patient is unable to unable to eat conventional or purée food it may still be possible to maintain metabolism by beverages alone. Such a diet must be acceptable and free from side effects. The reader would have no problem in downing seven drinks over a period of 12 hours and would probably complain of hunger, but a seriously ill patient may find a liquid diet difficult due to general weakness, apathy, or dyspnoea. Persuasion, praise, even bullying may be required to ensure that a 2-hourly regime succeeds, an example of a liquid diet providing about 2000 kcal and 80 g of protein is shown in Table 17.3.

Table 17.3 Example of a fluid diet. All seven drinks must be consumed to provide adequate nutrition

Time		Protein (g)	Energy (kcal)
8.00	Egg in 200 ml milk and sugar	12.8	320
10.00	Complan 30 g in 200 ml water	5.5	150
12.00	High protein soup 250 ml and/or	19.0	200
	milkshake 250 ml	15.0	350
14.00	150 ml fruit juice and 100 g Caloreen		400
16.00	Complan 30 g in 200 ml water	5.5	150
18.00	High protein soup 250 ml and/or	19.0	200
	milkshake 250 ml	15.0	350
20.00	Complan 30 g in 200 ml water	5.5	150
Total intake		60–90	1500–2200

4. Intra-gastric nutrition

This is easy to understand. When the gastrointestinal tract is working but the patient cannot swallow, i.g. nutrition is cheap and simple, and i.v. nutrition is unnecessary. Examples will be head injury, and Guillain Barré syndrome.

An early example of successful tube feeding was recorded by John Hunter in 1790. Mr. Hunter assisted by Mr. Cumming, a watchmaker, used a tube made from a fresh eelskin. At one end was fixed a bladder and pipe,

> '...to inject jellies, eggs beat up with a little water, sugar, and milk, or wine by way of food.'

(a) Materials.   We need to avoid side effects but ensure adequate nutrition. In the early days of intensive care side effects were numerous; diarrhoea due to excessive osmolarity, or intolerance to the sugar lactose, to name just two. Fortunately, these problems are now behind us. The patients who can be fed by this method have physiological requirements of energy and nitrogen, so that a diet for a healthy adult must be developed in liquid form. From the evidence it can be concluded that protein is better than amino acids (an elemental diet) and an obvious choice is casein. Carbohydrates is given in the form of a glucose polymer and vitamins and trace elements are added. At Whiston we used for 20 years a tube feed made up from milk powder (Complan, Heinz) and a glucose polymer (Caloreen, Clintec). This was shown to maintain metabolic balance and had few side effects. The materials are sterile, and when the diet is prepared hygienically, then no harmful bacteria will contaminate the food. Complan–Caloreen remains an entirely satisfactory liquid diet. During the last 10 years numerous commercial tube feeds 'ready to use' have been competing for a small market. The makers have resorted to hard selling techniques to convince hospitals of advantages that don't exist! Two examples of tube feeds are given in Table 17.4.

(b)   We now require an intra-gastric tube and a means of moving the liquid into the stomach. For intensive care a Ryle's tube is preferred to an enteric feeding tube. It is an easy job to pass the tube when the patient is conscious or drowsy but still capable of swallowing. In contrast, it may be very difficult when an oral endotracheal tube is already in position. In this case, it may be possible to pass the tube into the upper oesophagus by using a laryngoscope and McGill's forceps. When this method fails, the following method invariably succeeds. The operator places a finger in the patient's mouth and lifts the endotracheal tube anteriorly. The other hand is now used to pass a second endotracheal tube (without a cuff) into the oesophagus. About 3 cm of the tube is left protruding from the lips. The Ryle's tube is now threaded into the second endotracheal tube and passed into the stomach and the endotracheal tube is then removed. It then remains to change the position of the free end of the Ryle's tube from the mouth to a nostril. A suction catheter is passed through a nostril into the mouth and

Table 17.4 Standard intragastric diets

MATERIALS

A   refers to 'Fortison Standard' (Cow and Gate), widely used in the UK.
B   refers to Isocal (Bristol-Myers, Mead Johnson) used at the Royal Prince Alfred Hospital

Composition	A	B
Volume (ml)	3000	3000
Energy (kcal)	3000	3000
Nitrogen (g)	19	20
Electrolyte (mmol)		
Sodium	105	69
Potassium	114	102
Calcium	38	45
Magnesium	18	24
Chloride	66	84
Phosphate	144	144
Osmolarity (mosmol/l)	260	300
Trace elements (μmol)		
Copper	45	48
Iodine	1.5	1.8
Iron	40	480
Manganese	218	165
Zinc	15	459

then hooked out of the mouth with a finger or by McGill's forceps. The tip is firmly inserted into the free end of the Ryle's tube and the catheter is next pulled back through the nose, leaving the Ryle's tube in its final position. When suction with a syringe fails to produce gastric contents, the following test is carried out. An observer auscultates below the xiphysternum whilst 10 ml of air is quickly injected down the Ryle's tube. Air will be heard entering the stomach if the tube is correctly positioned. If the position of the tube remains uncertain, then a radiograph is taken to confirm its whereabouts. To reduce the likelihood of oesophageal reflux during the tube feeding, the bed is adjusted so that the head, neck and trunk are inclined at about 10° to the horizontal. The liquid food can be passed down the tube by gravity (no cost!) or by an infusion pump. The cheap method first. An aliquot of liquid diet is measured into a medicine glass and then poured into the barrel of a 20 ml syringe which is used as a funnel. Slight pressure by means of the plunger on the syringe may be needed to start the flow which will continue with the aid of gravity when the funnel is held about 15 cm above the nose. Tube feeding is started with aliquots of 40 ml each hour and the stomach is aspirated just before giving the next feed. When there is no significant aspirate, the aliquots are increased up to 125 ml each hour and the Ryle's tube is then aspirated only once or twice a day. The intake of liquid diet is entered on a simple fluid balance chart, together with any gastric aspirate of bowel action. The alternative is to pump the sterile liquid from a container by means of an infusion pump and adjust the controls to deliver the volume quoted above.

(c) Complications. The commonest complication, frustrating and often perplexing, is when the food refuses to go down the gastrointestinal tract. Despite bowel sounds being heard the stomach refuses to empty. The syndrome defies explanation although drug therapy is often blamed. The condition may be self-curing, or gastric emptying can sometimes be started by giving a few doses of metaclopramide or cisapride. Failure of i.g. nutrition means a change to i.v. food and this is never postponed for more than 24 hours. Regurgitation of the food into the pharynx will be recognised early by the expert nursing team. This requires immediate investigation to ascertain whether the food has entered the trachea, even when a cuffed tube is in place. In the early days of tube feeding diarrhoea was common and due to hyperosmolar food or lactose intolerance; both these problems were solved, but diarrhoea still occurs and cannot be explained. Treatment of the diarrhoea is empirical. One or two days' therapy with codeine phosphate syrup BPC can be tried, 10 ml of the syrup 6-hourly. An alternative drug is loperamide syrup given hourly in a daily dose of 6–16 mg. When these fail the best policy is to stop tube feeds and substitute an intravenous diet. The Ryle's tube can cause ulceration of the nostril when badly taped to the nose or roughly handled, or ulceration of the lower end of the oesophagus, especially if the patient is nursed continuously in a horizontal position. The authors have not seen any overt effects of damage to the oesophagus. The remaining problem of i.g. nutrition, although not strictly a complication, is that of bacterial contamination of the food. The materials are safe but bacterial contamination can easily occur during preparation. To reduce bacterial multiplication only sufficient food for 6 hours is prepared in the reservoir bag which is changed daily. We would again emphasize that the stomach is an important reservoir of infection and therefore it is important to make sure that gastric aspirate does not reach the feed, fingers or equipment.

III PARENTERAL NUTRITION

1. Materials

These are widely available to westernized medicine and have been thoroughly tested for safety. The materials can be grouped as 'main courses' and 'side dishes'. The former consists of glucose solutions, amino acids and fat emulsion. The side dishes are vitamins and trace elements. Insulin is often required and is given as a continuous infusion. The amino acid solutions consist of a mixture of essential and non-essential acids. The concentration of each is based on the structure of first class protein and the concentrations of amino acids present in the ECF of healthy subjects – the concept of the milieu intérieur again (Chapter 4). The fat emulsion is made from soya with an emulsifier and stabilizer. The emulsion resembles the chylomicrons of the lymph fluid in your thoracic duct after a nice fat lamb chop! The writers believe that the principle of standardized methods (Chapter 2) must apply to nutrition, a view backed up by their combined experience of a hundred years. This means that the shopping for materials is not made at random but is decided by the ICU team and then adhered to until such time that advances in nutrition make for a change. We recommend the choice of one or two amino acid solutions, one made of fat emulsion and glucose, as shown in Table 17.5

2. Design of the diet

For any application i.v. nutrition must provide a balanced diet – hopefully as taken by the reader enterally! For general intensive care the diet must be a liberal one because most of the patients have a high metabolic rate, even though they are at rest. Those patients with injuries or infections will have both increased metabolism and also metabolic failure. This follows the pattern known as the metabolic response to injury (Chapter 12). This harmful process cannot be 'treated' or switched off but is mitigated by giving a generous supply of both energy and nitrogen. For example a negative nitrogen balance of 14 g/day (equivalent to the loss of 400 g of lean muscle) can be reduced by half. A standardized diet will therefore be balanced and provide about 3000 kcal. (12.6 MJ) and 12.0 g of nitrogen. Such a diet would suit a hard labourer but not a navvy of the last century. The experts recommend that half of the (non-protein) energy should be derived from the fat emulsion and the remainder from glucose. Another essential point is to balance the energy intake against that of nitrogen. If you calculate the energy in kilo calories and the daily nitrogen in grammes, then a satisfactory ratio of kcal/gN would be 200 : 1.

Table 17.5 Standardized intravenous diets commonly used in the UK.
A; big bag system. B; paired infusions with lines X & Y. Both methods supply appropriate vitamins. Materials other than glucose, KCl and folic acid from Pharmacia and Upjohn

Materials for A			Materials for B		
Single line (ml)		*Time* (h)	*Line X* (ml)	*Line Y* (ml)	*Time* (h)
Vamin 14	1000			Vamin 14 500	
Glucose 50%	500			Additrace 10	8
Glucose 10%	500			15% KCl 10	
Intralipid 20%	500			Folic acid 1	
Addiphos	20	24	Continuous		
Vitlipid N adult	10		infusion of	Intralipid 20% 500	8
Additrace	10		glucose 40%	Vitlipid N adult 10	
Folic acid	1		at 40 ml/h		
Solivito N	1 vial			Vamin 14 500	
				Addiphos 20	8
				Solivito N 1 vial	

	Compositions			Trace elements (µmol/l)	
	A	B		A and B	
Volume (ml)	2541	2511	Iron	20	
Total energy (kcal)	2200	2536	Zinc	100	
Nitrogen (g)	13.5	13.5	Manganese	1	
Folic acid (mg)	15	15	Copper	20	
			Iodide	1	
Electrolytes (mmol/l)			Chromium	0.2	
Na	130	130	Selenium	0.4	
K	80	82	Molybdenum	0.2	
Ca	5	5	Fluoride	50	
Mg	8	8			
Cl	100	102			
PO_4	47.5	47.5			

A menu is next needed and there are two methods of constructing this. The first is to design a diet for each patient and to repeat this daily. In some hospitals this is done by a team of "ologists". The alternative is to design a universal diet and to add to this or subtract during the rest of the intensive care. This system was developed simultaneously at Whiston by MJT Peaston and by IHJ Johnson at Hammersmith. The materials used in the Peaston diet were updated, but the idea survived 24 years. Two examples of standardized diets are given in Table 17.5. The next problem to tackle is the strategy of starting, continuing and hopefully stopping with recovery.

Table 17.6 Overall plan for fluid therapy and nutrition (From *Essential Intensive Care*, with permission)

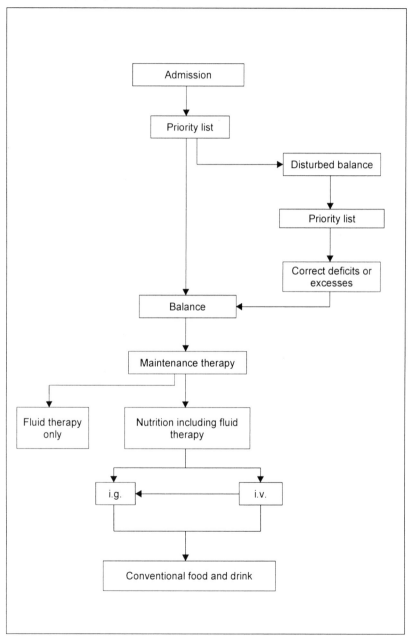

Nutrition must fit into the overall therapeutic plan. In particular, it follows resuscitation and the initial fluid therapy as shown in Table 17.6. Although nutrition is not urgent, it should be made a rule that a start is made within 48 hours of admission. Intravenous nutrition is not given when there is oliguria until this is sorted out by the methods described in Chapter 16. If the diagnosis is that of acute reversible oliguric renal failure, and if intensive therapy is to be considered (Chapter 22), and if the nutrition is to be given i.v., then this is started as soon as electrolyte balance is restored.

Having made a start, how to continue? The intensive care patients who need i.v. nutrition are those who also need a metabolic balance, an idea developed over 25 years ago. The monitoring of the electrolyte and nitrogen balance was described in Chapter 4 and summarized here: clinical observations of the tissue turgor, the intake and output of water, Na, K, and lastly, the plasma chemistry. The beginner must be told again that the plasma concentration of Na and K, Pi do not reflect total amounts in the body. The results of the external balance are 24 hours behind i.v. nutrition, but by the third day the question can be answered, is the standardized diet too little or too much? More will be required if paralytic ileus, ulcerative colitis or polyuric renal failure; less would be indicated in oliguric renal failure and haemodialysis or haemofiltration have not caught up. For the patient who needs more, this can be electrolyte solution or nutrients. The choice depends on the degree of catabolism. The intake is examined daily and the scheme adapted when the external balance shows this to be necessary. These principles are illustrated in the Appendix by observations on an injured patient.

To the basics described, supplements are essential, some routine, others according to the individual observations. The daily regulars can be grouped as follows: electrolytes, potassium and phosphate are reviewed daily according to the plasma levels and external balance; calcium, and magnesium and zinc are given daily but the dose may be varied according to the plasma concentrations; vitamins; all these and folic acid are given daily; trace elements; five of these are given each day and the amounts are assumed to suffice.

Last but not least is the control of the blood sugar. The dilemma is that the patients who need a high intake of energy, partly as glucose and partly as fat, are the very patients who develop glucose intolerance (Chapter 12) – the diabetes of injury. Severe hyperglycaemia is harmful or lethal, causing brain failure – hyperosmolar coma (Chapter 4); prevention is the order of the day. If hyperglycaemia develops then insulin is started without delay and given by a continuous i.v. infusion by a pump. A simple but effective scheme was published in 1980 by David McWilliam and is now described. We infuse the glucose for 4 hours before measuring the blood glucose to determine

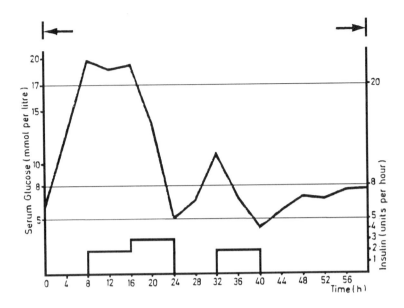

Figure 17.1 Example showing the control of the blood sugar (upper curve) by insulin (From McWilliam, 1980, with permission)

the dose of insulin required. When the glucose is 17 mmol/l or more, insulin is started at a dose of 2 units/h. If the blood glucose remains at or above 17 mmol/1 then the dose is increased by one unit/h when the syringe is recharged; this takes place at intervals of 8 hours. When the blood glucose falls to 5 mmol/1, or symptoms of hypoglycaemia develop, the insulin is stopped. When the blood glucose rises to 8 mmol/1 the insulin is restarted, but at a dose of 1 unit/h less than that previously used. This method of adjusting the insulin dose according to the blood glucose can be readily understood by reference to the example illustrated in Figure 17.1. In this case the insulin was started 8 hours after the start of the glucose infusion, because the blood glucose was over 17 mmol/l. At 16 hours the blood glucose was still above 17 mmol/l and the dose was therefore increased by 1 unit/h to 3 units/h. At 24 hours the blood glucose had fallen to 5 mmol/1, so the insulin was stopped. Eight hours later, i.e. at 32 hours, the blood glucose had risen above 8 mmol/1 and so the insulin was restarted at a dose of 1 unit/h less than the previous dose, i.e. 2 units/h. At 40 hours insulin was again stopped as the blood glucose was less than 5 mmol/1, subsequently 4-hourly results were all below 8 mmol/1, showing that the patient could tolerate the glucose without exogenous insulin. This method gives satisfactory control in most intensive care patients but in a minority it is necessary to adjust the dose by more than 1 unit/h, or alter the insulin dose at intervals of 4 hours rather than 8 hours.

3. Delivery

For the best results a little knowledge is required; the practical skills are learnt by apprenticeship and, in common with all therapies, organization is essential. The appropriate attitudes to intravenous nutrition have already been dealt with. To obtain the maximum utilization of the amino acids and fat, these are infused along with glucose. The various components of the diet can be delivered in one of two ways. The first system is to mix the day's nutrients in a big bag which is delivered through one line over 24 hours; a system ideally suited to a patient in a ward or at home. The diet is prepared in a sterile cabinet and the components are added in a controlled sequence. The alternative method is to infuse two or more of the components at the same time from individual containers. This system is run by the ICU nurses and has the additional advantage of flexibility, should modification become necessary. A word on practice. The addition to the nutrients of vitamins, potassium, phosphate, and trace elements are carried out with aseptic techniques which includes face mask and polythene gloves. The novice will require a check-list so that each additive is injected into the correct nutrient: fat soluble vitamins are added to the fat emulsion, and so on. Accurate labelling is essential. The diet is infused by gravity or pump into the vena cava using the central venous line already described. The polythene cannula used for resuscitation can be used for nutrition or a softer line of silicone rubber is substituted. The general ICU will have standardized on the materials of the basic i.v. diet and the delivery system. The organization, therefore, depends on the unit, policies, the nursing team, and the pharmacy. Nutrition then becomes a smooth running therapy in common with IPPV or dialysis. But even well organized systems must be protected by a few rules. In particular, the nurses must not be 'bombarded by conflicting instructions'. Hence one rule is that the diet for the day is not to be altered according to the whims of visiting specialists. Modifications to the daily plan are the sole responsibility of the one (and only one) service doctor.

4. Complications

The good thing is that most of the complications are preventable. The problems fall into two groups, those relating to the central line and the metabolic: (a) the puncture wound for the CVP line becomes colonized by bacteria which may cause the familiar chain reaction: local inflammation or bacteraemia. Prevention consists of: fully aseptic insertion, occlusive dressing, and bacterial monitoring. When local sepsis or bacteraemia develop the line is removed and a new one inserted at a fresh site. Bacteraemia is dealt with in other chapters. The mechanical complications of the central line are wholly preventable. Perforation of the vena cava leading to mediastinal haematoma or perforation of the right atrium causing cardiac tamponade. Likewise, pneumothorax during the cannulation. Bacterial endocarditis of the right heart can occur when a polythene cannula abrades the atrium, enabling bacteria to grow at the site and throw off emboli. (b) Metabolic and nutritional complications are due to omissions or ignorance. Vitamins, zinc, or trace elements are given routinely, and phosphate, potassium and so on according to the electrolyte balance and plasma analysis. Turning next to the excesses. Saline excess (Chapter 4) is avoidable and hyperglycaemia is easy to manage by continuous i.v. insulin. Too much glucose results in the production of huge amounts of carbon dioxide, the removal of which depends on alveolar ventilation. To quote from Victor Parsons: 'the lungs will dictate the amount of glucose'. Consequently, during respiratory failure completed with or without IPPV there is a risk of hypercapnia. This complication is prevented by giving the appropriate amount of glucose rather than practising glucose mania. When an excessive production of CO_2 fuelled by too much glucose is likely, it is a simple matter to confirm this by measurement. Expired gas from the ventilator is collected and analysed for CO_2, the control value is 250 ml CO_2/min.

APPENDIX: External balance following severe trauma; errors due to ignorance and a successful rescue

After helping to construct a few balance charts, the apprentice will soon learn the correct interpretation and also appreciate that appropriate nutrition is vital to recovery. An example is given in Figure 17.2; the format should now be familiar. 'A' is the control; 'B' the state of affairs 5 days after multiple injuries. Up to this time i.v. fluid therapy was saline and dextrose* – clearly the patient was not in an ICU! Comparing 'A' With 'B', the results are a positive

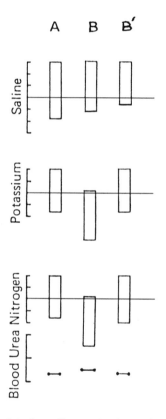

Figure 17.2 Balance data for saline, potassium, nitrogen and the blood urea.

---

* Starved into submission and drowned in sea water, to quote former Whistonian MJT Peaston

balance for saline and negative balance for potassium and nitrogen. Now the interpretation. The saline retention was either due to the hormonal changes which follow injury (Chapter 12 or a response to abnormal losses of saline due to continuing losses from the circulation-haematomas for example. The former might be harmful (oedema) but the latter would be beneficial. How to get the diagnosis right? – the plasma sodium? No. The CVP?; certainly not! The question can only be as answered by using the eyes and hands to assess the turgor of the skin, muscles and mucous membranes. The negative potassium balance is easier to interpret; none was given and the urinary losses would be high due to the metabolic response to injury. The newcomer should predict the likely total deficit of potassium and the consequences for the patient (Chapter 4). Lastly, the negative nitrogen balance, again due to starvation and the accelerated protein catabolism which invariably follows trauma; note that the blood urea was elevated.

The i.v. therapy was changed on day 6 to that which should have been started on the second day! A standard i.v. diet plus intensive potassium therapy (Chapter 16) was given and the state of balance 3 days later is shown at 'B'. The saline balance if the same as on day 7 requires the same interpretation. An intake of 500 mmol of potassium has restored the balance to normal. The disastrous negative balance for nitrogen was changed to a small negative state and the blood urea has returned to normal. In all, a satisfactory metabolic rescue. With increasing experience, the learner will delve deeper into the fascinating results obtained by metabolic balance; for example those found during IPPV used to treat injury (Gett *et al.*, 1971).

18

Respiratory therapy: first part

In ordinary cases the patient does not require pure oxygen but only a
sufficient addition to the air of oxygen to prevent anoxaemia.

J.S. Haldane, 1920

It is easier to delay cure than to deny rescue.   Bryan Jennett, 1979

I	THE UPPER AIRWAY
II	BRONCHOSCOPY
III	TRANSTRACHEAL VENTILATION
IV	TRACHEOSTOMY
V	HUMIDIFICATION
VI	OXYGEN THERAPY
VII	CHEST PHYSIOTHERAPY

I THE UPPER AIRWAY

1. Primary care

First aid for intensive care staff? Certainly, because resuscitation is taught
to so few and so infrequently, that the ICU staff must share in the crusade.
So, without apology, here is the first aid of the upper airway quoted from
the Resuscitation Council. 'Inspect the casualty's mouth and throat; remove
blood, vomit, loose teeth or broken dentures. Leave well-fitting full dentures
in place as it will assist in mouth-to-mouth resuscitation if this is necessary.
If there is doubt whether the casualty is breathing adequately, tilt the head
and support the jaw. This will open the airway. At this point check again to
see if the casualty is breathing'.

Restoring a clear upper airway may only need altering the position of the
head and jaw as just described. When a Brook or Guedel airway is available
then this should be inserted. And when equipment for intubation is on hand,
then an E-T tube is passed when the reflex activity allows. whether at the
site of an accident, at home, or in hospital, tracheal intubation should be
done by those trained and not by the partially competent. It is fortunate that
the mobile rescue services have portable suction machines to aspirate the
upper airway. Suffocation due to a foreign body means that the larynx is
completely obstructed by an object 3–4 cm across. This demands urgent
but pre-planned action. There is a choice of three techniques chosen

according to the state of consciousness and the results. (i) back-blows, (ii) manual thrust, (iii) finger probe and sweep. In the conscious patient (i) is tried first and if this fails then (ii) is used. In the unconscious (i) and may be (ii) are used, and when these fail, we resort to (iii). The three techniques are next described. (i) The back of the chest is thumped with the heel of the hand three or four times, once a second. These blows will produce a rapid increase in airway pressure, but only about one-fifth that of a cough. (ii) The lower chest and upper abdomen are compressed once a second. In the conscious patient the operator's arms encircle from behind. When unconscious the thrusts are applied to the lower sternum as for external cardiac compression. Alternatively, compression can be applied to the epigastrium – the Heimlich manoeuvre – but gastric regurgitation is a real disadvantage.

The inhalation – overt or suspected – of vomit calls for immediate tracheal intubation aided by a muscle relaxant. Following intubation, the bronchi are aspirated. A decision is next made whether or not prolonged IPPV is necessary. An antibiotic is not given prophylactically, and steroid therapy is of no value.

2. Intubation

(a) Equipment

The oral (or nasal) endotracheal tube (E-T tube), performed and fitted with an inflatable cuff is the first necessity. E-T tube can be made either of rubber or plastic and the cuff has a variable wall thickness. The thin-walled cuff (floppy) was perfected in 1973 and when inflated to produce an air-tight seal, the pressure is much lower than in the cuff of the standard E-T tube. The standard tube is safe for short term use – a few hours for anaesthesia or resuscitation; the tube with a low pressure (high volume) is essential for prolonged intubation, with or without IPPV. The remaining items required for intubation will already be familiar: laryngoscope, suction, a syringe to inflate the cuff, and possible anaesthetic agent or relaxant. The E-T tube is secured in place by a tape tied to the tube close to the lips and then passed round the neck and tied a second time.

(b) Technique

The skills are acquired during a proper training scheme. Nurses attending a basic course practice on a teaching mannequin before instruction in the anaesthetic room. The IC service doctors will already have been trained. The technical sequences depend on consciousness and the need for IPPV illustrated by two examples. An unconscious overdose needs airway protection but not IPPV; the sequence is gastric aspiration, cricoid pressure, pharyngeal suction under the vision provided by the laryngoscope, and intubation. Anaesthesia of the vocal cords by a lignocaine spray might be used as well. In sharp contrast, is the conscious asthmatic who needs IPPV. The standardized sequence is; informed consent, preoxygenation i.v. anaesthesia, i.v. muscle relaxant, cricoid pressure and intubation.

Immediately following intubation simple tests are quickly performed to ensure success. An anaesthetic reservoir bag is connected to the E-T tube by the catheter mount, and oxygen fed into the circuit. In our first patient the movements of the bag and thorax will confirm correct intubation. Manual IPPV with appropriate pressures (Chapter 19) and auscultation are the next steps in both examples. A decision is then made on the oxygen–air mixture delivered to the E-T tube. For both patients the gas must be humidified as described subsequently. Now that both patients are 'safe' the position of the E-T tube is determined by a chest X-ray; in part intubation of the right main bronchus can be corrected.

II BRONCHOSCOPY

A general ICU needs a fibre-optic bronchoscope (and the technical staff to care for same!) with light source and suction. A handful of the service staff are trained in the therapeutic uses and the occasional use in diagnosis. These indications are listed in Table 18.1.

III TRANSTRACHEAL VENTILATION (TTV)

The reader is unlikely to have seen this technique used, (Spoerel *et al.*, 1971) and may never have heard of it. Both the aim and the method are simple. When the upper airway is acutely obstructed and death is imminent but intubation is near impossible or will certainly take time (a minute is a long

Table 18.1 Indications for bronchoscopy in a general ICU
(From *Essential Intensive Care*, with permission)

Diagnostic	Suspected bronchial tear
	Exclude bronchial neoplasm
	To isolate pathogen in primary pneumonia
Therapeutic	Removal of foreign body
	Treatment of absorption collapse
	when physiotherapy fails
	Rarely in asthma to aspirate large mucous plugs

time) then ventilation can be restored and maintained by an emergency tracheostomy or, and, much easier, by TTV. This emergency, although very rare, can be due to an assortment of causes; facial injuries, foreign body, or laryngeal oedema.

The items required are immediately available in A & E, a ward, or ICU; a cannula with needle, tubing to connect to an oxygen outlet or cylinder, and lignocaine solution. In the hospital, commercial kits will be at the ready. Fifteen seconds is plenty of time to introduce the cannula below the vocal cords. Fit a syringe to the cannula needle and perforate the trachea just below the cricoid cartilage; check that air can be aspirated. The needle is then withdrawn slightly into the cannula which is next fully advanced, when the needle is removed. It only remains to connect up to the oxygen which is turned fully on. The tubing is obstructed by kinking and the flow interrupted at the normal rate of breathing. Although the chest does not move, gas exchange will be maintained until the airway problem is corrected, 'at leisure'. This type of ventilation is used daily in our hospitals during bronchoscopy.

IV TRACHEOSTOMY

A tracheostomy is a hole in the trachea; the term refers both to the operation and to the end result. The hole in the trachea is made by fitting a curved tube, which provides an artificial airway. The tube may or may not have a cuff, made from soft plastic, which lies in contact with the trachea and can be inflated or deflated with air via fine tubing which extends outside the tracheostomy. When the cuff of the tracheostomy tube is inflated, the trachea is sealed off above the level of the cuff. The lower airways are therefore protected from the entry of foreign material, and the lungs can be inflated artificially without the wastage of gas that would occur with a non-cuffed tube. The cuff of a tracheostomy tube therefore gives the same results as the familiar cuffed endotracheal tube, widely used for inhalation anaesthesia. We now have to decide when to carry out a tracheostomy; sooner or later? This is one of the few instances where practice differs, even 30 years on. (a) Early tracheostomy. The policy is to change from an E-T tube to tracheostomy within 72 h or earlier when it is predicted that IPPV will go on for weeks. (b) Late tracheostomy. An oral or nasal E-T tube is used for two weeks. If an artificial airway is still needed for IPPV or because of coma, then a tracheostomy is performed. For successful intensive therapy, tracheostomy is a planned operation arranged 'by appointment' with the surgeon, and carried out under general anaesthesia; therefore the operation is a safe one. It suffices to say that emergency tracheostomy appropriately referred to as 'kitchen table tracheostomy' is unnecessary and can be omitted.

Tracheostomy is most often performed so that the patient can be given prolonged intermittent positive pressure ventilation (IPPV) of the lungs, that is, for periods of three days to several weeks. Patients with respiratory failure due to chest injuries, acute non-specific lung disease, are most commonly treated, and more rarely, those with injuries to the brain or spinal cord. Secondly, the tracheostomy protects the airways from the inhalation of foreign material when the natural defences are absent or inadequate, for example, during prolonged unconsciousness due to head injury or hypoxia. The tracheostomy both protects the lower airways from aspiration and provides an artificial airway through which the trachea and bronchi can be kept clear by suction. In health, the cough mechanism and clearing action of the cilia will keep the trachea and bronchi clear of obstruction from inhaled material and mucus produced in the respiratory tract glands. In semi-coma or lung disease, the cough mechanism is lost or becomes ineffective, and many pathological processes damage the ciliated mucous membrane. In such cases, suction through the tracheostomy provides a substitute for the natural defences of the lung.

1. Tracheostomy tubes

We will keep to the essentials and describe two types only. The first type (Figure 18.1A) is for artificial ventilation and the portion in the trachea resembles a cuffed E-T tube. Indeed, the cuff has the same characteristics; thin walled, large volume and low pressure. The proximal end of the tube connects to the catheter mount, which in turn connects to the ventilator or reservoir bag. The tubes are supplied with internal bores of 7.0 to 9.0 mm; a large adult would probably need a 8.5 mm sized tube. Uncuffed tubes are used to replace a cuffed tube when IPPV is finished but endotracheal suction is still needed. An example is shown at Figure 18.1B. The example shown has a window cut in the tube (fenestrated). This window reduces the resistance to gas flow and can also enable a patient to speak. This will require a plug or one-way valve fitted to the proximal end. Then, during expiration, air will pass through the window between the vibrating vocal cords. Uncuffed tubes are made of plastic or silver; the latter was designed by Sir Victor Negus* in 1930 and is still used! A tracheostomy tube is secured in position by a loop of sterile tape as shown in Figure 18.1A. The wound is

---

* Sir Victor Negus, laryngologist extraordinary, 1887–1974

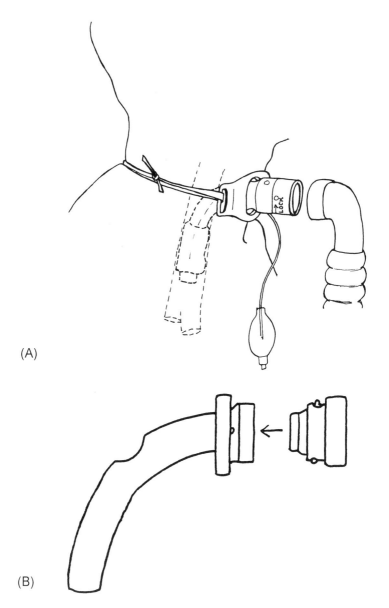

(A)

(B)

Figure 18.1 Examples of tracheostomy tubes. A, cuffed tube in position; B, uncuffed and fenestrated tube, with detachable plug

dressed with an absorbent material chosen from those available and according to unit protocol.

A brief addendum on percutaneous tracheostomy. This method is relatively new (1969) and the idea is to reduce the complications of the formal surgical tracheostomy and to carry out the procedure at the bedside. The technique is based on the percutaneous cannulation of blood vessels, now familiar to the reader. Firstly the skin is incised and the trachea is then punctured with a needle used to introduce a guide wire. The puncture is dilated to allow the insertion of a tracheostomy tube; a 9 mm tube for a large man. The authors do not use percutaneous tracheostomy because, during their combined experience of a hundred years, surgical tracheostomy has proved to be very safe and almost without complications related to the operation.

2. Care of the wound

On completion of the operation the wound is dressed with gauze cut to fit round the tracheostomy tube – a key-hole dressing. This dressing is changed when it becomes wet or blood-stained. After 24–48 h the dressing is removed and the wound left exposed. The exposure of the wound has two advantages. Firstly, it allows the tracheostomy tube to be under constant surveillance and secondly, as soon as exudate accumulates it can be removed quickly by suction or mopping with gauze. The continuing care of the tracheostomy is to maintain a clean wound by the use of techniques which are clean but not strictly aseptic and by keeping the wound as dry as possible. The latter requires occasional or frequent suction or mopping with gauze. Additional suction is required in patients who are unable to swallow saliva. In such cases, the secretions are dammed up in the pharynx and larynx above the cuff of the tracheostomy tube. Indeed they can leak past a cuffed tube and enter the larynx. The secretions will be observed leaking out of the tracheostomy wound but it is important to aspirate the pharynx as well as the wound. To do this the patient is tilted 10° head down. A laryngoscope is next used to visualize the pharynx and larynx which are cleared of secretions by suction. This technique is repeated according to the need. The wound sutures can be removed on the 7th to 10th day according to conventional surgical practice. The tapes which secure the tracheostomy tube in position are changed when soiled. Bacterial swabs are taken daily to determine and then record the bacteria which colonize the wound. The same bacteria may colonize the bronchial tree and cause pulmonary infection, so that the swabs taken from the tracheostomy wound serve as an early warning of possible sepsis. When it is clear that a

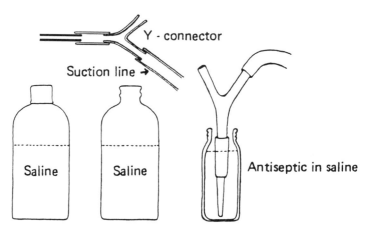

Y - connector

Suction line →

Saline

Saline

Antiseptic in saline

Figure 18.2 Accessories for endotracheal suction. Details are given in the text

tracheostomy is no longer required then the tube is removed and the wound thoroughly cleaned. The skin edges are next drawn together with adhesive tape. A small pad of gauze is applied to the site and kept in position with adhesive tape. This process is repeated 2 or 3 times a day when the sputum is copious. A week or so later the wound will have healed and the stoma closed, when dressings are abandoned. Occasionally the wound fails to heal by first intention and a fine stoma persists, requiring surgical closure at a later date.

3. Endotracheal suction

(a) A vacuum source is required.   This may come from a 'piped,' system with distribution points on the walls, or from a separate portable suction machine powered by a foot pedal or by electricity. Whatever the source, the apparatus must be cleaned each day, and collecting bottles and suction lines sterilized before use. From the collecting bottle, plastic tubing ends in a Y-shaped nylon connector (Figure 18.2). A rubber suction catheter is attached to one end of the Y-connector, and the remaining open end can be closed by the fingertip. This enables the operator to start and stop suction quickly. (b) Technique. We use the following technique based on studies carried out at the Radcliffe Infirmary. The oxygen concentration of the inspired gas is increased to 100% for a minute or two before starting. (i) The suction is switched on. (ii) A catheter is selected and the plastic envelope is torn across approximately 5 cm from the proximal (connecting) end. (iii) The catheter is next placed on a flat surface with the exposed end overhanging. (iv) The nurse now dons sterile gloves placing a paper towel flat at the side of the patient's head or on his chest. (v) The catheter is attached to the suction connector. (vi) Holding the catheter in the right hand the envelope is removed with the left hand and the catheter is looped around the right hand to prevent contamination. (vii) The left hand is used to disconnect the patient from the respirator; the Noseworthy connector is placed on the paper cover referred to. (viii) The catheter is inserted through the tracheostomy tube into the trachea or a bronchus. (ix) Suction is commenced by closing the open end of the Y-connector and the catheter is withdrawn slowly. (x) The patient is reconnected with the left hand. (xi) The catheter is cleared by sucking up saline from a 100 ml bottle attached to the suction machine. (xii) The catheter is discarded and the Y-connector is stored with its tapering and dipped into chlorhexidine in alcohol. (xiii) The polythene gloves are discarded and the hands washed. The time required for endotracheal suction must be reduced to the minimum in order to avoid dangerous hypoxaemia and distress; this is especially important to a patient with respiratory paralysis due to disease or muscle relaxant. The total time the patient remains disconnected should not exceed 30 seconds.

During resuscitation of a patient with a chest injury, asthma, chronic lung disease, or respiratory failure following surgery, endotracheal suction may be used every few minutes. Following a tracheostomy operation, suction is used to make certain that the airways are safely cleared. Except in these short-term situations, the suction should be made only when there are clear indications that it is needed. Endotracheal suction is restricted because the procedure inevitably causes some damage to the mucosa, and also there is a risk of introducing infection. During IPPV it is often possible to decide the frequency at which suction will be required during the following 24 h of treatment, and to give written instructions. The common indications for suction are: (i) The control of ventilation is difficult and the patient gets out of step with the machine (ii) Coughing. (iii) The minute volume falls. (iv) The air entry decreases, and crepitations are heard in one area of the chest. (v) The chest X-ray shows an opaque area, suggestive of absorption collapse.

The technique of endotracheal suction just described has potential drawbacks, three in number. Disconnection is necessary and can lead to the airborne spread of bacteria to other patients or staff; the catheter can be contaminated by the operator; artificial ventilation stops for the duration of the suction, which can cause hypoxaemia. A device to combat these problems was designed in 1985 and the system can be called a closed system. This apparatus remains in the circuit for 24 h and is then swapped for a new one. Disconnection is unnecessary and airborne spread cannot occur; the suction catheter is enclosed in a sheath to prevent contamination;

ventilation is continuous, thus avoiding hypoxaemia. After each suction, the catheter can be flushed through within the closed sheath. The results of systematic studies of this system are published.

4. Complications

The main ones are obstruction, tracheal damage and infection; the last two are detailed in the next chapter, which leaves us with obstruction. There are four main causes of airway obstruction. Extreme kinking of the neck of the tube may occur. It is usually due to drag of the respirator hoses, and is therefore easy to prevent. Secondly, a defective tube may obstruct the airway, and thirdly, sputum may obstruct the passage. Thick purulent sputum may seriously narrow the tube, or serum may harden like glue on the inner walls of the tube. This is the most common complication and can usually be prevented by adequate humidification of the inspired gas, by using correct suction techniques and by changing the tracheostomy tube at intervals of a few days when the sputum is thick and infected. Lastly, symptoms of tracheal obstruction may develop when the need for a tracheostomy has passed and the wound has closed and healed. This obstruction is due to stenosis of the trachea.

V HUMIDIFICATION

In health, the nose – more precisely the nasal passages and sinuses – is a most effective air conditioner; man-made substitutes are definitely third rate. During acute illnesses this system is commonly lost due to mouth breathing, intubation or tracheostomy. The result is that the mucous membranes of the trachea and bronchi lose the protection of the nose, dry up and the clearance function becomes ineffective. Things are made worse if compressed gases are given, because these contain less water vapour than does room air. The least we can do is to humidify the inspired gas when a patient is mouth breathing or intubated. The essentials are; there must be no bacterial growth in the apparatus, the droplets must reach the smaller bronchi and be at body temperature. The devices commonly used are based on one of two principles; to humidify with water vapour* or by means of droplets of water. The first two to be described use vapour.

---

* Gaseous form of a normally liquid or solid substance (*OED*)

1. Moisture exchanger

Your own expired air is warm and moist. Why not use this vapour to humidify the inspired gas? This can be done by a commercial device. During expiration the warm moist gas condenses on a filter and on inspiration the fresh gas picks up heat and water. The design can incorporate a bacterial filter. Small, simple and cheap are the strong points. There is a drawback, namely obstruction to gas flow by secretions. This will quickly be recognized and remedied by intensive care nurses, but not necessarily outside the unit. The moisture exchanger is used for the intubated patient breathing spontaneously.

2. Hot water

This is the best apparatus and has remained so for 30 years. The essentials are very simple. A cylindrical pot has an electric heater to keep the sterile water at body temperature. The pot is topped up from a drip set. We want the gas to pick up the maximum amount of water vapour. Two methods of doing so are illustrated in Figures 18.3 and 18.4. In the first type a spiral of absorbent paper is supported on a metal spiral. The gas enters the chamber and sweeps across the large surface of wet paper. The disposable part of the apparatus is pre-packed and sterile. At Figure 18.4 a humidifier is shown in which the entering gas bubbles through the warm water and then passes through a perforated disc to leave saturated with water vapour. This type is sterilized by heat and fed from a drip set of sterile water.

Finally, there are two ways of ensuring that the vapour reaching the patient is at 37°C . Firstly the water heated is set to 40°C and the temperature will fall by 3° by the time it reaches the patient. Alternatively, the heater is set at 37°C and a second heater fitted in the hose towards the delivery end. The hot water humidifier poses problems, but these are preventable; overheating, obstruction due to condensate and infection.

3. The nebulizer

The principle is familiar as the hand-held device for spraying the leaves of plants. A jet of gas sucks up fluid and propels this as fine droplets. The nebulizer is widely used in hospital wards and the ICU to humidify the inspired gas during oxygen therapy. In this case the device is combined with the venturi (Section VI) to mix the two gases in fixed proportion as shown in Figure 18.5. In addition, the nebulizer is an excellent way to give a bronchodilator.

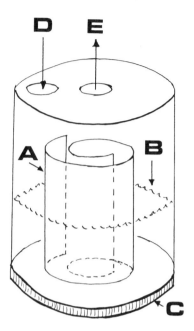

Figure 18.3 Hot water humidifier (Fisher and Paykel) utilizing a coil of absorbent paper A; B, sterile water; C, heater; D, entry port; E, exit port

VI OXYGEN THERAPY

This is so simple, rarely harmful, and yet so badly practised. In particular, the patients who might benefit from oxygen therapy are often denied it, and those who get this treatment often don't need it! Poor teaching must be the explanation, and certainly not shortage of the equipment. As with much intensive therapy, a nurse or doctor can give one or more treatments without understanding the 'how or whyfore' but the proper aim of training is to acquire more skills and knowledge and the appropriate attitudes. This justifies a short piece on the physiology.

1. Applied physiology

(a) Oxygen pressure

Fluids or gases move when force is applied to them as a pressure. The negative pressure generated in the thorax during inspiration draws air into the lungs. When the air reaches the alveoli, oxygen diffuses across the lung membrane into the capillaries and oxygenates the blood. In a healthy person at rest the blood leaving the lungs is more than 95% saturated with oxygen.

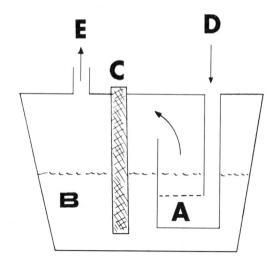

Figure 18.4 Hot water humidifier utilizing a perforated disc A; B, sterile water; C, heater; D, entry port; E, exit port

The diffusion of oxygen across the alveolar membrane occurs because the pressure of this gas in the alveolus is higher than in the capillary blood. Similarly, when oxygenated blood passes through the capillaries of the tissues, it gives up oxygen because the pressure of the gas in the blood exceeds that in the interstitial fluid. Since intensive therapy is frequently concerned with oxygen uptake by the lungs and delivery to the tissues, and since the pressure of oxygen in arterial or capillary blood is a common investigation, it is important to understand some elementary facts about the pressure of this gas. To obtain the pressure of a gas in a mixture is a matter of simple arithmetic, and obtained from the following equation:

$PO_2 =$ (atmospheric pressure – pressure of water vapour)
× per cent oxygen

The pressure of water vapour is dependent upon the amount of water vapour (humidity) in the air or gas mixture, and the temperature of the gas. For example, in a room of 20°C and a relative humidity 70% the water vapour exerts a pressure of 1.06 kPa (8 mmHg). Therefore, if the barometer reads 100 kPa (750 mmHg).

Inspired oxygen tension (PIO_2) $= (100 - 1.0) \times \dfrac{21}{100}$

$= 20.8$ kPa (156 mmHg)

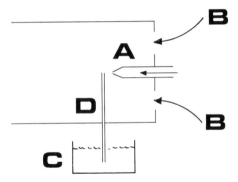

Figure 18.5 Principle of the nebulizer. A, jet of oxygen; B, entry ports for air; C, sterile water; D, aspirator tube

When inspired air reaches the trachea, its temperature is about 37°C and the pressure of water vapour has risen to about 50 mmHg. During its passage through the bronchi this warmed and humidified air meets with expired air which contains less oxygen, and the average PO_2 of gas in the alveolus, in health and at rest, is 13.3 kPa (100 mmHg). This value is referred to as the alveolar PO_2 and labelled PAO_2. It should be recalled here that, in health or disease, the PAO_2 of many alveoli will be below 13.3 kPa (100 mmHg). The PAO_2 cannot be measured directly but can quickly be calculated from the alveolar gas equation, which can be written in a simplified form:

$$\text{Alveolar } PO_2 \ (PAO_2) = \text{inspired } PO_2 \ (PIO_2) - \frac{\text{arterial } PCO_2 \ (PaCO_2)}{0.8}$$

In a healthy person at rest the $PaCO_2$ is 4.7–6.0 kPa (35–45 mmHg). Substituting a value of 5.3 in the alveolar equation, and an inspired PO_2 of 20.8, then $PAO_2 = 20.8 - 6.7 = 14.1$ kPa (106 mmHg). If the arterial PO_2 of our subject is 12.8 kPa (96 mmHg), then the pressure of oxygen, or the gradient, forcing this gas across the alveolar membrane is 1.3 kPa (10 mmHg). The value of the gradient increases with age and with the pressure of oxygen in the inspired gas. (Table 18.2) The alveolar oxygen gradient ($PAO_2 - PaO_2$) is a valuable estimation to make during the intensive therapy of respiratory failure; particularly repeated determinations help to decide the response of the patient to treatment. The tensions of oxygen and carbon dioxide in the arterial blood of a resting healthy subject are remarkably constant. This finding obviously applies to the blood in any artery. In contrast the PO_2 and PCO_2 of venous blood vary considerably from one vein to another. The blood

Table 18.2 Alveolar arterial oxygen pressure gradients in healthy subjects: variations with inspired oxygen concentration (F_iO_2) and age. (From *Essential Intensive Care*, with permission)

Age (years)	F_iO_2%	Gradient kPa	mmHg
20–30	21	0 to 1.73	0 to 13
	40	2.4 to 4.5	18 to 35
	60	2.9 to 6.0	22 to 45
	100	2.9 to 5.9	22 to 44
40–50	21	0.5 to 2.3	4 to 17
	40	2.5 to 7.1	19 to 58
	60	3.3 to 10.4	25 to 78
	100	4.3 to 10.9	32 to 82
60 and over	21	1.2 to 3.5	9 to 26
	40	3.9 to 10.9	30 to 82
	60	5.2 to 15.0	39 to 113
	100	3.6 to 14.2	27 to 107

The gradients were obtained from the means and standard deviations

leaving the right ventricle is truly mixed venous blood and its PO_2 and PCO_2 reflect the level of metabolism of the body as a whole. When sampled by means of a catheter and analysed, the results can be used to determine the oxygen consumption and carbon dioxide production of the tissues and the cardiac output.

(b) Assessment of tissue hypoxia

Tissue hypoxia may be localized or generalized. Local tissue hypoxia is recognized by its effects on organ function, for example acute myocardial infarction or pulmonary embolism. Laboratory measurements on the serum of the intracellular enzymes liberated from the ischaemic tissue help to confirm the diagnosis. Generalized tissue hypoxia is difficult to recognize. This is because significant hypoxia can occur without diagnostic symptoms or signs. Alternatively, we may fail to separate the symptoms of tissue hypoxia from those of the primary disease. The brain is the most sensitive organ to generalized hypoxia. An alteration in cerebration, such as restlessness, disorientation, confusion, or drowsiness should be assumed to be hypoxia rather than attributed to the primary disease. Unfortunately laboratory measurements do not help us to recognize moderate degrees of tissue hypoxia. In clinical practice, therefore, we are forced to infer that generalized tissue hypoxia is present during many acute illnesses and to give oxygen therapy empirically. Widespread tissue hypoxia always follows apnoea or cardiac arrest.

The conditions which frequently cause generalized hypoxia are listed in Table 18.3. The hypoxia is produced by hypoxaemia, inadequate tissue perfusion, or both as in cardiogenic shock. Hypoxaemia results from one or two mechanisms. Firstly, alveolar ventilation is reduced by a depression of the respiratory centre (head injury, sedative poisoning). The second mechanism concerns perfusion of the lung, either changes in total perfusion or in regional flow. For example, in severe hypovolaemic shock the total blood flow through the lung is reduced as is the cardiac output. By far the commonest mechanisms of hypoxaemia is a disturbed balance between ventilation and perfusion in one or more regions of the lung; this can result from obstruction to the airways, from oedema or embolism. Since hypoxaemia can be present without cyanosis, the PaO, is a valuable if indirect assessment of hypoxia. Furthermore the measurement requires arterial puncture and the monitoring is intermittent. Continuous monitoring of the oxygen saturation of the blood (SaO_2) is provided by the non-invasive oximeter (Chapter 6). When correctly used this instrument will display the SaO_2 to within 2%. The $PACO$ is the best measure of alveolar ventilation. When hypoxaemia is combined with shock a lactic acidosis occurs and this causes a fall in the plasma bicarbonate. Therefore, during shock or respiratory failure a metabolic acidosis signifies generalized tissue hypoxia. Serial measurements of the lactic acid in arterial blood, or the ratio of lactic to pyruvic acids can be used to follow the course of a disease during tissue hypoxia, but laboratory measurements are no substitute for clinical wisdom.

2. Uses

The single aim is simple in theory, difficult in practice. What we want to do is to correct hypoxaemia which can cause hypoxia of vital organs. The hypoxia, especially that of the brain, may be recognizable clinically but more often (it is hoped) the hypoxia is suspected rather than certain. To use oxygen scientifically the treatment would only be given to patients with acute hypoxaemia – or acute-on-chronic hypoxaemia. The widespread unselective measurement of the arterial blood gases would be the unjustified use of resources, but oximetry (Chapter 6) is non-invasive and valuable in diagnosis and monitoring. In the main, however, oxygen therapy is given or at least started on clinical grounds. The natural history of the disease will decide the issue. It is important to recall a few points on the recognition of respiratory failure (Chapter 6). Cyanosis is a late sign, except in severe chronic bron-

Table 18.3 Conditions causing generalized tissue hypoxia(From *Essential Intensive Care*, with permission)

Shock	hypovolaemia heart failure bacterial
Left ventricular failure	ischaemic heart disease hypertensive heart disease rheumatic heart disease cardiomyopathy
Lung disease	asthma pneumonia chronic non-specific lung disease chest injury
Respiratory paralysis	poisoning head injury spinal injury myasthenia gravis polyneuropathy

chitics; dyspnoea is often absent in the injured or surgical patient, when increased breathing pattern is the key observation. The indications for oxygen therapy in acute illness are summarized in Table l8.4. (a) Apparatus. For the patient breathing spontaneously, oxygen is given by disposable face masks. The first requirement is comfort; when a mask causes a feeling of suffocation or heat it will not be tolerated. Oxygen masks of two designs will suffice for treatment of the conditions shown in Table 18.4. The choice is easily decided by the concentration of oxygen (F_1O_2) required and whether this must be controlled, that is within narrow limits. A simple cheap mask giving 35–60% oxygen is appropriate for most of the diseases. Controlled oxygen requires a more complex device which will deliver the F_1O_2 and not allow the rebreathing of expired gas. An easy job for an engineer? It is worth recording that having achieved this specification 20 years lapsed before manufacture! It is nice to know how they work. The principle is called the venturi* which will mix a little oxygen with a lot of air, resulting in a high flow of the mixture to the face. If your car has a carburettor, this does the same with petrol and air. The proportioning of air to oxygen can be arranged in one of two ways. The original method was to make a venturi for each oxygen

* G.B. Venturi (1746–1822) Italian physicist.

Table 18.4 Indications for starting oxygen therapy (From *Essential Intensive Care*, with permission)

	Oxygen percentage
Acute hypoxaemia	
Cardio-pulmonary resuscitation	90
Acute severe asthma	35
Primary pneumonia	
Chest injury	
ARDS, suspected or overt	
Pulmonary oedema due to irritant gases	
Anaphylaxis	35–60
Bacteraemia or toxaemia, suspected or proven	
Shock, irrespective of cause	
Acute myocardial infarction	
Acute heart failure due to any cause	
Pulmonary embolism	
Acute-on-chronic hypoxaemia	
Severe chronic bronchitis	
exacerbation	
chest injury	24–28
following surgery	
rescue following medical errors	
Severe chronic heart failure	
acute worsening	35–60

concentration: 24, 28, 35 or 50%. The alternative is to fix the flow of oxygen through the jet but vary the amount of air to give the appropriate F_1O_2. In the diagram (Figure 18.6) two of the four ports are temporarily closed. (b) There are two complications, both readily avoidable. A mixture of room air and piped oxygen will dry the mucous membrane of the trachea and lung unless the patient breathes through the nose – the air conditioner. Hence when the patient mouth breathes, is intubated or has a tracheostomy, the inspired gas must be thoroughly humidified. This is easily done by using one of the methods already described. The second complication is that of carbon dioxide narcosis which can complicate the oxygen therapy given to a severe bronchitic, a familiar picture known as the 'blue bloater'. Recognized in 1948, this complication is due to the fact that the respiratory centre of such patients cannot (for reasons unknown), respond normally to a rise in $PACO_2$. The same phenomenon could be demonstrated if the healthy reader was given a dose of morphine or pethidine. Carbon dioxide poisoning can nearly always be avoided by giving 24–28% oxygen continuously and

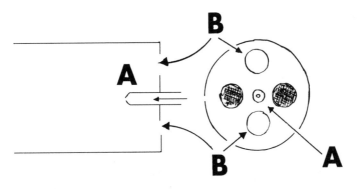

Figure 18.6 Controlled oxygen utilizing the Venturi principle. A, jet of oxygen; B, ports for air, of which two are closed off

combining this with assisted coughing carried out at regular intervals day and night. These treatments can be monitored with oximetry or blood gas measurements. (c) Oxygen during IPPV. During cardio-pulmonary resuscitation and when mechanical IPPV is started, then the lungs are ventilated with about 90% oxygen. During the ensuing ventilator programme the F_1O_2 is reduced to that which is just sufficient to oxygenate the blood. The reason for this policy is that high concentrations can damage the lungs. A brief degression will help the beginner to understand the problem. Since 1899 we have known that when small animals breathe 100% oxygen for some weeks a high pr proportion develop interstitial pulmonary oedema, progressing to fibrosis with hyaline membranes – a state of fibroplasia. Can high concentrations of oxygen cause similar damage to the human lung? The answer for healthy subjects is not known. During acute respiratory failure the indirect evidence suggests that inspired concentrations of about 60% given for more than two days can cause pulmonary fibroplasia. Oxygen is more strongly implicated in the pathology of the respiratory distress syndrome of the newborn when the lung is imperfectly developed and deficient in surfactant. When high values of P_1O_2, are required to correct hypoxaemia then the oxygen is an important cause of interstitial oedema and fibrosis. The adult respiratory distress syndrome was only recognized during the 1960s when prolonged IPPV became widely used to treat respiratory failure. In its fatal form the lung histology is the same as the infant type and the experimental animal; it was therefore natural to blame oxygen. The case is unproven but the evidence does suggest that during IPPV inspired concentrations above 60% will cause fibroplasia. Oxygen therapy ends on a crusade. The new medical graduate is badly taught and thinks that oxygen is bad for all patients with lung disease. To try and correct this, here are two quotes from our preaching: 'oxygen is good' and 'many patients given oxygen don't need it and most who need it don't get it'.

3. Continuous positive airway pressure (CPAP)

Basic physiology would predict that increasing the upper airway pressure and thus the alveolar pressure should improve gas exchange. Can this be done without resort to mechanical ventilation? The affirmative was demonstrated in 1938 by the American investigator Alvin Barach and then labelled positive pressure breathing; we now use the term CPAP. The technology is very simple and based on (i) a source of oxygen-enriched air at a flow rate of about 100 l/min, (ii) a device called a positive end-expiratory pressure (PEEP) valve, to partially obstruct the expired gas, (iii) air-tight face mask or E-T tube. The gas supply is generated by the venturi principle already described. The valve is ingenious in that the pre-set pressure (2.5 to 20.0 cmH_2O) stays remarkably constant irrespective of the expired flow of gas. CPAP can be given by any intensive care ventilator or by equipment designed solely for this purpose. The uses in acute illness are twofold. To improve gas exchange in acute respiratory failure, for example in pneumonia. Secondly, to prevent or treat absorption collapse; for example a patient with a tracheostomy breathing spontaneously but likely to develop absorption collapse.

4. Other methods

Alternatives to the methods described have been invented, some abandoned and others shown to be ineffective. These are mentioned out of interest rather than for intensive care application. Microscopic bubbles of oxygen given i.v. was a clever idea but abandoned. Cardio-pulmonary bypass is widely used for open heart surgery, and the oxygenator maintains the PaO_2 for the duration of the surgery. It was natural to try this out when IPPV failed to maintain a safe PaO_2. A multi-centre control trial showed that the treatment did not influence the outcome. Lastly, hyperbaric oxygen may be available in the unit where you are training. For intensive care this treatment is valuable in the treatment of carbon monoxide poisoning.

VII CHEST PHYSIOTHERAPY

Last but by no means least. Almost every patient in a general ICU needs chest physiotherapy given every day (or several times a day) by a team of specially trained and allocated therapists. The techniques of vibration, percussion, positioning, bagging and suction will soon become familiar to the nurse or trainee doctor, and are described in monographs (Webber and Pryor, 1993). The workload on the physiotherapy department is considerable. At the RPA hospital each patient is assessed and treated at 7.00 a.m. and the day's programme formulated. For one patient there can be four treatments in the day and one at night; for another case, two treatments per 24 h will suffice.

19

Respiratory therapy: artificial ventilation

Never use artificial respiration, always give the real thing.
Found in a Christmas cracker

'Like other discoveries, it is not only elementary in its simplicity, but the fundamental ideas involved in this important suggestion have been lying idle before the eyes of the profession for years.'   Matas, 1899

I   PHYSIOLOGY
II   PRINCIPLES OF THE MECHANICAL VENTILATOR
III   VENTILATORS FOR GENERAL INTENSIVE CARE OF THE ADULT
IV   PRACTICE OF IPPV
V   COMPLICATIONS DURING VENTILATOR TREATMENT
        APPENDIX: THE APACHE SYSTEM

Artificial ventilation (respiration) is frequently needed for resuscitation (Chapter 21) and in the hospital is commonly given by means of a bag and facepiece. When trained staff are available, artificial ventilation is best continued by means of intermittent manual inflation through a cuffed endotracheal tube. This simple technique permits more effective inflation of the lungs and protects the lungs from the entry of foreign material. When artificial ventilation and the other treatments quickly succeed, for example in cardiac arrest or poisoning, artificial ventilation can be stopped when it is certain that spontaneous respiration is adequate. When artificial ventilation is necessary for hours, days or weeks, then it is best given by a machine powered by an electric motor, or compressed gas. The ventilator (or respirator) simulates to some extent the action of the doctor or nurse inflating the lungs by intermittent pressure applied to a bag or bellows. This method of mechanical artificial ventilation is known as intermittent positive pressure ventilation or ventilator treatment. IPPV is one of the many treatments used in the general ICU and in respiratory and thoracic surgical units. When skilfully used to treat selected patients, excellent results are obtained. In some diseases such as sedative poisoning, asthma or crushed chest, it is evident that the treatment saves life, even without the proof of a controlled trial. Following brain injury, whether due to trauma or hypoxia, following the inhalation of vomit or pulmonary fat embolism, to quote just a few examples, it is much more difficult to prove that IPPV reduces the death rate or the duration of the illness. An inherent problem of IPPV is that it is very easy to start, but much more difficult to stop – with a live patient! In the general ICU the patients treated by IPPV are nearly always conscious and one should never forget that this treatment is at the very best unpleasant. Its more disturbing and distressing features are endotracheal suction, frustration in communication and lack of sound sleep. Ventilator treatment, like other advanced skills, can only be learnt by apprenticeship at the bedside. The aim of this chapter is to provide background knowledge.

I PHYSIOLOGY

Only a very elementary knowledge of physiology is required for the success-ful practice of IPPV in the general ICU. This short account starts with normal breathing and then proceeds to artificial respiration. Consider yourself at rest and reclining on a back rest in bed (Figure 19.1); a Ryle's tube is swallowed so that the distal end lies in mid-oesophagus. The proximal end is connected to a pressure recorder and the tube filled with water: the pressure readings (P_{oes}) will represent intrathoracic pressure (cm water). A mouthpiece or rubber facepiece is fitted and the flow of air (l/min) in and out of your lungs recorded, pressure changes (cm water) in the mouth are also recorded (P_{aw}) and it will be assumed that they parallel those in the trachea; the result can then be compared with those obtained during IPPV. The minute-volume ventilation and frequency of breathing are observed. You are requested to increase the depth of your breathing and records are then taken of the air flow and the two pressures. The results (Figure 19.2) show that during inspiration, air flows into the trachea and the intratracheal pressure shows a small drop of 10 cm below that of the atmosphere. The pressure in the oesophagus mirrors the small decrease in the intrathoracic pressure which normally occurs during inspiration. During the expiratory phase, the flow changes direction; P_{aw} shows a trivial rise above the base line and the P_{oes} returns to atmospheric pressure. The reference point for pressure in this experiment is the sternal angle. Normal breathing then, is negative (sub-atmospheric) respiration and the pressure changes in the thorax are small. A second experiment is next carried out to observe the tracheal and oesophagus pressures during the Valsalva manoeuvre. At the end of an inspiration, a pressure of 50 cm (positive, that is above atmos-pheric) is maintained in the mouth for 10 s; during this time there can be no air flow. Both the tracheal and the intrathoracic pressure show a considerable rise. If haemodynamic measurements were to be made at the

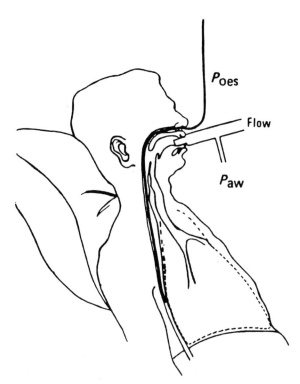

Figure 19.1 Diagram showing arrangements for demonstrating pressure–volume relationships during spontaneous breathing. P_{oes}, pressure in oesophagus; Flow, flow in the trachea; P_{aw}, pressure in the trachea (From *Essential Intensive Care*, with permission)

same time, the blood pressure in an artery, the central venous pressure and the cardiac output, we could readily appreciate how the Valsalva manoeuvre affects the circulation.

When the pressures P_{aw} and P_{oes} were sustained at raised values, the blood pressure fell for a few seconds but quickly recovered and then overshot the normal (Figure 19.2). What happened during the Valsalva was as follows. The rise in pressure in the airways and thorax impeded venous return and impeded the filling of the heart; the cardiac output fell, the blood pressure fell and the subject might faint. By spinal reflexes, a compensatory mechanism was rapidly brought into action, that of the arteriolar constriction, and this restored the blood pressure. An understanding of this train of events is essential to those using ventilator treatment. In disease, the compensatory mechanism may fail – for one or more reasons. Commonly

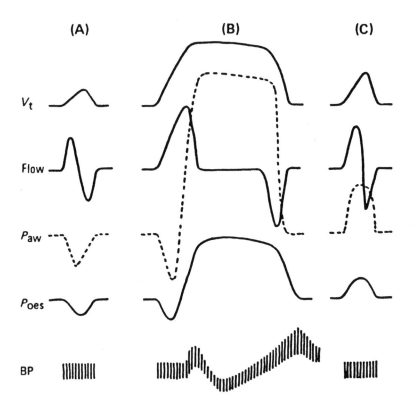

Figure 19.2 Pressure–volume relationships in the thorax. borax and blood pressure readings. V_t, tidal volume; Flow, tracheal flow; P_{aw}, tracheal pressure; P_{oes}, oesophageal pressure. A, control; B, Valsalva manoeuvre; C, during IPPV (From *Essential Intensive Care*, with permission)

because of hypovolaemia or left ventricular failure and rarely because the reflex is interrupted (blocked) by polyneuropathy. These are important relationships between the Valsalva response in health and disease and IPPV, and these are considered next. Consider first the healthy subject, anaesthetized and then given a muscle relaxant; the lungs are ventilated manually from a bag or bellows. The measurements made during spontaneous breathing are repeated during IPPV (Figure 19.2). The flow of air or air/oxygen mixture is similar to that in the previous experiment. In contrast the P_{aw} and P_{oes} are both positive (above that of the atmosphere), instead of negative. A minor Valsalva manoeuvre has been produced but with the important difference that the duration is short and the manoeuvre is repeated time and again – that is IPP. In most patients requiring IPPV, including the intensive care patient, the compensatory mechanisms are operational, and the circulation is maintained. On the other hand, IPPV can quickly cause serious hypotension. This occurs when the tracheal pressures are high, and usually when a high pressure is unnecessary; this situation is exactly the same as Valsalva manoeuvre. Alternatively, the IPPV is performed with modest tracheal and intrathoracic pressures but the circulation is unable to compensate; this is seen in hypovolaemia, LVF or polyneuropathy. The beginner will now realize that the adverse effects of IPPV are both important and inescapable. IPPV is just un-physiological! This applies equally to all methods from the kiss of life to the latest computerized ventilator from 'Star Trek'. Since mechanical IPPV is commonly used, both in anaesthesia and in the various types of intensive care, it is obvious that the beneficial effects outweigh the adverse effects, and they were reduced by important features in the design of a mechanical ventilator. The information required haemodynamic studies, which were made in the late 1940s by H.L. Motley and his co-workers. The first essential was to make the duration of expiration approximately twice that of inspiration. Referring again to Figure 19.2, it will be seen that the flow of gas from the ventilator resembles a sine wave. Other ventilators have different wave forms or these can be adjusted at will. For most diseases the wave form is not critical.

Having stressed the adverse effects of IPPV, what of the beneficial results in terms of gas exchange in the lung and of the mechanics of breathing? The beneficial results, some real and some speculative, are given in Table 19.1. These aspects of IPPV will be considered later and only a few general remarks are necessary at this stage. What happens to gas exchange? In most situations exchange can be quickly restored to normal. When ventilation is reduced and the lungs are normal (poisoning) then both total ventilation and alveolar ventilation can be quickly restored to normal. At the same time a reduced PaO_2 will be restored to normal by using IPPV with air or a modest increase in F_IO_2. In the case of lung disease, or during combined lung and heart disease, IPPV can improve gas exchange by one or more mechanisms. Consider alveolar ventilation. Firstly the ventilator can restore and then maintain alveolar ventilation when the patient is unable to do so; this is the situation in asthma, crushed chest or chronic bronchitis, and in some cases of pulmonary oedema. The result in terms of blood gases is that a raised $PaCO_2$ is brought down to normal. The mechanism by which IPPV restores $\dot{V}_A$ varies from patient to patient; relief of respiratory fatigue; clearing of obstructed or narrowed bronchi; improvement in the balance of ventilation and perfusion. What of oxygen exchange in the lung? When oxygen therapy fails to correct dangerous hypoxaemia (4.0–6.5 kPa), IPPV can often succeed. Again, the mechanisms are usually several in number.

Table 19.1 Results of IPPV (From *Essential Intensive Care*, with permission

Increases V_T and $\dot{V}_A$ carry on line

(a)	in normal lung gas exchange is restored.	Sedative poisoning Chest injury
(b)	in diseased lungs gas exchange is improved	Pulmonary oedema Asthma Chronic bronchitis
	Relieves the work of breathing and relieves fatigue.	Asthma ARDS Following thoracic surgery
	Permits analgesia and sedation without danger of hypoventilation	Crushed chest ARDS Asthma Chronic bronchitis
	Relieves mechanical stresses on the circulation	Asthma Crushed chest Following thoracic surgery
	Stabilizes a flail segment	Crushed chest
	'Opens up' collapsed (closed) alveoli and improves regional ventilation perfusion balance.	Pneumonia ARDS Crushed chest
	Maintains pulmonary gas exchange when muscle relaxants are required to control spasms or convulsions	Tetanus Epilepsy

It is an easy matter to employ very high inspired concentrations of oxygen. But IPPV with much lower concentrations of oxygen can correct hypoxaemia by alternative mechanisms, by restoring $\dot{V}_A$ to normal or by using hyperventilation; by enabling narrowed or obstructed bronchi to be cleared by suction; by improving the balance of ventilation and perfusion, by reducing the oxygen consumption of the body by taking over the work of breathing. It is an easy matter to postulate the mechanisms, but impossible or difficult to demonstrate them in the critically ill patient. The mechanics of IPPV, which are quite abnormal in comparison to normal breathing, can, in two diseases benefit the patient. The two diseases are a crushed chest with a flail segment and severe asthma. In the former the IPPV stops the paradoxical movement of the flail segment and thus stabilizes the thoracic cage and enables the fractured ribs to unite. In asthma, our Whiston colleagues demonstrated that IPPV relieves life-threatening stresses on the circulation.

The last result of IPPV to be considered at this stage, is that ventilator treatment makes it quite safe to use powerful analgesia or sedation, without risk of impairing gas exchange. It should be emphasized that in respiratory failure there is no safe analgesic or hypnotic; all affect the carbon dioxide response of the respiratory centre and such drugs can also prevent clearing of the bronchi by coughing.

II PRINCIPLES OF THE MECHANICAL VENTILATOR

The modern mechanical ventilator is a box with knobs on and hoses attached; a very expensive box. The newcomer to intensive care is usually bewildered by the controls which increase year by year as 'new' techniques evolve. Take heart, the principles are easily grasped. Imagine that the lungs (Figure 19.3A) are being inflated from a pair of bellows (B). Air and oxygen are fed to the bellows and the concentration of oxygen can be read off the meter (C), this is labelled the $F_1O_2\%$. When the bellow is compressed gas will flow through the inspiratory hose provided that the clamp (D) is open. The pressure in the hose and the trachea will rise and can be noted on the meter (E); this is the peak airway pressure P_{aw}. At the end of inflation (inspiration) the clamp D is closed and the clamp (F) on the expiratory hose is opened. The elastic recoil of the lungs will then expel gas to waste and the volume of gas is recorded by the meter (G). This volume is the expired tidal volume and when measured over one minute is labelled the expired minute volume ventilation $\dot{V}_E$. So far so good. If you yourself are operating the bellows then the ventilation of the lungs can readily be adjusted in three ways. You can make slow or rapid inflations (frequency, f) You can increase or decrease the volume (V_T) delivered at each compression of the bellows. Lastly, the handles of the bellows can be moved quickly or slowly; thus this will alter the rate at which the given tidal volume enters the lungs – inspiratory flow rate. Now refer back to Figure 19.2. In the normal subject (A) gas volume of flow in the trachea represents wave forms of mechanical ventilation and these can be altered as just described. It is an easy matter to transpose the IPPV given by fireside bellows to a modern machine. The V_T frequency and the $F_1O_2\%$ are just 'dialled in' by twiddling the knobs and the $\dot{V}_E$ is measured for you. The machine has other controls (too many) which will alter the inspiratory flow rate – the wave-form. We have nearly completed the beginner's guide to IPPV. The next step is to get an overall picture of ventilation and to define the essential types. This can readily be done by referring to Table 19.2. Artificial ventilation branches into continuous positive airway pressure (Chapter 18) and IPPV just described. The latter is next subdivided into three modes. So far we have assumed that the patient

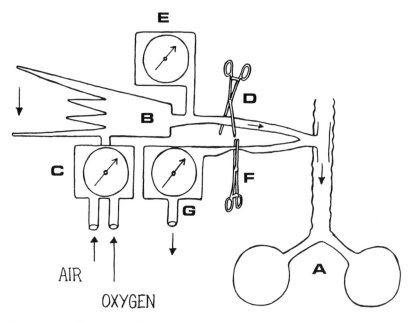

Figure 19.3 Diagram to illustrate the principles of the mechanical ventilator. A, lungs; B, bellows; C, meter to record F_1O_2; D, valve to control inspiratory gas flow; E,upper airway pressure; F, valve to control expiratory gas flow; G, meter to record volume expired

will allow you to ventilate the lungs at a chosen depth and rate. This is only possible if the patient has respiratory paralysis due to disease (Guillain–Barré), myasthenia), because a muscle relaxant has been given, or because the respiratory centre is severely depressed by a drug, accidentally or deliberately. This method of abolishing the patients.' voluntary breathing is called controlled IPPV or continuous mandatory ventilation. Is there an alternative? Yes, there are two. The first (1946) is patient-triggered IPPV. The inspiratory effort made by the patient triggers (sends a message to) the machine which inflates the lungs more fully; this 40-year-old method is very valuable. The other choice is labelled intermittent mandatory ventilation (IMV) The machine of Figure 19.3 is readily modified so the patient can breathe air and oxygen humidified and warmed to 37°C whenever they want. But, their spontaneous respiration is supplemented by mechanical inflation of the lungs at a predicted rate known as the mandatory frequency and volume. (Figure 19.4). Inevitably from time to time the machine will inflate the lungs when the patient is breathing in or out without causing distress.

Table 19.2 Overall view of pulmonary ventilation

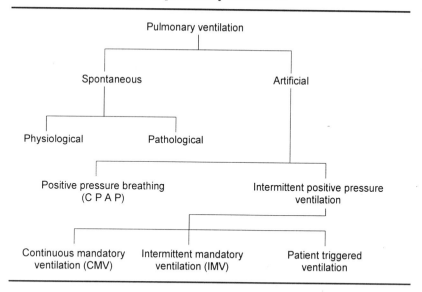

When setting the ventilator controls, there is a choice of pre-setting the tidal volume (V_T) or the peak airway pressure (P_{aw}). When the is V_T is pre-set, then the P_{aw} will vary according to the lung compliance; when P_{aw} is pre-set the V_T will vary in the same way. In adult practice there is little evidence that one technique is better than the other. When using a pre-set V_T and the P_{aw} is very high, then pre-set P_{aw} might be beneficial. In paediatric practice pre-set pressure is often the first choice. The techniques of CMV, IMV, and SIMV can be used when either volume or pressure are pre-set.

This section is concluded by describing two further tricks of the trade. Refer again to Figure 19.2. At the end of each lung inflation the P_{aw} returns to atmospheric. A simple device can be incorporated to obstruct the expired gas and thus raise the end-expiratory pressure above atmospheric called positive This is naturally labelled Positive End-Expiratory Pressure. In practice, the PEEP is varied from 5 cm water pressure to 30 cm. PEEP is used when controlled IPPV with high concentrations of oxygen fail to oxygenate the blood, that is correct dangerous hypoxaemia. PEEP can act on the circulation adversely or to the patient's benefit. Two examples will illustrate this principle. In the hypovolaemic patient PEEP will reduce the cardiac output; in left ventricular failure with pulmonary oedema the addition of PEEP can increase the cardiac output and improve gas exchange.

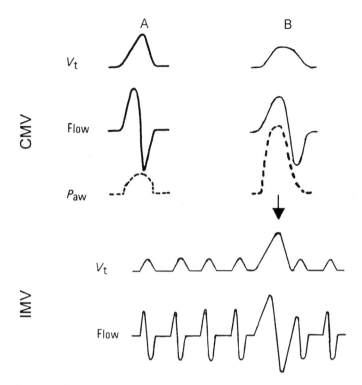

Figure 19.4 Two commonly used modes of artificial ventilation. Upper trace; CMV with A, standard wave-form and B, modified wave-form in a case of asthma. Lower trace; IMV showing spontaneous breaths and a single mandated inflation (arrow)

Finally, the manner of inflation, that is the wave-form, can be altered. Referring back to Figure 19.2 the wave-form shown is fixed so that the inspiratory time is nearly twice that of expiration; an I/E ratio of 1.8/1.0. This is satisfactory for many of the conditions treated in the ICU; chest injury, paralytic respiratory failure, but is not the optimum for asthma, for example. The explanation is quite simple. The asthmatic who needs IPPV to survive has extreme obstruction to the movement of air, both during inspiration and expiration. In some instances the ventilator can only match the patient's previous efforts! In this desperate situation, the optimum ventilation is best achieved by using a longer inspiratory time, that is a lower gas flow. The results from a patient are illustrated in Figure 19.4.

III VENTILATORS FOR GENERAL INTENSIVE CARE OF THE ADULT

Should you be tempted to open the best reference book on mechanical ventilators (Mushin, 1980) there you will find dozens of machines; fortunately, for general intensive care one type will suffice! Looking back over 30 years of ventilator practice the pioneering results were obtained using one of six machines. Ventilators in common use have a few advantages over their precursors but many are unnecessarily complicated and they cost many times more. It is worth noting that too many manufacturers are chasing a relatively small market of which over half is already captured by Nellcor Puritan Bennett of the USA.

The requirements of the general ICU are: reliability which guarantees safety; sterilization by heat rather than the complex methods of formaldehyde or ethylene oxide; provision of bacterial filters; versatility to enable ventilation to be controlled, patient triggered, IMV, or PEEP; pre-set oxygen concentration. When re-equipping the unit, there are advantages and disadvantages in using only one make or in diversifying. The advantages are that training is simplified and servicing is easier; the only disadvantage is that experience is restricted to one ventilator. The use of the mechanical ventilator is learnt by apprenticeship at the bedside, not in a classroom. However, before driving a strange car it is essential to have a good idea of the controls – where they are and what they do! The controls of the machines can be classified into two kinds: those you pre-set, for example frequency, and those which measure things, like upper airway pressure (Table 19.3).

IV PRACTICE OF IPPV

The skills of IPPV are learnt by apprenticeship in the anaesthetic room, operating theatre, recovery room and ICU (Table 19.4). Some general knowledge on the practice of IPPV is now described to help the novice. By far the most frequent use of IPPV is in general anaesthesia. During a general anaesthetic the patient's own respirations may be adequate for gas exchange or, when inadequate, ventilation is increased by synchronized manual inflation of the lungs. Alternatively after inducing anaesthesia, the patient's own respirations are deliberately abolished by a muscle relaxant and gas exchange then maintained by IPPV. This technique is called controlled IPPV. At the end of the surgical operation the anaesthesia is stopped and the action of the muscle relaxant is neutralized (reversed) by the drug neostigmine so that normal respiration is restored. The patients admitted to the general ICU with sedative poisoning resemble in some respect the deeply anaesthetized surgical patient. Respiration can be

Table 19.3 Operating an intensive care ventilator: the controls set by the operator and the measurements by the machine

Pre-set controls	Measurements by the machine
Frequency	
Tidal volume	Tidal volume: by the ventilator and that by the patient
Inspired oxygen	Peak airway pressure
Positive end-expiratory pressure	Plateau airway pressure
Inspiratory flow rate	Inspiratory to expiratory ratio
Pause time	
Sensitivity level for triggered ventilation	...and lots more!

Table 19.4 Some of the skills to be learnt on the practice of mechanical IPPV (From *Essential Intensive Care*, with permission)

Ventilator	Positioning of the machine for observations
	Positioning of the hoses
	Drainage of the condensate
	Gas leaks in the patient circuit
	Machine failure
Patient	Communication
	Turning the patient
	Hygiene
	Signs of distress

severely depressed or absent altogether, the drug taken as an overdose has depressed or completely stopped ventilation. IPPV is essential to maintain gas exchange until the poisoning wears off and spontaneous respiration is adequate. Acute sedative poisoning accounts for the commonest use of mechanical IPPV in the general ICU. The remaining patients who require mechanical IPPV bear no resemblance to either anaesthesia or poisoning. Obviously, acute respiratory failure is the common denominator; most patients are conscious, and breathing can be increased rather than decreased! The diseases with which we are concerned are: chest injuries, asthma, acute non-specific lung disease, and various types of pulmonary oedema. When one of these conditions requires prolonged IPPV the doctor must know how to start, how to continue and how to stop. These topics are now briefly considered; the steps can be quickly grasped by referring to Table 19.5.

1. How to start

Unless faced with an emergency situation – apnoea, cardiac arrest or severe hypotension – two important preliminaries should be undertaken. Firstly, the patient is given high concentrations of oxygen to breathe from a facepiece fed from the anaesthetic machine, and secondly, a Ryle's tube is passed and the stomach aspirated. The conscious patient is next anaesthetized by means of an intravenous agent.

The principles require emphasis; firstly, to use a minimal amount of agent, and secondly, to be patient, because a low cardiac output can prolong the arm-to-brain time. Suxamethonium (1.0 to 2.0 mg/kg) is given intravenously and the trachea next intubated with a preformed plastic E-T tube. Manual IPPV with 100% oxygen is started and the trachea and pharynx cleared by suction. An assistant observes the pulse closely and takes the blood pressure every few minutes unless the patient is already fully monitored. The treatment of hypotension occurring at this stage will be described later. After a short time both consciousness and spontaneous respirations will return. Before this event occurs a plan of action (Table 19.5) is necessary. One of two courses is possible: to continue with controlled ventilation or to use patient-triggered IPPV. The choice depends largely on the disease to be treated and is partly a personal one. Whichever technique is chosen a clear therapeutic programme is essential. This programme consists of the ventilator settings, the composition of the inspired gas and the skilled use of methods to control ventilation. The writers only use the IPPV to treat cases of sedative poisoning or head injury who show inadequate breathing; the mode chosen would be IMV or triggered IPPV. The remaining conditions are initially treated by means of controlled IPPV. The ventilator programmes for asthma, crushed chest, tetanus, myasthenia gravis, polyneuritis, pulmonary oedema, or pneumonia nevertheless vary. Common to each is the use of one or more methods of controlling ventilation.

2. Methods used to control ventilation

IPPV may be necessary to treat respiratory failure in patients who are making powerful respiratory efforts which are ineffective in maintaining gas exchange. This is the situation in asthma, pneumonia, and in the critically crushed chest. When the ventilator is used to give artificial respiratory support the result will be a dangerous and ineffective combination of

Table 19.5 Overall plan for prolonged ventilator therapy (From *Essential Intensive Care*, with permission)

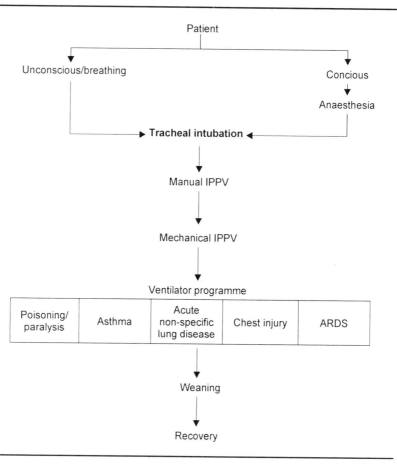

artificial and spontaneous respiration. The patient will be unable to allow the machine to breathe for him, that is, synchronize his breathing with that of the ventilator. A continuous state of fighting the respirator will occur, alveolar ventilation will fall rather than increase and the cardiac output and blood pressure may also fall. It is clear that when IPPV must be used to treat these conditions, some method must be used to control respiration and thus allow the ventilator to take over all the work of breathing. Muscle relaxants are widely used (and misused) to control IPPV since curare (tubocurarine) was introduced. Pancuronium bromide may be used when a

Table 19.6 Examples of intravenous muscle relaxants used to control IPPV in the adult

Pancuronium bromide	2–6 mg every 1–2 h or
	1–4 mg/h by infusion
Atracurium besylate	25–50 mg every 30–60 min or
	30–50 mg/h by infusion
Vecuronium bromide	5–10 mg every 30–60 min or
	3–6 mg/h by infusion

more prolonged action is required. This drug is given intravenously in aliquots of 2–6 mg. Alternative relaxants are given in Table 19.6. A muscle relaxant is the easiest and most effective method of controlling respiration: it is also the most unpleasant and the most dangerous. The patient is conscious and may hear discouraging remarks about his condition. He is unable to communicate pain, to cough or swallow. The rule therefore is to sedate the patient receiving muscle relaxants. The loss of muscle tone reduces the venous flow from the limbs and the skin is more susceptible to pressure. The conjunctivae are liable to trauma or infection. Saliva accumulates and may track past a cuffed tube and enter the lungs. If the endotracheal or tracheostomy tube becomes dislodged or disconnected from the respirator, the patient will quickly suffocate unless the fault is remedied. By no means the least important nor the last disadvantage of muscle relaxants is that they are used as a substitute for medical skill! Large and repeated doses of a muscle relaxant – intensive relaxant therapy – are occasionally needed to treat tetanus, when diazepam and chlorpromazine have failed to control the muscle spasms. With rare exceptions intensive relaxant therapy has more disadvantages than advantages. The writers advocate the use of muscle relaxants, (i) to obtain control of respiration during the first few hours of IPPV and (ii) to regain control of respiration when the patient fights the respirator, but only when all other techniques have been tried and have failed. These objectives can be obtained with doses of relaxants which are short of those required to produce total muscle paralysis. (b) Analgesics. Repeated doses of morphine sulphate will depress respiration and therefore allow controlled IPPV. During IPPV it is important to get the patient moving his body at regular intervals or sitting out of bed. This process of progressive rehabilitation helps to prevent thromboembolism, bed sores, and depression. Sedatives and hypnotics hinder this important part of the treatment. Morphine also causes nausea and vomiting. We use morphine to relieve pain but not to control ventilation. The powerful analgesic phenoperidine hydrochloride (Operidine, Janssen) is used in place of morphine. This drug relieves pain and in large frequent doses (2.0–4.0 mg) depresses respiration. Phenoperidine is given intravenously at intervals of 2–4 h, alone or together with pancuronium. Synthetic narcotic agents such as fentanyl or alfentanyl are often used, particularly in renal failure. These latter agents, especially alfentanyl, are 'clean' and do not produce large quantities of toxic metabolites. Naturally, they are much more expensive!

3. How to continue

How to continue prolonged ventilator treatment, that is for weeks or months, is much more difficult to practice than a short period of IPPV. The chief reason for this is that high standards can only be attained by continuous care by specifically trained nurses with the appropriate skills, and staff with the appropriate skills and attitudes are often in short supply! 90% of the observations and treatment are carried out by the nursing team and the clinician is correctly delegated to regular assessments and the investigation of complications. Each patient needs one trained nurse at all times. When turning the patient, carrying out hygiene or physiotherapy, two nurses are required. In the general ICU about half the patients require prolonged IPPV. This treatment in common with many of the other practices requires standardized facilities and the techniques which are now briefly described.

(i) Patient accommodation. When possible the patient is treated in a single room having a floor area of about $20\,m^2$. In theory this reduces the incidence and spread of infection but there is little scientific proof that this occurs. Following the discharge of each patient, the room is emptied, the walls and floors are washed and disinfected. Similarly, the bed, mattress and pillows are disinfected. The treatment room is ventilated by conventional windows or by a system of air conditioning which greatly reduces the concentration of airborne bacteria. When air conditioning is not available, the spread of air-borne bacteria from the lavatories and sluice can be reduced by fitting extraction fans to these rooms. Pharmaceuticals, dressings and disposables are stored in the treatment room to reduce the traffic in and out of the room.

(ii) Basic hygiene (Table 19.7) is of cardinal importance in reducing the complications of ventilator treatment. Our methods are based on standard practice used in the management of infectious diseases and on the technique of endotracheal suction developed in the Respiration Unit of the Churchill hospital. On entering the treatment room the nurse or doctor dons a clean apron. The hands are next washed with the aid of chlorhexidine and dried on an efficient paper towel. The hands are again washed immediately

Table 19.7 Prevention of infection

1. *When to wash the hands*
   Personnel should wash their hands between all patient contacts and when otherwise indicated. Sinks should be provided at convenient locations throughout the ICU and in each of its isolation rooms or alcoves to encourage handwashing. Antiseptics, when indicated, should be easily accessible for hand-washing.

2. *When to wear polythene gloves*
   Endotracheal suction
   Preparing and giving intravenous or intramuscular injections
   Connecting, disconnecting or adjusting ventilator fittings

3. *When to wear a mask*
   Vascular cannulation, preparing and giving infusions or injections
   Oral or endotracheal suction
   Introducing or changing drainage systems; urinary, chest or peritoneum
   Wound care
   Taking blood or bacteriological samples

4. When to wear an apron
   Nurses, doctors, in the treatment rooms and in the dialysis area.

---

before leaving the area of room and the gown is left behind. A face mask is worn when in close proximity to the patient. Polythene gloves are worn when carrying out one of the following procedures; preparing or giving intravenous or intramuscular injections; endotracheal suction; connecting or disconnecting ventilator fittings, any contact with the body fluids. Disposable items such as towels, gloves, face mask, suction catheters are dropped into a pedal-operated plastic bag which is sealed before leaving the room or area. Bed linen taken from the bed is handled according to classical fever hospital practice. A linen skip is fitted with a bag and the soiled linen placed in the bag which is closed prior to removal. The staff must appreciate that excreta are more often a danger to the patient rather than to the nurse.

(iii) Ventilator, humidifier and suction apparatus. It is obvious that IPPV is started with a clean ventilator having a sterile patient circuit. There is also a strong case for changing the ventilator at intervals, when treatment is prolonged, because of contamination from the patient. The air entering the ventilator should be filtered through a bacterial filter. The gas exhaled from the ventilator may contain pathogens from the patient's respiratory tract, and this gas should also leave the machine via a bacterial filter. The humidifier is either pre-packed sterile or sterilized by heat. Suction apparatus is dealt with on the same lines as ventilators. The tubing and the connector attached to the suction catheter are intermittently flushed with saline and chlorhexidine in alcohol; details of this will be found in Chapter 18.

(iv) Prolonged use of E-T tube versus tracheostomy. When IPPV is required for more than 72 h there is a choice of airways; IPPV can be continued via an oral or nasal E-T tube with a low pressure cuff. Alternatively a tracheostomy is carried out and the ventilator connected to a tracheostomy tube. Both methods can work well (Chapter 18). The decision to use one or other is based on habit rather than science.

(v) Physiotherapy is given by members of the hospital department who have received specific training in chest physiotherapy.

The service is co-ordinated by the nurse manager to the ICU and the superintendent physiotherapist. Treatment is given at least twice a day every day. The actual treatments are tailored to each ventilator programme and also to the stage of IPPV. The commonly used skills are postural drainage, vibration and percussion of the chest wall and 'bagging and suction'. Each of these skills is now briefly described. Postural drainage means that the patient lies flat with one pillow and the bed is tipped head down about 15°. After an hour in this position the physiotherapist and nurse carry out manual IPPV, vibration, percussion and suction. Drainage is especially important when the cough reflex is absent or weak. 'Bagging and suction' is a treatment designed to simulate an explosive cough. Firstly, IPPV is changed from mechanical to manual from a reservoir bag supplied with oxygen. A few slow but deep inflations of the lungs are made. Immediately following a maximum inflation, the bag is quickly released and the physiotherapist vibrates the chest wall; this is followed by suction and the procedure is then repeated. When the aspirate is thick and tenacious, 5.0 ml aliquots of saline are injected down the trachea in order to facilitate clearing of the bronchi. Clearly, the treatment is more effective when the cough reflex is present. The role of the physiotherapist in the treatment of absorption collapse will be described later.

(vi) Monitoring. IPPV requires specific knowledge and skills and is largely the responsibility of the nursing team. The medical staff are required to start ventilator treatment, to deal with complications and to carry out the routine assessments, twice a day, every day. The observations which make up monitoring are, in the order of their significance: clinical observations of the patient, readings taken on the ventilator, respiratory measurements taken during spontaneous breathing oximeter readings, the chest radiograph, and lastly, the analysis of the arterial blood. The clinical picture is monitored continuously by the nurse, the readings on the ventilator are made hourly, a chest radiograph is taken daily, or on three days during a week and the blood gases are measured with about the same frequency. Should complications develop, many more radiographs and arterial samples will be necessary. Long experience has shown that the more competent the nursing team the fewer the X-rays and blood gases. When IPPV is started, manual IPPV with oxygen is invariably used and the monitoring differs from that used during mechanical IPPV. Manual ventilation is also used when, during the course of prolonged mechanical IPPV, complications develop such as shock, absorption, collapse or tension pneumothorax. In these situations monitoring is essentially clinical in nature; the colour of the inside of the lips, the compliance judged by the feel of the anaesthetic bag and the expansion of the chest, and observations of the radial pulse. Monitoring during mechanical IPPV also depends on clinical observations, supplemented by routine recordings. The overall scheme is given in Table 19.8. The values for frequency, tracheal pressure, $V_T \dot{V}_E$ readings are taken hourly and entered on a chart, table or in a computer. A word in the interpretation of P_{aw}. The hope is that the pressures are normal or will return to normal. Since we were unable to find control values, Dr. R.G. Clark made observations when at Whiston in 1975. The values in Table 19.9 are easy to use.* Note the tidal volume and frequency of the ventilator and read off the control value. For example, if volume tidal = 1200 and frequency = 12, then the P_{aw} should lie between 26 ± 4.0 cmH$_2$O. Assessing progress during IPPV depends on the signs listed in Table 19.8, and the recovery or otherwise, that is the prediction of outcome, is very dependent on experience. But as with brain failure, experience can mislead and quantitative monitoring is preferable.

A predictor which has wide application during intensive care is the APACHE. This system was devised in 1981 by W.A. Knaus and his colleagues of the George Washington University and has been tested out on thousands of cases. The APACHE score is described in the Appendix to this chapter.

Monitoring consists of observing, recording, interpreting, and then taking action when necessary; trends are more important than isolated results. The problems of interpretation depend on the particular disease under treatment and this in turn requires a ventilator programme.

---

* These observations were made using a machine with an inspiratory–expiratory ratio of 1.8/1.0. We cannot find similar results using other ventilators; will healthy volunteers please step forward!

Table 19.8 Monitoring progress during prolonged IPPV (From *Essential Intensive Care*, with permission)

Pressure–volume relationships on the machine, i.e. compliance	
Breathing pattern when off the machine	
Cough power	(no reflex – expulsive cough)
Sputum	Volume, colour, bacteria Retained secretions – heard or felt by physiotherapist
Chest X-ray	Clearing of oedema, consolidation, pulmonary haematomas
Pneumothorax	Lung expanded, no leak on chest drain, decreasing surgical emphysema
Gas exchange	PaO_2 rising for constant or decreased values of $\dot{V_E}$ and F_IO_2, $PaCO_2$ falling at constant or decreased value of $\dot{V_E}$ (i.e. decrease in venous admixture or dead space effect)

4. Ventilator programmes

It has already been emphasized that prolonged IPPV has to be tailored to each disease. The only condition which has similarities to the IPPV of general anaesthesia is sedative poisoning. The other diseases treated in the general ICU require quite different ventilator programmes. Each programme has a scientific basis and an empirical component based on previous experience. Some knowledge and skills are common to each programme and can be separated at this stage; these are an artificial airway and endotracheal suction; humidification of the inspired gas and methods used to control ventilation. When treating patients with paralytic respiratory failure due to acute poisoning, polyneuropathy or myasthenia gravis, the IPPV can be continued without having to resort to the use of a sedative, or a muscle relaxant. In contrast the patient with a crushed chest, asthma or bacterial pneumonia will require one or more of these methods of controlling ventilation. The writer hopes that the beginner will remember the dictum – the drugs are no substitute for skill!

(a) Programme for asthma. The aim of the programme is two-fold. Firstly, to restore gas exchange – the difficult part – and then maintain exchange until the airways obstruction is relieved by nature aided by drugs. The second aim is to relieve mechanical stresses on the circulation caused by the

Table 19.9 Control.values of peak upper airway pressure, P_{aw} (cmH$_2$O)
(From Smith and Gordon, 1986, with permission)

Tidal volume (ml)	Frequency of respiration					
	10	12	14	16	18	20
500	11.4	12.0	11.6	12.4	13.0	13.6
600	12.8	12.9	13.4	14.0	15.2	16.5
700	14.6	15.5	15.7	16.8	18.0	19.7
800	16.6	17.2	18.0	18.9	20.8	22.7
900	18.3	18.5	20.4	21.8	23.6	26.3
1000	20.7	21.4	22.4	24.0	26.9	29.8
1100	22.4	23.8	24.9	26.7	30.2	32.9
1200	23.8	25.5	27.7	30.5	33.2	36.4
1300	25.9	27.8	30.2	33.9	36.7	39.6

extreme swings in the intrathoracic pressure; IPPV quickly removes these stresses, as was clearly demonstrated in 1966 at Whiston. The step-by-step technique is given in Table 19.10. The only difficult part of the programme is during the first hours or so of mechanical IPPV, when despite sedatives, relaxant and high inflation pressures, it can be well-nigh impossible to increase alveolar ventilation; skill and patience are always rewarded.

(b) Acute non-specific lung disease. This label is unsatisfactory when compared with primary pneumonia or pneumothorax, but we can't think of a better one. After a few weeks of experience, the beginner will see IPPV used to treat patients with respiratory failure, the pathophysiology of which seems obscure to say the least. The starting point of the illness is so variable: non-thoracic trauma, peritonitis, inflammatory bowel disease, pancreatitis. The patient's breathing is increased but dyspnoea can be absent. As might be expected, the pathophysiology is variable and multiple factors lead to the respiratory failure. In the lung there may be absorption collapse (the syndrome of the lung bases), consolidation or oedema. Some of these patients are in the early phase of ARDS or go on to develop this syndrome. Fatigue, especially muscle fatigue is important. Oxygen therapy and physiotherapy have failed and IPPV holds out the only hope. For success, there must be an early start (the right patient in the right bed at the right time!) and the primary disease must be curable; IPPV is not to be used to treat the

Table 19.10 Ventilator programme for asthma (From *Essential Intensive Care*, with permission)

Preparation	Communicate the plan
	Gastric suction
	Correct metabolic acidosis with i.v. $NaHCO_3$
	X-ray for pneumothorax
Start	Pre-oxygenate
	Induce anaesthesia
	Intubate with suxamethonium
	Manual IPPV. Polygeline i.v. if BP falls
Continue	CMV using pancuronium and phenoperidine or papaveretum
	Low V_T, low frequency, low inspiratory flow rate
	Rarely bronchial lavage to dislodge mucous plugs
	Slowly increase V_T as P_{aw} falls. Aim for fall in $PaCO_2$ from high to normal over 24–48 h
	Triggered IPPV 12–24 h
Stop	Extubate
	Offer patient a better out-patient care in future!

lung disease caused by a hole in the colon without sewing up the hole. The ventilator programme uses sedatives and relaxants and perhaps an early tracheostomy and the IPPV lasts weeks rather than days. The programme should be simplified as much as possible so the other systems can be dealt with – heart failure, renal failure, metabolic failure.

(c) Crushing injury of the chest. The scientific basis is to stabilize the flail segment of the chest wall and at the same time ensure gas exchange. This programme depends on an advantage of the unphysiological principle of IPPV. The change from negative pressure spontaneous breathing to positive pressure artificial respiration prevents the flail segments from moving paradoxically. The lungs then act as an internal splint – 'internal pneumatic stabilization' as the originators called their method (Avery *et al.*, 1959). The programme is summarized in Table 19.11.

(d) Paralytic respiratory failure. The causes seen in the general ICU are sedative poisoning, polyneuropathy, myasthenia gravis and 'failure to reverse' after general anaesthesia. Obviously with the unconscious overdose, IPPV is started and continued without anaesthesia, sedative or relaxant. In the other patients anaesthesia is used to start IPPV which is then continued without relaxants. In this group of patients the lungs are usually normal and

Table 19.11 Ventilator programme for chest injury (From *Essential Intensive Care*, with permission)

Resuscitation	Relief of pain Intravenous infusions Anaesthesia/manual IPPV with O_2 Chest drainage	BP and CVP every few minutes Skin temperature Hourly urine volume Chest X-ray ECG
First 48 h of mechanical IPPV	Controlled IPPV Tracheostomy Chest drainage Endotracheal suction i.v. nutrition physiotherapy	Hourly BP and pulse Ventilator readings Blood gases once or twice daily Chest X-ray daily and immediately after tracheostomy Metabolic balance for water, sodium and potassium Blood count Chemistry Bacterial monitoring of nose, throat and tracheal aspirate

Subsequent
mechanical IPPV
	Controlled IPPV
	Later triggered IPPV
	Endotracheal suction
	Physiotherapy
	Tube feeding
	Treatment of the
	  complications, e.g.
	  antibiotics or diuretics
	Pleural aspiration
		Reduce BP recordings
		Otherwise as above
		Chest X-ray alternate days

gas exchange is easily maintained. The ventilator programme therefore includes steps to prevent hyperventilation and hypocapnia. In polyneuropathy IPPV can cause alarming hypotension due to a blocked Valsalva response. Intermittent mandatory ventilation is the ideal mode to treat such a condition; the patient breathes as they like, but the machine will ensure that total ventilation is always maintained. IPPV buys time until a poison is excreted or metabolized, until myasthenia is brought under control with drugs, or until the respiratory muscles recover; thus the duration of the programme varies from a few hours to many weeks.

5. How to stop

As with starting, the stopping process, known as weaning, is tailored to the individual disease. The weaning process can be very simple (poisoning, cardiac arrest, asthma), difficult (crushed chest, myasthenia, polyneuritis) or very difficult (chronic bronchitis with emphysema). The weaning process can take a few minutes or a few weeks. In the difficult case the technique consists more of an art than of a science and is learnt by apprenticeship. A few points on the practice of weaning are made here. To consider the *When* the *How* of weaning. When to start weaning is decided after examining the checklist for monitoring of IPPV (Table 19.8). When the signs show the progress is favourable, then weaning is contemplated. Prior to weaning the patient is dogmatically reassured and his favourable progress is emphasized. The second parameter for monitoring progress, that of the breathing pattern, requires comment. The first thing to do is to stop the relaxant and analgesic and delay the examination for some hours until the drugs have been metabolized. To observe the pattern of spontaneous breathing the machine is adjusted to IMV. This means that the patient can breathe spontaneously but mechanical inflation is continued at a slow rate – the mandatory frequency. The observations are easy. The interpretation difficult for the first five years! Spontaneous breathing which is either very rapid or shallow or those requiring great effort are unfavourable signs, but require a different interpretation if the patient is afraid. When the overall picture has been weighed up, and we see again that the blood gases are the least important – then there is a choice of four techniques. When the assessment shows that spontaneous ventilation is normal and the patient's breathing does not tire, then IPPV is simply stopped, a method known as the crash wean (what a horrible label). This is the routine in the recovery room but rare in the ICU where it can be used on recovery from acute poisoning. The second technique is patient triggered IPPV, already described on page 258. The method requires: communication skills to reassure the frightened patient and experience in adjusting the trigger sensitivity and flow rate. Weaning by patient-triggered IPPV may turn out to be plain sailing or fail, and have to be postponed or IMV used. If the machine is set to IMV the patient can breathe spontaneously at any depth or frequency, the spontaneous $\dot{V}_E$ is measured and the mechanical ventilation adjusted to supplement the spontaneous. Depending on the progress of the patient, the mandatory frequency is re-adjusted eventually to zero; weaning is then achieved. In some diseases (e.g. Guillain–Barré) IMV is a beneficial feature of the ventilator programme itself and is started soon after intubation.

   Ventilator treatment is finally concluded when the patient can breathe normally or more precisely, as well as he/she did before the acute illness or injury. At this state the clinical signs are the most valuable. The breathing pattern should be normal or only moderately increased (hyperventilation); there must be no signs of tiring, that is respiratory fatigue; there should be an expulsive cough; cyanosis (of the inside of the lower lip) should not develop. In the case of the crushed chest, the flail segment is stable and breathing and coughing should cause only moderate pain. The next decision is when to extubate the patient. This depends on whether there is still a need for an artificial airway. An E-T or tracheostomy tube will be required if the patient is unconscious (poisoning) or when the larynx is incompetent (myasthenia). In other patients who are conscious, and able to cough and swallow (poisoning, asthma), the E-T tube is removed without delay. A further group of patients require the tracheostomy for a few days in order to ensure that the bronchi are kept clear with the aid of suction; chest injury is an example. A stage is reached when suction only is required without the need for a cuffed tube to protect the airway. We then substitute an uncuffed fenestrated tracheostomy tube. Removal of a cuffed E-T or tracheostomy tube is carried out by a standardized technique. Firstly, explain the procedure to the patient. Lie the patient flat and clear the mouth and pharynx by suction. Deflate the cuff; carry out endotracheal suction; and then request the patient to cough out the tube. A tracheostomy wound is closed by pulling the edges together with adhesive tape.

In some diseases, e.g. asthma, successful IPPV is followed by a few days of controlled oxygen. During the convalescence period the patient is able to catch up on lost sleep and try to forget a life-saving ordeal. Unhappily in other conditions not all the patients will recover as they should in asthma. In patients with ARDS progress is monitored as already described. In some patients the lesions resolve, gas exchange and compliance improve, and the radiological signs regress. When the signs show that the syndrome is following this favourable course, the ventilator programme can again be adjusted and the necessary steps should be obvious. In the remaining patients the pulmonary oedema shows relentless progression and kills in days or weeks. In these patients the desperate state is worsened by bacterial colonization and sometimes infection of the trachea, bronchi and lung parenchyma. The train of events is as follows: The overall clinical picture is worse; there is cyanosis and hypoxic sweating; the pulmonary shadowing spreads and air bronchograms appear; the blood shows acidosis – metabolic and respiratory; oliguria occurs and will not respond to frusemide; the blood urea rises. How will you cope with failure? No matter where you work, the death rate from ARDS is 50%. Experience with a few such tragedies will teach the service doctor when the syndrome has reached an irreversible stage, and he can then switch off the machine and thus avoid needless distress to the patient and relatives. To stop IPPV in the absence of brain death, without feelings of guilt or remorse, but with sadness and inadequacy, implies that attitudes appropriate to the situation have previously been developed. The terminal care of the patient and the consolation of the relatives taxes the best intensive care team, stopping the machine is easy. Adequate sedation is ensured and the oxygen to the ventilator then turned off; hypoxic arrest quickly follows.

V   COMPLICATIONS DURING VENTILATOR TREATMENT

The side-effects and complications of IPPV can harm the patient, or directly result in his death. Some knowledge of the complications is essential to enable the clinician to off-set the risks against the possible benefits. For the purpose of description the side-effects and complications are grouped under five headings.

1. Pain, discomfort, fear and sleep deprivation

Leaving out the overdose patients, the remaining admissions to a general ICU who need IPPV are nearly always conscious. To them, IPPV is invariably unpleasant and can resemble a prolonged nightmare. The E-T or tracheostomy tube causes discomfort and suction is very unpleasant. On the other hand, inadequate or unskilled suction produces a feeling of suffocation. Unless the patient has paralytic respiratory failure, IPPV supplied by the machine causes the patient to fight the respirator and the drugs needed to gain control of the ventilation are themselves unpleasant. Indiscreet conversation in the treatment room can disturb and depress. These side-effects can be reduced to the minimum by a competent and confident team of nurses. The patient then feels that everything is under control and that no harm can come to him. Short visits by close relatives and clergymen also maintain morale. Radio or television is arranged according to the patient's wishes. Natural sleep is completely impossible and it is a rare occurrence for the patient to obtain adequate sleep. The IPPV itself is sufficient to prevent sleep but the problem is compounded by all the other disturbances; recording the blood pressure, turning of the patient, to mention only two. Our own practice to facilitate sleep is on the following lines. At night recording is reduced to the safe minimum; lighting is adjusted to give the minimal intensity and is reflected rather than direct; noise is rigorously frowned upon; the patient is nursed in a single treatment room; all injections are intravenous, rather than intramuscular and via a central venous catheter thus avoiding thrombophlebitis; the bladder is catheterized only when this

Table 19.12 Drugs given intravenously to induce sleep during IPPV and a guide to the dosage

Midazolam	5–15 mg
Papaveretum	7.7 –15.4 mg
Droperidol	5–15 mg
Phenoperidine	2–4 mg
Chlormethiazole (Heminevrin 0.8%)	8–32 mg/min
Morphine	5–10 mg
Propofol	20–200 mg/h

is essential; sedation at night is increased. Unfortunately, there is no ideal drug to induce sleep and each sedative shows a striking variation in response. It is therefore necessary to try one and observe the results and change if necessary. A list from which to choose is given in Table 19.12. Sleep deprivation can be very serious, causing confusion, restlessness and depression; this should be remembered in the differential diagnosis.

2. Mechanical complications

These consist of failure of the ventilator or the lifelines to the patient. When the ventilators and other machines belonging to the unit are carefully maintained, the mechanical failures rarely occur. Should machine failure pass unnoticed then the patient will quickly suffocate. A mechanical fault is quickly recognized by the experienced nurse, who wastes no time in exchanging the machine, but substitutes manual IPPV and then replaces the ventilator. The change of manual IPPV is made quickly, but with equanimity. Disconnection most commonly occurs at the junction of the tracheostomy tube with the Noseworthy connector and unless quickly rectified the patient will die. A leak of gas in the circuit leads to defective gas exchange in the lungs. Prevention depends on testing the machine before use, high nursing standards and repeated checks of the ventilator and the hoses. A significant leak in the circuit is detected by finding a discrepancy of more than 1000 ml between the inspired and the expired minute volume. When a serious discrepancy is found the nurse checks the hoses and listens for a leak around the E-T or tracheostomy tube. Unless the leak is readily stopped then the ventilator and hoses are exchanged. Excessive traction by the ventilator hoses can pull out a tracheostomy tube. In a paralysed patient the nurse should make one, but only one, attempt to replace the tube. If this is not possible she quickly intubates the trachea with an E-T tube, continues IPPV, and then summons aid. When, on the other hand, the patient can breathe spontaneously oxygen therapy is given via the tracheostomy and the doctor is summoned to replace the tracheostomy tube. On rare occasions the patient – usually in the recovery phase of acute self-poisoning – pulls out his own E-T tube. In this situation the nurse gives oxygen via a face mask and a doctor then decides whether IPPV is still required.

3. Pharynx, larynx or trachea

The pressure produced by an E-T or tracheostomy tube on the lips, pharynx, vocal chord or trachea can damage the mucous membrane. Ulceration at the angle of the mouth can usually be avoided by taking care. Should ulceration occur, it is painful although temporary. Oedema or ulceration of the vocal chords can lead to dysphonia; the voice can recover in weeks or is permanently affected due to the development of a granuloma. These pressure sores of the mouth, pharynx, larynx are avoided by the use of a tracheostomy tube, but this can be followed by a train of complications. These are wound infections, dilatation or ulceration of the trachea and rarely the formation of a fistula between the trachea and oesophagus (ulcerative tracheo-oesophageal fistula). The complications in this group occur only during IPPV, unlike tracheal stenosis which can develop long after the tracheostomy is closed.

Tracheal damage requires further information, so that this can be minimized in practice. All cuffed tubes damage the tracheal mucosa by obstructing the capillary blood flow to the mucous membrane. It follows that the lower the pressure the less the damage. Even with the current methods and materials the ciliated epithelium is lost for ever, replaced by a non-ciliated lining. As little damage as possible is achieved by using a 'low pressure, large volume thin-walled cuff', and for prolonged IPPV no other cuff tubes should be allowed. To reduce mucosal damage the pressure in the cuff must not exceed 30 cmH$_2$O. (22 mmHg, 2.9 kPa) and it is important to learn that even this pressure threatens the mucosal blood flow; a pressure of 50 cmH$_2$O is bound to cause serious harm. There are two ways of setting the cuff. The more reliable is to measure the pressure on a gauge – and repeat the measurements regularly. Alternatively, the user may put their faith in the safety valve built into the inflation tubing. The safety valve is set to release air when the cuff pressure reaches 30 cmH$_2$O.

4. Circulatory

Enough has already been written about the pulmonary mechanics during IPPV for the reader to understand that a fall in the cardiac output can occur.

This complication is more likely to occur when one or more of the following are present; hypovolaemia, left ventricular failure, or when polyneuropathy or spinal cord injury block the Valsalva response. Consequently, it is often possible to anticipate or prevent a fall in the cardiac output and hypotension by maintaining the CVP and by giving an infusion to correct hypovolaemia. An important additional principle is to go slowly when starting IPPV, using a small tidal volume low bag pressure when using manual IPPV. When, despite these measures, the blood pressure falls the first consideration is: Is the hypotension causing harm? This question can partly be answered by the patient's circulation, skin temperature, and urine flow. When the fall in blood pressure is only moderate and organ function appears satisfactory, treatment can be delayed for an hour or so because the hypotension may prove to be self-correcting. On the other hand the fall in blood pressure may be quite severe and the other signs suggest deficient blood flow to the brain, kidney and muscle. The step-by-step treatment is carried out as follows: lie the patient horizontally, reduce the V_T to the minimum value necessary to maintain alveolar ventilation; measure the CVP – if normal or low, infuse 200 ml of dextran 70 in 5% dextrose and observe the blood pressure frequently. If the CVP is high, give intravenous inotropic agent to increase the cardiac output, in polyneuropathy give a vasopressor, such as methoxamine or metaraminol. These treatments are repeated as dictated by the result of monitoring. Two specific examples may help the beginner. (i) A patient acutely poisoned with a phenothiazine has hypotension, oliguria and the skin temperature of 20°C; the CVP is 10.0 cm. An infusion of inotrope is started and there is a dramatic improvement of the circulation and urine flow. (ii) Soon after starting IPPV for a crushed chest the blood pressure falls, there is sweating of the face, and oliguria. After excluding a tension pneumothorax, the CVP is measured and found to be zero. One unit of polygeline is infused over 10 minutes and the blood pressure is restored, but oliguria persists. The CVP is 6.0 cm. A further infusion of 200 ml polygeline in 5% dextrose is given but without an increase in urine output. Following 40 mg of frusemide intravenously, there is a brisk diuresis.

5. The lung

Thirty years ago the pulmonary complications of prolonged IPPV were both common and serious. This gloomy picture was changed largely by centralizing the care of such patients and by the training of a nursing team aided by chest physiotherapy. The prevention of pulmonary complications was considered under 'How to Continue', but absorption collapse, infection and pulmonary oxygen toxicity require individual consideration.

(a) Absorption collapse occurs because the normal defence mechanisms or bronchial clearing mechanisms are ineffective; these are summarized in Table 19.13. The cough reflex or the mechanisms of coughing can be defective for one or more of the reasons shown. The second most important cause of absorption collapse is that of retained bronchial secretions. The obstruction can be caused by normal bronchial mucus, especially when this is thick and tenacious or when endotracheal suction is of poor quality; the remedy is improved humidification and a larger or better nursing team. In many conditions abnormally large quantities of material are present in the bronchi. This is seen in chronic bronchitis, inflammatory lung disease or during oedema, when the alveolar fluid tracks up the bronchioles. Consequently, in these diseases the bronchi can only be kept clear by frequent skilled suction and chest physiotherapy. Absorption collapse will also occur when foreign materials (Table 19.13) enter the bronchial tree from above the E-T tube or tracheostomy tube. Here is an eminently preventable cause. The correct inflation of the cuff, effective oral and pharyngeal suction, postural drainage of the pharynx, are the techniques and these depend on the quality of the nursing team. The prevention of absorption collapse has been stressed repeatedly; recognition and treatment follows. Absorption collapse of the whole lung can be due to mucus, blood clot and also occurs when an E-T tube is accidentally passed into the right main bronchus. Fortunately the signs are obvious; decreased expansion and feeble breath sounds on the affected side and a high inflation pressure. Treatment is a simple matter of removing the plug or shortening the E-T tube. To remove the mucus, blood or other material, the IPPV is first changed from mechanical to manual. The treatment known as bagging and suction is next employed and when possible help is obtained from a physiotherapist. Since the procedure is unpleasant, the patient is given an analgesic agent or is lightly anaesthetized. The posture of the patient is adjusted so that when 5 ml of saline are injected down the trachea it is likely to enter the obstructed bronchus. After injection has been made the lungs are inflated slowly but deeply; at the end of an inflation the reservoir bag is suddenly released to simulate an expulsive cough. At the same time the physiotherapist squeezes and vibrates the chest or percusses the obstructed side. At the end of expiration suction is performed. The catheter is carefully – but quickly – directed into the obstructed lung. One or two treatments will usually clear the bronchus and mechanical IPPV is then resumed; an X-ray should be taken to confirm the clinical evidence; the aspirate is cultured yet again. In our experience bronchoscopy is rarely necessary. Absorption collapse of a lobe or segment is more difficult to recognize. The condition should be suspected when one or more of the following signs appear; unexpected rise

Table 19.13 Pulmonary complications of IPPV (From *Essential Intensive Care*, with permission)

Pathological process	Prevention/treatment
Drying of the airways	Humidification/intratracheal saline
Retains secretions → absorption collapse	Efficient suction, physiotherapy Oral/pharyngeal suction
Inhalation of saliva, nasal secretion, vomit	Postural drainage of the pharynx nasal secretions, vomit Correct cuff inflation Frequent small tube feeds Efficient gastric suction
Oedema	Prevention of early treatment of bacterial toxaemias Monitoring balance for sodium and water Diuretics Maintaining serum albumin Using minimal O_2 concentration
Bacterial infection	High standards of patient care especially endotracheal suction and tracheostomy care Bacterial monitoring Selective use of antibiotics

in body temperature, shadowing on X-ray linear atelectasis or a larger homogeneous opacity. The radiographic appearances of linear atelectasis are characteristic, but homogeneous shadowing is non-specific and can also be caused by oedema or pleural effusion. In our experience the only method of differentiating these causes is to observe the changes in the X-ray after various treatments. We have adopted the policy of assuming that homogeneous shadowing with or without an air bronchogram, is caused by absorption collapse. Intensive efforts are then made to clear the bronchi and the lungs are then re-assessed. If the shadowing is reduced then absorption collapse was the correct diagnosis; when the radiograph is unchanged then an alternative explanation is pursued. A second policy relating to absorption collapse occurring during IPPV, is to regard this complication as an emergency and never to delay the treatment.

Table 19.14 Sources and transmission of hospital acquired infection

Patient	Nostrils, mouth, pharynx,
	Skin
	Sputum, gastric aspirate, faeces
	Wounds, drains, burns
Staff	Nostrils, expired air (talking, coughing)
	Skin, fingers, hand-cream
	Clothing
Immediate environment	Air, dust
	Walls, floors, trolleys
	Bed linen
	Handbasins, taps, lotions, soaps
	Shaving equipment, toothbrushes
	Thermometers
Equipment	Suction apparatus
	Ventilators, anaesthetic machines
	Dialysers, filters
	Catheters
Nutrition	Beverages, ice-cubes, food
	Intragastric feeds
	i.v. infusions

(b) Bacterial infection is considered next. It seems logical to start with the sources of infection and these are summarized in Table 19.14. The pathogenesis is of two kinds. Firstly, erogenous, that is transmitted by the staff and equipment directly into the patient without previous carriage. Secondly, endogenous which means that the patient is his own source of infection by previously harmless commensals carried in the oropharynx, stomach, colon, and on the skin. Another generalization is that the clinical experience has taught us that the patient needing IPPV has a lowered defence to bacterial infection. Exogenous infections transmitted from the ventilator or suction apparatus were an important source in the early days of ventilator treatment but is now almost unknown. Until the late 1960s it was assumed that bacterial infection during IPPV invariably originated from the staff, the patient excreta or equipment and was therefore an example of the familiar hospital cross-infection. Systematic studies by clinicians and microbiologists showed this to be only true for some patients. In the remainder, the patient infected himself or the origin could not be traced. How did the patient's own enterobacteria and pseudomonads reach the respiratory tract despite meticulous standards of hygiene? This problem remained unsolved until it was discovered that Gram-negative carriage in the naso-pharynx and stomach was a major source of micro-organisms causing lung infections. Aspiration of these bacteria led to colonization and infection of the bronchi and alveoli. In 1970 research at Whiston showed that the patient's stomach was a reservoir of infection. Bacteria – Gram negative and positive and fungi reached the stomach from the gut, multiplied there and migrated up the oesophagus and Ryle's tube to colonize the throat. Gastric aspirate is therefore bacteriologically a lethal fluid! The bacterial colonization of the stomach is very common during IPPV starting in a few days, but especially so when there is paralytic ileus. It is important to learn that the bacteria can not only move up the Ryle's tube into the collecting bag but also colonize feeding bags even when the nutrient is fed via a pump unless the latter occludes the tubing. From this it is hardly necessary to tell you to culture the gastric aspirate daily. This important discovery almost reads like science fiction. The information obtained from bacteriological studies in burns units, cardiothoracic and renal units as well as general intensive care units has helped us in a number of ways. One result is a working hypothesis of how infection spreads; secondly, how to 'contain' bacterial infection during the IPPV and lastly, to use antibiotics in a rational way.

Infection of the respiratory tract during IPPV is preceded by colonization. Bacteria uncommon in the nose, throat, and not normally found in a tracheostomy and wound or tracheal aspirate are isolated but do not appear to be causing home, that is, infection. These bacteria can be Gram positive, e.g. *S. aureus* or Gram-negative enterobacterial and pseudomonads. In many instances, daily cultures will show the progression of the bacteria down the respiratory tract. Likewise, the IPPV can be continued without signs of infection and the treatment is successfully concluded without the use of antibiotics. In contrast, the bacteria, many often having a relatively low pathogenicity, can cause infection (sepsis). The infection shows itself in one or more ways; inflammation and exudate in the tracheostomy wound, a thick yellow or green tracheal aspirate, as shadowing on the chest X-ray with associated changes in lung compliance or gas exchange, or lastly, as the systemic manifestations of infection. The latter are fever, leucocytosis and a rise in blood sugar due to glucose intolerance (stress diabetes). There may be a bacteraemia or sepsis. It follows that the bacterial infection is recognized by clinical and laboratory criteria defined in Appendix 15.2. The presence of bacteria in the stained film of the tracheal aspirate or in the culture does not by itself imply infection. If the stained bacteria are seen to be intimately mixed up with pus cells, then infection is probable. Similarly, copious thick aspirate probably means infection but should be confirmed by quantitative culture. Shadowing on the radiograph must be carefully distinguished from the shadowing of oedema or absorption collapse.

Turning next to the interpretation of the systemic signs of infection. During prolonged IPPV most patients have a low grade fever even though the primary disease is not caused by infection. A rapid rise in temperature can indicate infection (respiratory tract, bacteraemia or both, but also occurs when a segment of lung collapses due to mucus plug. Despite these obvious limitations we always recognize that a core temperature of 38.5°C or more probably signifies respiratory infection or bacteraemia or both. Changes in the white cell count are also of value in diagnosing infection, although these are subject to similar limitations. A white cell count of $11 \times 10^9/l$ or above usually signifies dangerous infection but could equally be caused by the extensive inflammation of acute pancreatitis or ulcerative colitis. Daily measurements of the blood sugar are needed for metabolic care, and also help in the diagnosis of bacterial infection, because the latter causes glucose intolerance. When a previously stable blood sugar rises to 11.2 mmol/l (200 mg/100 ml) then other signs of bacterial infection should be quickly sought. Severe bacterial infection of the respiratory tract during IPPV is invariably serious and sometimes fatal; every effort is made at prevention. This applies to all patients and includes the occasional use of IPPV to treat a patient with a lung infection. In this instance the danger is one of secondary infection. Prevention depends on the thorough application of several principles. Firstly, high standards of hygiene of the individual patient, based largely on the routines of the infectious diseases hospital. Secondly, on clean techniques of endotracheal suction and care of the tracheostomy. Treatment of lung infection, if it is to be effective, consists of intensive parenteral antibiotic therapy which must be started at an early stage; too little, too late, is useless. The patients run a high risk of life-threatening infection and the beginner might therefore be tempted to give systemic antibiotics to all, in the hope of preventing infection during IPPV. Such a policy has led to disastrous results and is accordingly condemned. Prophylactic parenteral antibiotics invariably lead to super-infection by resistant bacteria and the morbidity of mortality is increased; the opposite results to the objective. Prophylaxis based on sound principles and tested out by trials can abolish Gram-negative carriage in the throat and stomach; this is called selective decontamination of the digestive tract (SDD) and is described in Chapter 27.

Early recognition depends on clinical and laboratory monitoring. Core temperature is measured hourly, and the white cell count and blood sugar are measured at least once each day. Bacterial monitoring consists of taking daily swabs from the nose, throat, tracheostomy wound, surgical drains, tracheal aspirate, rectum etc. Films and cultures of the tracheal aspirate are made daily and the laboratory is requested to report the results quickly and directly. The urine and gastric aspirate are cultured daily. The faeces is tested for the isolation of *Proteus* spp. *Pseudomonas* spp, and *Klebsiella* spp. Blood cultures are taken at the least suspicion of infection. These bacteriological results are charted on a table. Antibiotic policies are drawn up for Gram-positive infections *S. aureus*, *S. pneumoniae*, and Gram-negative infections (*Klebsiella* spp., *E. coli*, *Proteus* spp., *Pseudomonas* spp.) In general terms, a short delay in treating the former is less serious than delaying the treatment of infections by Gram-negative bacteria. When the evidence indicates that Gram-positive infection is producing harmful effects then an antibiotic is started. A different policy is required for Gram-negative infections. The reason for this is that such infections readily cause fatal toxaemia (endotoxaemia). By the time damage to the kidney, heart, brain or lung is clinically evident antibiotics rarely, if ever, save life. It follows that early warning signs are necessary, which indicate the need to start intensive antibiotic treatment. We found changes in core temperature, white cell count, or blood sugar were valuable 'red alert' signs of bacterial toxaemia. Consequently, we use these signs, along with others, as indications for starting antibiotics (Chapter 27).

(c) Pulmonary oxygen toxicity. Although essential for life, oxygen can also act as a poison. Oxygen can harm the lungs in a number of ways. If dry oxygen is used to inflate the lungs for any length of time it will impair the cilial action in the bronchi. Since 1899 we have known that when animals breathe 90% oxygen for days or weeks they develop interstitial oedema and fibrosis, a pathological process known as the Lorraine Smith effect. Whether this would occur in normal man is quite unknown. Of relevance to intensive care is the possibility that high concentrations of oxygen used during prolonged IPPV may harm the lung; circumstantial evidence points to the possibility. When IPPV was used – initially without success – to treat premature infants with the Respiratory Distress Syndrome of the newborn, increasing concentrations of oxygen were needed to maintain the PaO_2, but the interstitial pulmonary lesion was due to oxygen toxicity. We now know that the immature lung was deficient in surfactant, and that this is more important than oxygen toxicity. Now the pulmonary lesion in the adult syndrome of ARDS is very similar histologically to that of neonatal syndrome, so that it was natural to deduce that oxygen was a cause of the pulmonary lesion when this developed during IPPV. High concentrations of oxygen from the Bird ventilator were especially blamed. The Bird ventilator is powered by compressed gas. It is very compact, portable and ideal for IPPV. The

Table 19.15 The golden rules of ventilator therapy (From *Essential Intensive Care*, with permission)

Don't start until you have answered the questions
     Is this in the best interests of the patient?
     Would you wish this treatment on yourself?
Don't ventilate a corpse, namely a patient with brain death
Don't use IPPV on a respiratory cripple
Don't use relaxants without a sedative
Always start with manual IPPV
Don't connect a breathing patient to a ventilator unless you intend to use
  assisted ventilation
Remember healthy lungs are easily overventilated by a machine
Remember to communicate with the patient – often!

---

design is ingenious and dates back to 1946. It is now recognized that there are several causes of interstitial oedema developing during the course of IPPV, including saline excess (sodium retention) and capillary leak due to bacterial toxin. So far as our patients are concerned, we do not know whether high concentrations of oxygen during IPPV harm the lung and in man suitable experiments are clearly impossible. The practical implication of these observations is to use the minimal concentrations of oxygen which will maintain a safe PaO_2 and to monitor the F_IO_2.

This introduction to ventilator treatment ends with a set of golden rules (Table 19.15); their aim is to help in patient selection and to avoid unnecessary suffering or stress to patients, their relatives or the nursing team.

APPENDIX   The APACHE system

To use the method three packages of information are required, and these results are used to calculate the APACHE score. To start with the familiar, the Glasgow coma score (Chapter 10). The result for a patient is subtracted from 15 to give us the first result. Next comes the acute physiological assessment for each day. This consists of the 12 observations listed in Table 19.16. Most of these routine measurements are familiar but two require explanation. Oxygenation is assessed (fifth measurement) as follows. When the inspired oxygen exceeds 50% then calculate the oxygen gradient $(P(A–a)O_2)$ and thus obtain the score. If on the other hand the F_1O_2 is less than 50%, then use the arterial oxygen tension alone. When a patient has acute renal failure (reflected in the serum creatinine) then the score in this column is doubled. The system mirrors the fact that the more severe the changes are in the ECF the worse the outlook – back to the milieu intérieur (Chapter 4).

It will be no surprise that the second part of the predictor deals with pre-existing disease; this is the CHE which stands for chronic health evaluation. The first component is easy, the patient's age (Table 19.17), and the chronic diseases are defined as follows:

(i) Liver: Biopsy proven cirrhosis and documented portal hypertension, episodes of past upper GI bleeding attributed to portal hypertension, or prior episodes of hepatic failure, encephalopathy or coma.

(ii) Cardiovascular: New York Association Class IV (Chapter 6, Table 6.5).

(iii) Respiratory: Chronic restrictive, obstructive or vascular disease resulting in severe exercise restriction, i.e. unable to climb stairs or perform household duties or documented chronic hypoxia, hypercapnia, secondary polycythaemia, severe pulmonary hypertension (mean pulmonary artery pressure 40 mmHg) or respiratory dependency.

(iv) Renal: receiving chronic dialysis.

(v) Immuno-compromised: the patient has received therapy that suppresses resistance to infection, e.g. immuno-suppression, chemotherapy, radiation, long-term or recent high-dose steroids, or has a disease that is sufficiently advanced to suppress resistance to infection, e.g. leukaemia, lymphoma, AIDS.

One or more of the preexisting diseases is next given points depending on whether or not the patient has undergone surgery. For non-operative or emergency post-operative patients, assign 5 points; for elective post-opera-

Table 19.16 The acute physiological assessment for APACHE II (From Knaus and Zimmerman, 1998, with permission)

Points	4	3	2	1	0	1	2	3	4
Core temp (°C)	>41	39.0–40.9		38.5–38.9	36.0–38.4	34.0–35.9	32.0–33.9	30.0–31.9	<29.9
Mean BP (mmHg)	>160	130–159	110–129		70–109		50–69		<49
Heart rate	>180	140–179	110–139		70–109		55–69	40–54	<39
Respiratory rate	>50	35–49		25–34	12–24	10–11	6–9		<5
$F_iO_2\% >50$ $P_{(A-a)}O_2$ kPa	>66.5	46.6–64.9	26.6–46.4		26.6				
$F_iO_2\% <0.5$ P_aO_2 kPa					9.3	8.1–9.3		7.3–8.0	<7.3
Arterial pH	>7.7	7.6–7.69		7.5–7.59	7.33–7.49		7.25–7.32	7.15–7.24	<7.15
Nap (mmol/l)	>180	160–179	155–159	150–154	130–149		120–129	111–119	<110
Kp (mmol/l)	>7.0	6.0–6.9		5.5–5.9	3.5–5.4	3.0–3.4	2.5–2.9		<2.5
Creatinine p (µmol/l) Double score for ARF	>309	177–300	133–168		53–124		<53		
PCV (%)	>60		50–59.9	46–49.9	30–45.9		20–29.9		<20
WBC × 10^9/l	>40	20–39.9		15–19.9	3.0–14.9		1.0–2.9		<1.0

Table 19.17 Age points; assign points to age as follows
(From Knaus and Zimmerman, 1988, with permission)

Age (years)	Points
less than 44	0
45–54	2
55–64	3
65–74	5
over 75	6

tive patients assign 2 points. The grand total score is now quickly obtained by addition of these components; the APACHE score can vary between 0 and 71. The various pieces of information can be recorded in tables or stored in a computer, which can also be programmed to calculate and display the final APACHE score. Having gone to the trouble of obtaining a predictor, what of its value? It must be stressed that the system only allows comparison between groups of patients with the same disease or condition. Thus, a patient in diabetic keto-acidosis may have the same score as a case of bacterial toxaemia, but the predicted outcome in the former is much better than in the latter. The results on the individual patient for any day can be compared with values obtained on huge numbers of patients whose outcome is known. The following is a rough guide: a score of 27 means a 50:50 chance of recovery; if the score is over 35, the chances of recovery are remote. This comparison can help to decide whether a patient will benefit from intensive care, or in another situation, whether or not to stop the intensive therapy.

20

Therapy of shock

I AIM OF THERAPY

The aim of therapy is to restore the circulation, in particular the transport of oxygen. The physiological basis of therapy is to increase the cardiac output and the blood flow to the tissues; another aim difficult to achieve is to adjust the distribution of the cardiac output in order to minimize damage to vital organs. The three essentials in treating shock are: rapid intravenous infusions and blood transfusions; the use of drugs acting on the heart and circulation; the treatment of the cause (specific therapy). Clearly the first two are non-specific. These therapies are now briefly described.

II INTRAVENOUS INFUSIONS AND BLOOD TRANSFUSIONS

The aim of intravenous therapy is to restore the circulating blood volume. To achieve this the fluid infused must remain in the circulation for some time and such infusions are collectively known as plasma expanders. This highly important therapy is best considered as follows: When to infuse? What to infuse? How much should be infused?

To infuse or not to infuse? When the shock is clearly of the hypovolaemic type (Table 7.1) then infusions are started as soon as possible; prompt action is more important than the choice of fluid. In contrast for shock due to heart failure (Table 7.1) infusions are definitely contra-indicated or used only after thorough assessment including measurement of the CVP and maybe the PAWP. In the cardiogenic shock due to acute myocardial infarction infusions are not given. When the shock is again due to heart failure caused by poisoning or bacterial toxin then infusions may be required but are secondary to drugs. Our plan is as follows. Having decided that the shock needs therapy then a drug is given to increase the cardiac output (Section III). If this is successful and the CVP falls from a high value to a normal or low value then 250 ml of a plasma expander is infused to 'top up the circulation'. Infusions are sometimes given to prevent a recurrence of hypovolaemic shock. For example in burns, acute pancreatitis or haemorrhage when the blood pressure has been restored but the CVP is falling. Rather than wait for hypotension a plasma expander is infused to restore the CVP to normal. We would emphasize that this method must not delay the surgical arrest of haemorrhage.

What to infuse? There is no universal fluid for the treatment of shock, and if there is an ideal fluid for any particular case it is rarely possible to get it quickly! To understand the choice of intravenous fluid requires knowledge of any preceding deficits and of the applied physiology of intravenous fluid therapy given in Chapter 4. To deal with the easier problems first. Saline depletion is best treated with gelatin or dextran 70 in saline; burns by the use of protein, gelatin or dextran 70. When haemorrhage is obvious or a strong probability, blood transfusions are clearly necessary but with rare exceptions should await crossmatching. The exceptions are leaking aneurysm of the aorta, ruptured ectopic pregnancy and severe bleeding from the upper gastrointestinal tract. In the meantime, an intravenous infusion should be started, gelatin in saline is our personal choice. Normal saline or Ringer-lactate (compound lactate injection, BP) are considered second best. Normal saline, dextrose-saline and 5% dextrose are grouped as crystalloids, in contrast to the colloids, blood, albumin, dextrans and gelatin. Circumstantial evidence suggests that large volumes of crystalloids used in the treatment of shock can cause interstitial oedema and they are therefore best avoided. Having said this, it should be recalled that during the Vietnamese War thousands of shocked patients were treated with the aid of Ringer-lactate! Some side-effects or complications of individual infusions are given in Table 20.1.

The volume and rate of infusion is often more important than the choice of fluid. Tardy replacement in the early stages of therapy, under- or over-infusion can cause serious harm and lead to the death of a patient. Fortunately, a few simple measurements will, in most cases, enable the rate and volume of infusion to be adjusted correctly. Two measurements are of little immediate value in monitoring infusions, they are the haemoglobin level and the packed cell volume (PVC) and they do not alter until haemodilution occurs 6–8 hours after the fluid loss. Estimates of apparent blood or body fluid has been useful only as a guide to the minimum that must be replaced and may seriously under-estimate the actual loss incurred. Large or massive blood transfusions (Chapter 28), which have serious side-effects, can usually be avoided by the right operation carried out at the right time by the right surgeon. When the clinical signs indicate severe hypovolaemic

Table 20.1 Plasma expanders used in the treatment of shock

Infusion	Effects
Blood	Delay. In short supply. Cooling of the heart. Lactic acidosis or citrate toxicity with whole blood Incompatibility. Damage to the lung by micro thrombi
Plasma protein or albumin	The ideal, but expensive
Degraded gelatin (Haemaccel, Gelofusine)	Excellent plasma substitute. Few adverse effects
Dextran 40	Short stay in the circulation, improves blood flow, obstructs renal tubules in oliguria
Dextran 70	Excellent plasma substitute. Anti-coagulant action, attracts fluid from interstitial fluid

shock then 500–1000 ml of a plasma expander should be rapidly infused. The doctor should then decide whether or not CVP measurements are necessary. This decision is usually an easy one. The CVP line will be essential in the patient with multiple injuries, chest injury, closed trauma to the abdomen and during IPPV. In the remaining patients the amount of fluid to be infused and the rate of administration can be controlled by the clinical signs described in Chapter 7. Readings on the CVP are used to control infusions or transfusions in the following way. The infusion or blood transfusion given in aliquots of 200–500 ml run in as quickly as the system will delivery. After each aliquot the infusion is stopped and the circulation re-assessed. When the blood pressure, pulse volume, temperature and urine flow indicate a good response and the CVP is normal then rapid infusions are stopped, at least for a time. On the other hand a low CVP indicates the need for a further rapid infusion of 250–500 ml. When a poor response to rapid infusion is found together with a normal CVP a further aliquot should be infused and this will often restore the circulation. In other cases of hypovolaemic shock infusions will elevate the CVP to above normal but shock persists. This means that heart failure also exists and further infusions are dangerous. The use of the CVP in this way prevents under-transfusion and helps to avoid over-transfusion leading to acute circulatory overload and pulmonary oedema. This practice will not do for the syndrome of shock and pulmonary oedema. We need to determine whether infusions will improve the cardiac output or worsen the lungs and this can only be determined by measuring the pressure in the left atrium. This key value is obtained by measuring the PAWP as described in Chapter 7. The result is used as follows. When the PAWP is normal (mean value 8 mmHg) or less than 15 mmHg it is safe to infuse an aliquot of fluid, say 200 ml. On the contrary, when the mean pressure is over 15 mmHg then an infusion is potentially dangerous and drug therapy holds out the only hope of improving the circulation. These guidelines are rules of thumb for the inexperienced. A more precise method for determining the optimum value for PAWP is as follows. A colloid solution is infused to elevate the PAWP, and at each value of PAWP the cardiac output (CO) or left ventricular stroke work index (LVSWI) is obtained. There will come a time when increasing the PAWP does not improve CO or LVSWI. This plateau value represents the optimum wedge.

III DRUGS TO INCREASE THE CARDIAC OUTPUT

The drug therapy has one of two aims: to restore sinus rhythm when a dysrhythmia is causing shock; the alternative aim is to increase the cardiac output of the heart in sinus rhythm. The use of drugs to treat dysrhythmias is an extensive topic and is outside our scope. A handful of drugs are available which increase the cardiac output by increasing the rate (chronotrope) or by raising the stroke volume (inotrope). Such drugs can restore the circulation in heart failure over a period of minutes, hours or even days but the heart muscle must recover if the patient is to survive. The indications are acute heart failure and in our experience the best results are obtained when this is caused by one of the following: acute poisoning (overdose); bacteraemia or bacterial toxaemia; multiple injuries or acute pancreatitis. In cardiogenic shock due to acute myocardial infarction the results of drug therapy are so poor that we have abandoned their routine use. In treating heart failure our practice is to use dopamine or dobutamine singly or together. The drug is diluted in saline, glucose or lactate (not bicarbonate) and infused from a pump. At first, a dose at the lower end of the range (Table 20.2) is tried in the hope that this will improve the cardiac output. The dose of one or both drugs is adjusted to achieve the optimum effects on blood pressure, urine flow and skin temperature. At pre-determined intervals of a few hours the dose is reduced to determine whether or not the circulation is drug dependent. Should the performance of the heart improve, then drug therapy can be phased out in a planned way. Two other drugs used in acute heart failure are adrenaline and noradrenaline. These are used less frequently than the preceding agents and haemodynamic monitoring is essential.

Table 20.2 Drugs used to increase the cardiac output in shock

Dopamine hydrochloride	At doses between 5–20 μg/kg/min it is inotropic, increasing cardiac output with a negligible effect on the heart rate. At doses in excess of 20 μg/kg/min, stimulation of alpha receptors may cause peripheral vasoconstriction and tachycardia.
Dobutamine hydrochloride	Selective beta-agonist, increasing cardiac output with negligible effect on the heart rate. Usual dose range is between 2.5–10 μg/kg/min.
Isoprenaline hydrochloride	Non-selective beta-agonist, producing increased cardiac output, tachycardia and peripheral vasodilatation. Dose range 0.5–10 μg/min. Useful in states of shock associated with bradycardia. Isoprenaline may precipitate ventricular arrhythmias.
Adrenaline tartrate	Both alpha and beta adrenergic action. Used in anaphylactic shock and when increased myocardial contractility is needed. Dose range is 2–10 μg/min.
Noradrenaline acid tartrate	Predominantly alpha adrenergic action. Used in shock with vasodilatation, e.g. bacterial toxaemia. Dose range is 4–8 μg/min.

IV VASODILATORS

Having decided to use a vasodilator drug then a choice is made from the list shown in Table 21.3. Low dose dopamine given by continuous intravenous infusion is such an effective renal vasodilator that this drug is now used routinely by some in the shocked patient to prevent oliguria; acute myocardial infarction is an important exception. The dosage is shown in Table 20.3. The drug glyceryl trinitrate (nitroglycerine, dynamite), widely used to treat the angina patient, is a potent dilator of constricted vessels in the muscles and skin. This drug can be given by continuous intravenous infusion or through the skin using a known quantity in the form of a cream applied to the skin as an adhesive patch. Other vasodilators such as chlorpromazine, nitroprusside and prazosin are currently out of favour.

V EXTRACELLULAR FLUID

Severe disorders of the extracellular fluid can reduce the cardiac output and adversely affect the vascular trees. Such changes in the extracellular fluid can be caused by the disease which itself causes the shock, but can also be a consequence of the shock; a sort of hen and egg phenomenon. Examina-

Table 20.3 Vasodilator drugs used to treat shock

Dopamine	At low doses, 1–5 μg/kg/min, dopamine selectively dilates the renal and mesenteric vessels; improved renal perfusion can be expected in all 'shock' cases, with consequent improved water clearance. Its role as a 'protector' of the kidney is less clear cut.
Glyceryl trinitrate	Predominant venous dilator; reduces elevated left ventricular filling pressure in patients with heart failure. Myocardial oxygen consumption is decreased. Dose range 10–200 μg/min. May worsen hypotension.
Phentolamine	Alpha-receptor blocker acting directly on vascular smooth muscle; stimulates insulin secretion. Dose range is 0.1–2 mg/min. Adverse effects include hypotension and tachycardia.
Sodium nitroprusside	Arterial and venodilator by direct action on smooth muscle. Reconstituted with the diluent provided and added to 500 ml of 5% glucose. Protect from light. Dose range 0.5–6 μg/kg/min.

tion of the extracellular fluid should be made as soon as circulatory resuscitation is underway; concentrating on pH, oxygen and then proceeding to plasma potassium and calcium. The methods for correcting deficits or excesses are given in Chapter 16.

For many years it was postulated that the adrenal gland did not respond appropriately in shock – a stress state; this remains a theory, but also the basis of giving huge doses of corticosteroids during shock, especially of the bacterial type.

VI SPECIFIC THERAPY

Specific therapy means treatment directed to the cause of the shock. In most instances both non-specific and specific measures are used concurrently. (i) Tension pneumothorax urgently requires the insertion of a chest drain connected to an underwater seal. Release of the intra-thoracic pressure leads to a prompt improvement in the circulation. Should the patient be moribund, then no time should be lost in inserting a needle into one or both pleural spaces in the second or third rib spaces in the mid-clavicular line. An explosive escape of air will confirm the diagnosis. Perforation of the oesophagus can sometimes cause a tension hydro-pneumothorax needing drainage. Following this the patient is transferred to a regional thoracic centre for repair of the oesophagus. (ii) Pericardial tamponade is rarely seen outside units for cardiac surgery. Causes other than operations on the heart are: haemopericardium due to a combination of pericarditis and anti-co-agulant therapy. The pericardium can be drained in one of two ways; either at thoracotomy or in an emergency by aspiration of the pericardial sac. (iii) Surgical arrest of haemorrhage. In treating shock, we sometimes omit or delay the arrest of haemorrhage by a direct surgical assault. The timing of a laparotomy is decided after weighing up the dangers of operating on a hypotensive subject and of delaying inevitable surgery, together with the complications of massive blood transfusions. This is a situation calling for the surgeon and anaesthetist with the appropriate experience. Blunt injuries can result in continuing haemorrhage from the spleen, liver or mesentery. Such haemorrhage may be suspected because of tenderness or muscle guarding found during initial assessment, or may become evident later following resuscitation. Signs which suggest bleeding are easily found when sought; pallor, hypotension, falling CVP, abdominal distension and an increased tension. Further evidence can sometimes be obtained by aspiration of the peritoneal cavity or peritoneal lavage. The latter is now used exclusively. Equipment for peritoneal dialysis is prepared and the puncture site is anaesthetised with lignocaine with adrenaline. The PD cannula is next inserted and 1.0 litre of dialysate run into the peritoneal cavity. The patient is next turned from side to side and the abdomen gently massaged. The fluid is next run out. Haemoperitoneum will be obvious but it is the quantity of blood which will decide whether or not a laparotomy is required. (iv) Bacterial infections which cause shock are almost invariably Gram negative. The shock is probably due to the release of endotoxin and has a very high death rate. It is a depressing fact that the death rate remains high despite expert circulatory resuscitation and intensive antibiotic therapy. Personal experience has taught us that if antibiotics are given when the diagnosis is suspected rather than clear cut, then and only then, can more patients recover (Chapter 27). When such a policy is adopted it is inevitable that antibiotics are sometimes given unnecessarily. When patients show the cold hypotensive phase of endotoxaemia, intravenous infusions of colloid and vasodilators are given. In the warm phase, the arterial and central venous pressures can sometimes be maintained with the aid of intravenous plasma protein and inotropes. (v) Shock following pulmonary embolism, especially when it persists for hours, is one of the ominous signs. Some modifications to the non-specific therapy are required. The top priority is oxygen therapy. Intravenous infusions are given to keep the CVP within the range of 5–10 cm; dopamine or dobutamine is used for its inotropic effect on the heart. Three specific treatments are available and are used singly or in a sequence. The first choice lies between intensive heparin therapy or thrombolytic therapy with streptokinase or urokinase. We use heparin by continuous intravenous infusion from a powered syringe. The dose is adjusted to prolong the clotting time to within the range of 20–40 min. The heparin is continued for a week and then replaced by warfarin. The third treatment is emergency embolectomy carried out by a thoracic surgical team. (vi) In hospital practice, shock due to anaphylaxis is usually caused by drug hypersensitivity. Specific treatment takes priority over non-specific treatment and the following drugs are given as quickly as possible: adrenaline injection BP, 1.0 ml intravenously; hydrocortisone, 100 mg intravenously. (vii) During 21 years of general intensive care at Whiston, two cases of Addison's disease required circulatory resuscitation; both recovered and remained well. The specific treatment is hormone therapy and is given concurrently with intravenous infusions and oxygen therapy. Hormone therapy consists of intravenous hydrocortisone, 100 mg 2-hourly. Finally, we must emphasise the prompt and correct treatment of shock outside hospital. The patient is removed from danger. When this has to be delayed because the subject is trapped in a vehicle or otherwise immobilized, then pain is relieved and intravenous infusion started at the site of the accident. External haemorrhage is controlled by a dressing and serious fractures or dislocations given first-aid treatment. Heat loss from the patient's body is reduced as much as possible. Pain is relieved either by drugs or nitrous oxide. We use morphine and nitrous oxide 50% in oxygen, rather than pethidine or pentazocine. Nitrous oxide, has been shown to be both effective and safe. Oxygen therapy (Chapter 18) is started as soon as possible. The shocked patient travels badly, a fact established by the tragic wars in Korea and Vietnam. It follows that whenever possible the shock should be treated before transferring the patient to hospital or from one hospital to another. The patient should be kept horizontal during transport and never tilted head-up.

21

Resuscitation

Breathe on me breath of God, fill me with life anew.
Hymn 671, Ancient and Modern

Quite surely it is not too much to ask that British medical schools teach resuscitation to the same standards as the Girl Guides.
W.R. Casey, 1985

I INTRODUCTION

Resuscitation centres on treating the arrest of breathing or the circulation, usually both. Because of this we use the term cardio-respiratory resuscitation (CPR). Apnoea requires artificial ventilation and cardiac arrest or the pulseless state is treated by cardiac compression until equipment or drugs are available to re-start the heart. Acute circulatory failure without cardiac arrest – shock – requires resuscitation, but this type is separated off from the management of cardiac arrest. Resuscitation mirrors some of the principles of acute medical care and it is worth reflecting on these. Choosing the patient is essential for reasons of humanism and good results; the priority list is virtually the same for all situations and should be recalled instantly under all conditions; action must be prompt and this means thorough training and standardized methods; the intensive care nurse and trained paramedic can carry out intubation and defibrillation, thus improving outcome and extending their role. To round off this brief section: it must be stressed yet again that the staff of an intensive care unit are negligent unless they teach others the avoidable disasters, that is, treating a disease before apnoea or cardiac arrest.

II INDICATIONS

Although cardiac arrest calls for instant – 'reflex' – action, this must not lead to its misuse. Selection is essential for reasons of humanism and to obtain results which justify the treatment. Remember that it is easier to act as a technician and start resuscitation rather than as an experienced humanistic nurse or doctor and call off an inappropriate rescue! Guidelines will help the beginner to work out for themselves how to be selective. Resuscitation should be given when arrest follows acute myocardial infarction but there are reservations. Respiratory or cardiac arrest in the asthmatic, crushed chest or myasthenic demands resuscitation, but is eminently avoidable! The contraindications to resuscitation exceed the indications. Disseminated malignant disease, extreme age and most important, when chronic disease – renal, cardiac or pulmonary – has caused intolerable disability. Hopefully the hospital staff will know the individual patient and have already decided whether resuscitation is appropriate. The newcomer to intensive care will know that in most cases cardiac arrest is a merciful release from intolerable suffering.

III ARTIFICIAL VENTILATION

This cannot be started until the upper airway has been cleared which should only take a few seconds. The mouth is cleared with a finger and the head extended at the neck to enable IPPV to be started by one of the methods given in Table 21.1. The choice will depend on the equipment available at the time and the training of the operator. When the equipment is at the ready and a person trained in tracheal intubation is at the scene, then IPPV should be given by means of a cuffed E-T tube and reservoir bag, hopefully supplied with oxygen. Rarely the airway cannot be cleared in seconds; examples are a hunk of meat wedged in the pharynx or the clenched jaw of a patient with status epilepticus. These desperate situations call for instant action and the right action. In the first case the Heimlich manoeuvre is tried and when failure is obvious then transtracheal ventilation is given rather than waste precious time trying to intubate the patient. Transtracheal ventilation sounds rather grand, but is simple in extreme and has been available for 30 years. The minimum equipment is a 16 S.W.G. cannula and plastic tubing to connect the proximal end to an oxygen supply. The trachea is perforated by the cannula just below the cricoid cartilage, the stylette withdrawn slightly and the cannula then directed towards the carina. The stylette is withdrawn as the cannula is advanced to its full length. Alternative equipment can be used. The well-tried Seldinger method for cannulating blood vessels employs the sequence of needle, guide wire and cannula. A choice exists for

Table 21.1 Methods of IPPV for resuscitation

Mouth-to-mouth
Mouth to Brook airway
Mouth or bag to oesophageal obturator airway*
Ambu bag   ⎫
                 ⎬ to face mask or E-T tube
Anaesthetic bag ⎭
Transtracheal ventilation

*see Don Michael *et al.*, 1968

the next step. Oxygen can be insuflated as a continuous stream down the trachea. This will oxygenate the blood – the essential thing – but not ventilate the alveoli. Alternatively oxygen at a pressure of 2000 p.s.i. is squirted through the cannula intermittently. To do this means interrupting the flow to give 10 insufflations per minute simply by folding the tube on itself to stop the flow. Transtracheal oxygen or ventilation buys the time needed to remove a foreign body or carry out a planned tracheostomy.

Intermittent positive pressure ventilation given by face mask or E-T tube is described in Chapter 19. It is worth repeating the two common errors – too rapid frequency and too high an inflation pressure.

IV TREATMENT OF CARDIAC ARREST

If the patient with cardiac arrest is to have any chance of survival then three essentials are required. Treatment must be prompt, given by trained personnel and properly organized.

1. Aim

The aim of treatment (Table 21.2) is to maintain a sufficient flow of blood to the brain to prevent irreversible brain damage (brain death). A cardiac output is achieved by rhythmic compression (massage) of the heart, using either external cardiac compression (ECC), or manual compression of the heart (internal cardiac compression) made possible by a thoracotomy. During cardiac compression pulmonary gas exchange is maintained by artificial ventilation, preferably with oxygen. The combined cardiac and respiratory resuscitation can only succeed when three conditions are fulfilled. Firstly, when resuscitation is started within 3 or 4 minutes of the signs of cardiac arrest, because brain death is inevitable after this time interval. Secondly, the artificial respiration and cardiac compression must deliver sufficient oxygen to the brain to prevent fatal hypoxic damage. Failure to maintain oxygenation of the brain can be due to poor techniques, but in

Table 21.2 Overall plan for treating cardiac arrest (From *Essential Intensive Care*, with permission)

Respiratory	Circulatory	Metabolic
Clear the airway	Thump on sternum	
IPPV	ECC	Give 100 mmol $NaHCO_3$ if delay in starting
Mouth-to-mouth Brook airway Face mask plus bag E-T tube plus bag		
	Restore sinus rhythm defibrillation drugs cardioversion pacing	
		Correct acidosis hyperkalaemia hypokalaemia hypothermia

other instances perfect methods fail. Lastly, the patient cannot recover unless additional treatment restores an effective heart-beat by using electrical energy or drugs.

2. External cardiac compression

The member of the ward staff who diagnoses cardiac arrest starts treatment without delay, whilst a colleague or an ambulant patient telephones the cardiac arrest call. A witnessed cardiac arrest is always treated initially with a pre-cordial 'thump' with the closed fist; this may restore a normal cardiac rhythm. If the patient has collapsed on the floor, he remains there, and if small and manageable the bed patient is transferred to the floor. Otherwise a board is placed behind the patient's chest. The lone therapist alternates five external compressions with two inflations of the lungs, but with the arrival of the cardiac arrest team these tasks are divided. To carry out ECC the operator stands or kneels at the patient's side opposite the sternum. When a single therapist has to perform both ECC and artificial respiration he stands or kneels above the shoulder opposite the head. The heel of one hand is placed dead centre on the sternum and the other hand rests firmly on the top to increase the pressure. The correct site for pressure is the junction of the upper two-thirds with the lower third. The arms are kept rigid at the elbows and downward pressure is transmitted to the sternum by the weight of the operator, pivoted at the hips (Figure 21.1). Pressure is exerted rhythmically about one compression per second and the sternum is depressed downwards about 2.5 cm (1.0 inch). When correctly performed ECC will in most cases produce carotid and femoral pulses. Indeed, haemodynamics studies have shown that an intra-arterial blood pressure of 90 mmHg can be produced. The nurse or doctor carrying out the artificial resuscitation team will provide the apparatus necessary to determine the cardiac rhythm and the treatment. When the patient is not already lying on a firm surface the team quickly arrange this. Four tasks have to be performed prior to the treatment of ventricular fibrillation or other dysrhythmia: the initial operator is relieved; the trachea is intubated and the lungs are inflated with oxygen; an intravenous drip is established, the ECG is monitored. Should we assume a severe metabolic acidosis is invariable and therefore routinely give intravenous sodium bicarbonate? Answer, no. Current recommendations are to give bicarbonate when cardio-pulmonary resuscitation was delayed for more than ten minutes or it is probable that a metabolic acidosis preceded the arrest.

3. Restoring cardiac rhythm

The stage has now been reached when the cardiac rhythm is known and when it may be possible to restore a spontaneous heartbeat. Ventricular fibrillation requires defibrillation. The direct current defibrillator is prepared by applying jelly to the electrodes and charging to 200 Joules. The nurse or doctor (3) in Figure 21.1 stands opposite the colleague (2) giving ECC, and at a given signal 'NOW', the operators (1 and 2) quickly remove their hands from contact with the patient or bed and (3) firmly passes the electrodes on to the chest wall and discharges the defibrillator. One electrode is placed centrally over the sternum and the second in the mid-axillary line roughly in the same horizontal plane. Further shocks of 200 J, then 360 J are given, with a check on the carotid pulse before each shock. If VF persists operators 1 and 2 immediately restart artificial respiration and ECC whilst 3 studies the ECG. When debrillation has restored sinus rhythm then ECC is stopped to see whether the spontaneous heart action produces a pulse; if so, the EEC is suspended but the artificial respiration continued. When sinus rhythm is short-lived because VF quickly returns, then defibrillation is repeated time and time again until the sinus rhythm is stable or the team feels that resuscitation has failed. Defibrillation is more often successful when the VF

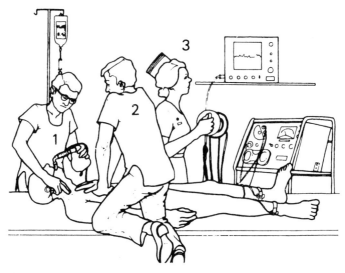

Figure 21.1 Position of personnel during resuscitation. Operator 1 gives IPPV and feels the carotid pulse. Operator 2 carries out external cardiac compression. Operator 3 observes the ECG and prepares the defibrillator (From *Essential Intensive Care*, with permission)

is of large amplitude, (referred to as coarse), in contrast to a low amplitude wave form (fine). Adrenaline can be used in an attempt to convert fine fibrillation into coarse. At this point we should state our view that intracardiac injections are dangerous and unnecessary. The management of VF requires a pre-determined plan and we teach and practise that published by the European Resuscitation Council (1994). It is shown as an algorithm in Figure 21.2. In asystolic cardiac arrest no QRS complexes appear on the ECG monitor. When P waves are also absent the rhythm is sinus arrest; if regular P waves are seen the diagnosis is complete heart block with ventricular asystole. Again the treatment must be based on current knowledge which is summarized as the flow chart of Figure 21.3.

4. Electro-mechanical dissociation

This label describes the situation where the QRS complexes appear normal, but there is no cardiac output. Cardiac resuscitation continues while a search is made for the causes. This includes hypovalaemia, tension pneumothorax, pericardial tamponade, myocardial rupture, hypokalaemia, hypocalcaemia and drug overdose. Successful outcome depends on identifying and treating the cause.

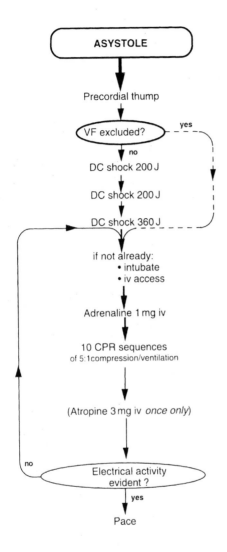

Note: If no response after 3 cycles consider high dose adrenaline: 5 mg iv.

Figure 21.2 Algorithm for the treatment of ventricular fibrillation or pulseless ventricular tachycardia (1997 resuscitation guidelines for use in the UK)

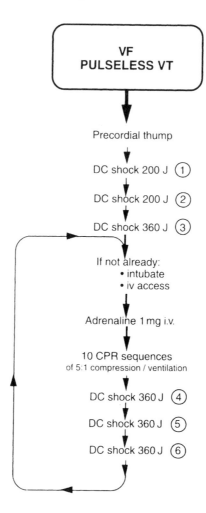

Notes: (i) The interval between shocks 3 and 4 should not be > 2 mins.

(ii) Adrenaline given during loop approx every 2 - 3 mins.

(iii) Continue loops for as long as defibrillation is indicated.

(iv) After 3 loops consider:

 • an alkalising agent

 • an antiarrhythmic agent.

Figure 21.3 Algorithm for the treatment of aystole (1997 resuscitation guidelines for use in the UK)

5. Metabolic

When artificial ventilation and ECC have been established then thought must be given to the possibility of a metabolic disturbance. The latter could be the cause of the arrest or render the treatment more difficult. The relevant disturbances are acidosis, hyper or hypokalaemia and rarely severe hypothermia. Recognition depends on information of the illness and laboratory tests. Thus hypokalaemia might be suspected in a surgical patient with prolonged ileus; hyperkalaemia in the patient known to have renal failure; acidosis in a diabetic. On the other hand cardiac arrest following acute myocardial infarction is unlikely to be associated with a disturbed metabolic balance. One or more of these disturbances requires blood analysis to establish the diagnosis; treatment was described in Chapter 16. Severe hypothermia requires rapid warming of the body.

6. Assessing progress

The 'well' coronary patient may recover dramatically from cardiac arrest and about 50% of such cases are discharged from hospital. Equally successful is the restoration of respiration and circulation in the pulseless case of acute poisoning. Other patients may show no immediate response to resuscitation and a systematic assessment must be carried out in order to determine whether resuscitation should be stopped or should continue. The same scheme of assessment (Table 21.3) may be used to detect the sequelae of cardiac arrest. When interpreting the neurological signs it should be emphasized that brain damage may have occurred before the cardiac arrest. Nevertheless such damage may recover during the following hours, days or weeks. On the other hand, when it is certain that resuscitation was started promptly, as during coronary care, then the unfavourable signs are truly ominous. When resuscitation restores spontaneous cardiac rhythm as seen on the ECG, the effectiveness of the heartbeat is assessed from the blood pressure, pulse, skin temperature, colour of the lips, and formation of urine. A persistent metabolic acidosis indicates inadequate tissue perfusion and is therefore an unfavourable sign. Determining the prognosis can be made more accurate by utilising information gathered on large numbers of patients. This information was published in convenient tables (Levy *et al.*, 1981).

When should circulatory resuscitation be stopped? The obvious indication is when it is successful! But when an effective spontaneous heartbeat cannot be restored, and other unfavourable signs are present, the resuscitation should be stopped after a time-limit set by the therapist. A total time of one hour should not be exceeded. During resuscitation it may or may not

Table 21.3 Assessing the response to resuscitation (From *Essential Intensive Care*, with permission)

Favourable signs	*Unfavourable signs*
Returning consciousness	Prolonged coma
Spontaneous respiration	Apnoea
Decreasing pupil size	Fully dilated pupils
Eyelash reflex	No eyelash reflex
Muscle tone present, struggling	Flaccid paralysis
Stable rectal temperature	Unstable rectal temperature
Good pulse, warm extremities, urine flow	Shock
Normal arterial pH	Acidosis
Stable cardiac rhythm	Unstable cardiac rhythm
Well oxygenated	Cyanosis on 100% O_2

be possible to keep the patient's relatives informed, but in either case they are subjected to great stress. Resuscitation also makes large demands on nursing and medical manpower and this should be considered when the signs almost certainly indicate failure.

V RESULTS

Of those who bother to collect results a few have courageously published their findings and these make depressing reading. A clear deduction is possible and important to our hospitals; do not treat the wrong patient. Not only will you cause pain and distress, but the patients cannot survive. When the right patient is resuscitated at the right time by the right people – the staff in the area at the time – the results justify the service. In hospital the essentials to obtain good results are: continuous training programmes made mandatory for nurses and doctors; standardized procedures; a clear-cut objective for each disease. For example, ventricular fibrillation in the well (non-shocked) coronary patient, over half should survive the arrest. In acute poisoning, Guillain-Barré, myasthenia, asthma, all should survive.

VI SEQUELAE

If cardio-respiratory resuscitation succeeds in restoring a heart beat, then a period of intensive care is advisable. Of course, the patient may already be in a unit for coronary care. The intensive care unit is necessary because

Table 21.4 The sequelae of cardiac arrest: cross references

Acid–base balance	5
Respiratory failure	6
Shock and heart failure	7
Renal failure	9
Brain failure	10

of the risk of a further arrest, because of a need for care of the airway or for artificial respiration, and to detect and treat any sequelae. The general measures are as follows: the patient is transferred to the unit and nursed in a suitable bed. The ECG is monitored and the intravenous line is checked. When there is hypotension, a CVP (central venous pressure) line is substituted. In the conscious subject, pain or fear are relieved by morphine, papoveretum or diazepam. The thoracic cage is examined for fractures of ribs or the sternum. A portable chest radiograph is taken and examined for oedema or absorption collapse and pneumothorax. When an endotracheal tube is still necessary, the position of the distal end is checked on the X-ray. Oxygen therapy is continued by means of an MC mask except in the severe bronchitic, when 35% oxygen is given. If the patient is breathing spontaneously the pattern of breathing is studied and the minute volume ventilation ($\dot{V}_E$ is measured by means of a Wright's spirometer. The oxygenation of the blood is monitored by an oximeter.

Failure of one or more body systems follows the method described elsewhere and Table 21.4 facilitates cross reference. Although brain failure is dealt with in Chapter 10 this does not include near-death experiences. The novice should appreciate that the patients who survive cardiac arrest unscathed by paralysis, coma or intellectual impairment, may recall experiences of the arrest. In a near-death experience the patient may look on the scene from outside themselves; they can describe in minute detail the members of the resuscitation team. These experiences are not unnecessarily unpleasant and you and I have failed to learn of them because we never asked! Fenwick and Fenwick (1995) investigated over 300 such cases.

APPENDIX
EQUIPMENT TO FACILITATE TRAINING IN
CARDIO-PULMONARY RESUSCITATION

BASIC

Function	*Equipment*
Tracheal intubation Ventilation Suction	Airway management trainer
Ventilation External cardiac compression	Training manikin e.g. Resusci Anne (Laerdal)
External cardiac compression Defibrillation	Manikin has carotid pulse, and rhythm simulator: SR, VF or asystole

WITH ADDED FACILITIES

Ventilation External cardiac compression Recording of results	Training manikin with monitor and recorder
Dysrhythmia recognition Intravascular pressure waveforms Defibrillation	Dysrhythmia training system. Manikin has carotid pulse, 7 QRS rhythms and 5 intra- vascular waveforms and pressures

22

Intensive care of renal failure: first part

'Begin at the beginning', the King said, gravely,
'and go on till you come to the end: then stop'.

Lewis Carroll

I   **STRATEGY**
II   **AIMS**
III   **INTENSIVE NURSING**
IV   **FLUID THERAPY AND NUTRITION**
V   **BLOOD AND DRUG THERAPY**

I STRATEGY

Strategy is essential to get the best out of intensive care. Strategy is made up of four parts; criteria for admission, criteria for stopping high technology medicine, the nursing process, and medical attitudes. The objective is the same for all hospitals and for all divisions of the hospital; the right patient in the right bed at the right time. But for renal failure the strategy is more complicated than that necessary for other conditions or diseases. A brief digression will change a vague concept into certain action. Severe acute asthma need neither kill nor maim. The criteria for urgent admission to hospital are easy; the pulse rate alone will suffice. Ward or ICU? another easy decision (Chapter 3) as is the indication for starting IPPV. The strategy results in a near zero death rate. We should remember that this strategy is rarely needed when the community care is good – educational feedback again! A return to the central theme, the individual patient. Using Figure 22.1 consider the patient already receiving intensive care who develops renal failure acutely. The cause? The failure will probably be attributed to preceding trauma, burns or to bacterial infection or toxaemia – or a mixture. Drugs – the therapeutic ones – must never be forgotten in the diagnosis. We sincerely hope that hypovolaemic shock was not allowed to occur. It follows that the diagnostic programme is answered, if not very accurately. Much of the therapeutic programme will be in operation. There will be no deficit or excesses and nutrition will be appropriate. This means that replacement therapy can be planned; dialysis or filtration or both. Is this strategy to apply to all patients? No. Brief experience will teach that acute failure of other organs or systems spells doom: brain failure, persistent heart failure, ARDS, and so on. The assessment must include chronic pre-existing disease. This will already be to hand as the APACHE II score (Chapter 19). For example a chronic health evaluation, (CHE) greater than 5, or a total score over 40 means that survival is improbable (Maher *et al.*, 1989) but not impossible. These figures can help to decide whether replacement therapy is justified. When dialysis/filtration is to be used then the other treatments are continued; IPPV, prevention and treatment of infection (Chapter 27) and so on. It is vital to learn that the right surgery at the right time by the right surgeon can decide the outcome; replacement therapy does not cure intra-abdominal abscesses!

The patients outside the ICU also need the right treatment at the right time, following alternative strategic pathways (Figure 22.1). A visit to all six hundred beds of a district general hospital would be long and unnecessary. The circumspect assessment can be limited to those patients with a raised urea or creatinine. We can soon find fifty patients with renal failure who do not require intensive therapy; following acute myocardial infarction, chronic heart failure, paralytic ileus due to any cause, stroke, and so on. In some of this group the renal failure is reversible. In contrast our hospital round will discover those with disseminated malignant disease or the frail elderly who have renal failure, but it will be quite wrong to offer these intensive therapy. Wrong, because there is no chance of long-standing benefit. Our survey now concentrates on renal failure which is a high priority and may require intensive therapy. This failure can be acute-on-chronic and pre-existing renal disease may or may not have been diagnosed. The patients in this group can be discovered in any of the wards; trauma, surgery, medicine or obstetrics. In the medical ward the disease can be restricted to the kidney or involve several other organs as in vasculitis or connective tissue disease. The common denominator of this conglomerate is the severity of the renal failure. Some in this group will show classical symptoms of uraemia (Chapter 19). The term uraemic emergency is an appropriate label since this implies the need for rapid and effective decisions. A decision will be needed whether or not to advise intensive therapy. As with resuscitation it is easier to say yes than to say no. When transfer is recommended never omit to ask the patient's consent, unless delirium prevents this. A fresh assessment is made, intensive care monitoring started, and additional diagnostic investigation is planned. The deficits or excesses are estimated in a priority list or triage. The therapeutic programme (Figure 22.1) entails intensive nursing, restoring and then maintaining the ECF and the prevention and treatment of infection. Failure of other organs is treated concurrently. It may be essential

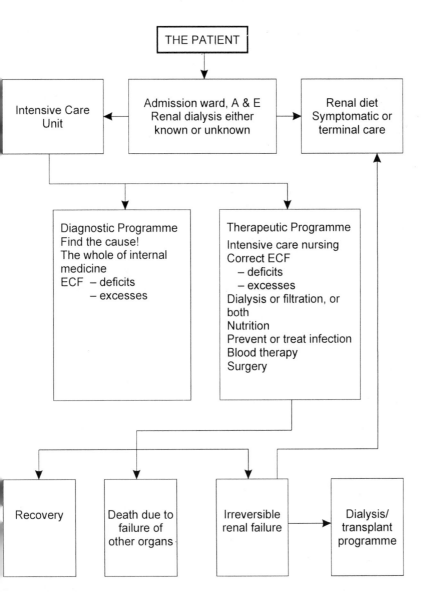

Figure 22.1 Strategic pathways in renal failure

to start dialysis in minutes rather than hours. This is medicine back to front – treatment before diagnosis. But then you don't investigate the lungs of the patient who has stopped breathing. Having 'pressed the button' even after hesitation, there must never be any delay in 'calling off the rescue' (Jennett, 1986) when new evidence shows that survival is impossible. This decision-making will be expanded in Chapter 25, but it is so important that a brief statement was made early on.

II AIMS

When the right patient with acute renal failure is admitted to intensive care at the right time the single aim is survival; preferably survival with adequate renal function. Unfortunately, this objective may not be attained because of hospital-acquired infection or haemorrhage from the gastrointestinal tract. On the other hand, the patient with acute-on-chronic renal failure is rescued and hopefully life then maintained by diet, dialysis and transplantation. Recovery depends on the thorough application of five packages of intensive care outlined later. Some, but not all, of the therapy has a sound physiological basis, which was described in some detail earlier in our book. To remind the reader of the two fundamentals; the restoration and maintenance of the milieu intérieur (Chapters 4, 5, 16 and 17) and the vital (literally) need to assess and maintain an external balance for water, electrolyte and nitrogen. Indeed, whatever the illness you cannot escape from these fundamentals.

To facilitate learning the treatment can be broken down in the following five modules; intensive nursing, fluid therapy and nutrition, dialysis and filtration (Chapter 23) blood and drug therapy, prevention and treatment of infections (Chapter 27). Three of these are next briefly described.

III INTENSIVE NURSING

This must be directed to each organ or system of the body, including the psyche. Such total care provides a challenge to the skill and knowledge of the nursing team (and some of the doctors!) and the necessary monitoring – clinical, biochemical, and bacteriological – must be obsessional. It should be emphasized that even a slight error or omission can rarely be rectified. In practice the numerous facets of care and therapy must be integrated, but have to be separated for the purpose of description. In any individual patient the facets are arranged in the appropriate order of priority but this will change during the illness.

We won't insult the nurse's expertise by describing the daily routines which follow the standardized practices, but there are a few points to emphasize. The mouth needs frequent care to reduce colonization by bacteria or fungi. In addition to oral hygiene, salivation should be stimulated by pieces of fresh orange and sweets; lozenges of amphoteracin *B* are prescribed routinely. Every effort is made to manage the illness without a urethral catheter. In the oliguric form, this cannot be done unless the bladder or urethra has been injured. Should urinary tract infection occur during the oliguric phase, then we wash out the bladder with noxythiolin, removing the catheter afterwards. Early mobilization is the order of the day, unless fractures or dislocations prohibit this, when bed exercises are instituted. When haemodialysis/filtration is employed, then all the blood samples are taken from the vascular access and venepunctures are prohibited. Bacterial monitoring includes the shunt, central venous line, the nose and mouth, and any wounds. In addition, the faeces are tested for the isolation of *P. aeruginosa*, *Klebsiella* spp. and *Proteus* spp. Fluid balance naturally includes the careful charting of the intake and output of urine (if any), gastric aspirate, ileostomy fluid, over 24 h periods. In addition, the weighing bed is used to determine the fluid removed by dialysis/filtration. The patient usually needs a sedative to aid sleep; brandy or whisky are safer than drugs! Confusion or disorientation often defy biochemical explanation and are therefore treated empirically. The battle to main morale may assume the same importance as that for the milieu intérieur. Support comes from relatives, a hospital chaplain and possible via entertainment by the radio or television.

IV FLUID THERAPY AND NUTRITION

Gone are the dark old days when the patient suffered thirst, was kept as dry as a prune, or became bloated as in the Michelin man and starved into the bargain! Also behind us is the more recent period of glucose mania. The materials for appropriate nutrition have been available for 25 years. There remained the difficulty in some patients of removing the excess water and electrolytes; haemofiltration has solved this one. Fluid therapy and nutrition must be integrated with dialysis/filtration to firstly restore the milieu intérieur and metabolic balance, and then to maintain both. In the patient recently admitted to the ICU the first job is to draw up a triage of therapy using Figure 22.1. At the top of the list there may be oedema or hyperkalaemia or even saline depletion. The predicted requirements of electrolyte and fluid for the next few hours or a day are committed to paper and the nutrition next planned. Starvation worsens renal failure and harms all the other systems. By now the reader will be familiar with the assessment of electrolyte balance (Chapter 4) and the correction of deficits or excesses (Chapters 16 and 17).

How do dialysis or filtration fit into the plans? To take the milieu intérieur first. The dialysate or replacement fluid is chosen to restore the ECF to normal; for example increase the bicarbonate or lower the urea and potassium. This objective is readily achieved as will be described in the next chapter. Of course, the treatment has to be repeated or even continuous until the kidney recovers. The second treatment is to substitute for the normal excretion or water and electrolyte. The first step is to restore the body fluid volume (Chapter 4) to near normal; the oedema is cleared by dialysis or filtration. From then on, the external balance is maintained until the diuretic phase develops. How this is achieved is left to Chapter 23; suffice to say here that a daily programme will be one of the essentials.

The energy requirements will be commonly the same as yours, 2600 kcal (10.9 MJ), or more rarely 3700 kcal (15.5 MJ). Insulin may be necessary to ensure that the substrate are burnt up. So far so good. The nitrogen balance needs additional explanation. The intake of nitrogen is already known – the standard enteral or i.v. diet; say 14 g/day. That lost each day will vary and will need to be calculated, albeit roughly. The output will be present in the urine, dialysate and filtration. When there is any urine, the volume over twenty-four hours is measured and an aliquot sent for urea concentration; the urea in g/l is converted to gN_2/day as follows:-

$$\text{Urinary urea (g/l)} \times \text{volume/day} \times \tfrac{1}{2} \text{nitrogen}$$

The nitrogen lost by dialysis or filtration is predictable and depends on the equipment and how this is used. Both variables are described in Chapter 23. Getting excess urea out of the body is a vital objective. Unfortunately, nitrogen in the form of amino acids is removed at the same time; a figure for bedside calculation of the balance is 3.0 g/h of haemodialysis. It can be argued that the nitrogen balance obtained in this way is too crude and does not justify the work involved. If this policy is chosen the nitrogen intake is based on the predicted needs and the dialysis/filtration programme adjusted to keep the ECF within acceptable limits.

V   BLOOD AND DRUG THERAPY

Blood therapy is a small but essential part of the overall plan of treatment. The patient's haemoglobin should be kept at about 10 g/dl by blood transfusion using one of the products of Table 22.1. The next essential is to maintain the concentration of plasma protein – about 30 g/l – by infusions of 4.5% human albumen. In renal failure with oliguria the volumes of the blood products must be added to the fluid and electrolyte balance. Hence

Table 22.1 Blood products used during intensive care

Citrated whole blood
Red cell concentrate
Red cell concentrate diluted with nutrient
Platelet concentrate
Fresh frozen plasma (FFP)
Cryoprecipitate
Dried factors VII, VIII, IX and XIII
Stabilized plasma protein solution (SPPS)
Albumin solutions: 4.5, 5, 20 and 25%

it is common practice to infuse blood or albumen during the dialysis/filtration. An additional advantage of this practice is that the dialysis will remove unwanted substances from the banked blood. When the disease causing renal failure also causes DIC, the other blood products will be necessary, coagulation factors and platelets (Table 22.1).

As with all hospital patients a close scrutiny should be kept on the prescription sheet. During renal failure drugs normally excreted by the kidney are potentially hazardous. But necessary drugs may or may not be removed from the body by dialysis/filtration so rendering the treatment ineffective. A nice challenge for the newcomer! It follows that when an unnecessary drug is both nephrotoxic and removed by dialysis the only logical practice is to monitor the dose by measuring the blood levels; these measurements are made seven days a week. This would apply to antibiotics, tobramycin and gentamicin. An example will illustrate the point. A patient of 62 kg requires dialysis and filtration and the antibiotic tobramycin. The latter was started at a dose of 120 mg, 8-hourly i.v. The blood level just prior to the injection was $2.0 \mu g/ml$ and that 30 minutes after the bolus was $8.0 \mu g/ml$. These results are satisfactory.

23

Intensive care of renal failure: haemodialysis and haemofiltration

I PRINCIPLES

1. Haemodialysis

The idea of using an artificial membrane to 'remove diffusing substances from the blood of living animals' was conceived in 1914. Repeated attempts at haemodialysis failed due to lack of suitable membranes and an antico-agulant. Success finally came in 1943 in Nazi-occupied Holland, to Willem Kolff. The first successful haemodialysis in the United Kingdom took place in Leeds on September 30th, 1956 and was performed by FM Parsons and his colleagues.

The artificial kidney is based on physical chemistry and mechanics. The chemical principles are three in number. (1) When blood is separated from an artificial physiological solution (dialysate) by a thin artificial membrane, small molecules and ions will diffuse across the membrane. This exchange depends solely upon the concentration gradients of each substance. For example, if the blood urea is 25 mmol/l (150 mg/100 ml) and the dialysate contains none, urea will diffuse across the membrane roughly according to the curve shown in Figure 23.1. Such clearance curves can be obtained for potassium, creatinine, uric acid and so on. (2) Water will move across the membrane in either direction depending on two forces; osmotic force and hydrostatic pressure. The movement of water in either process is called ultrafiltration. In years gone by osmotic force created by a high concentration of glucose, was used in the treatment of the 'overhydrated' patient, and is still employed during peritoneal dialysis (Chapter 24). Currently, hydrostatic force removes water from the blood and hence the other body fluids. How

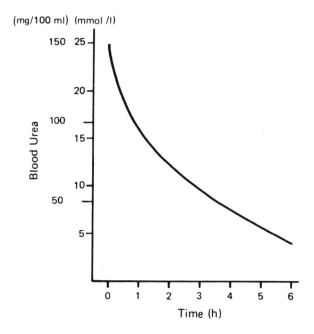

Figure 23.1 Diagram showing the fall in blood urea during dialysis (From *Essential Intensive Care*, with permission)

best to produce a pressure gradient between the blood and dialysate? The answer is to leave the blood pressure generated by the blood pump and to lower that in the dialysate. This is achieved by a hydrostatic pump similar in principle to that which the beginner will have used for wound drains. To summarize the mechanics of the artificial kidney: to keep blood the dialysate in continuous motion to make diffusion an efficient process; to apply a variable pressure to the dialysis fluid circulating through the artificial kidney; to remove any bubbles of air from the blood before it is returned to the patient. Haemodialysis can be used by itself or in combination with haemofiltration.

2. Haemofiltration

This process is a relative newcomer and the technique was discovered by L.W. Henderson in 1967. How the writers wish the invention had been made in 1960! The principle is simplicity itself. Imagine a membrane with holes through which the solutes of the blood can pass leaving behind the plasma proteins. The amount of solute (like urea) removed depends solely on the volume of fluid which passes through the membrane. Further, no dialysate is required, the filtrate just pours out of the system. The system is therefore extremely efficient at removing ECF from the patient without causing hypotension. The rate of removal of ECF depends on the blood flow and the pressure in the filter, but the aim of therapy is to remove waste products like urea, and excesses of potassium or acid; haemofiltration will remove the lot! Part of the system is to replace the beneficial electrolytes simultaneously using a replacement fluid which is very like protein-free plasma.

II ACCESS TO THE CIRCULATION

Is common to both therapies, and the components are made from high-tech materials, polyurethane, silicone rubber (silastic) and PTFE (Teflon). There are two ways of approaching the problem of getting blood to and from the vessels. (1). The simplest is to use the Seldinger technique of needle puncture – guidewire – cannula as previously described in Chapter 7. A cannula is thus placed in a large vein, the subclavian or femoral, or a femoral artery, a technique which goes back to 1961. There is now a choice of either using two cannulae in two veins – veno-veno – or one in a vein and the second cannula in an artery – arteriovenous access. Why not one cannula, but impossible! A double lumen cannula (Figure 23.2) is inserted into a large vein with the entry and exit holes spaced so that there is little mixing of the blood removed from that returned. We can go one further and use a single lumen catheter in a vein or artery. This technique of single cannula dialysis or filtration certainly needs a little explanation. In Figure 23.3 blood from the cannula (C) is removed from the vein by pump P_1 and enters the blood line and dialyser or filter; this only takes a few seconds. The pressure (shown on M) rises to a pre-determined level, the pump P_1 stops and V_1 closes. Valve V_2 now opens, pump P_2 returns the treated blood to the patient and the pressure at M returns to the original value. The cycle is then repeated over and over again. Of these varied techniques, the double lumen catheter is probably the most popular. (2). The Teflon–silastic shunt. Repeated dialysis became a relatively simple treatment following the design of an artificial shunt between an artery and vein which could be broken at will. This vitally important device was perfected in 1960 by B.H. Scriber and his colleagues in Seattle. Cannulae (referred to as vessel tips) of Teflon are inserted into the radial or tibial artery and an adjacent vein and connected by two lengths of silastic tubing joined by a Teflon connector. The authors fit the shunt in its original form with pre-formed elbows implanted in the tissues. Vessel tips of three sizes are available and the largest size is chosen which can be fitted into the vessel. The pre-formed silastic tubes for artery

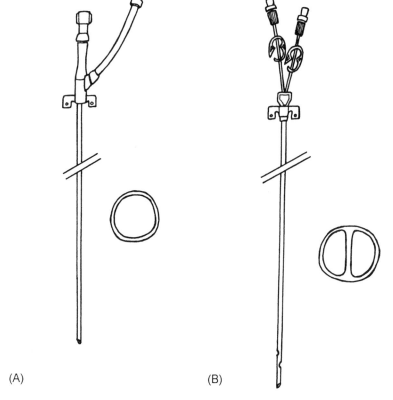

Figure 23.2 Cannulae used for haemodialysis or filtration. A, single lumen; B, dual lumen

and vein are shaped for the right or left arm or leg. The components of the silastic shunt and the surgical procedure are given in the Appendix.

III HAEMODIALYSIS: EQUIPMENT AND METHODS

The components can be assembled like building blocks.

(a) The dialyser. The bigger the area of membrane the better the diffusion. The dialysers used for intensive care are either plate or hollow fibre types. In the former, small sheets of membrane are held one on top of the next to form a sort of sandwich. Blood passes into a thin layer in one direction and the dialysate in the opposite direction. Both fluids are made to flow down

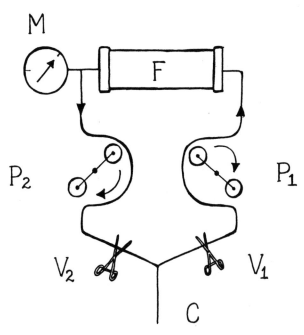

Figure 23.3 Diagram of single cannula dialysis or filtration. C, cannula; F, hollow fibre filter or dialyser; M, pressure gauge; P_1 and P_2, blood pumps; V_1, V_2, valves to control blood flow

wavy channels to increase the diffusion and reduce clotting. A typical plate dialyser in compact form provides a surface area of $1.0\,\text{m}^2$.

Dialysers made from sheet material and arranged into plates or coils have served us well for 30 years. A newer form of membrane became available in the late 1970s and is a wonder of modern technology. The membrane is formed into a tube, so fine it is called a hollow fibre. Each hollow fibre has a lumen of about $200\,\mu\text{m}$ across and a wall thickness of $10\,\mu\text{m}$. Thousands of such tubes can be housed in a compact casing fitted with connections for the blood and dialysate, and shown in Figure 23.4. Hollow fibre dialysers are available with surface areas of $0.2\text{--}2.0\,\text{m}^2$, and have a priming volume of between 35 and 120 ml.

(b) We now turn to a box which pumps the blood under electronic control. The pump is of the roller type and a miniature version of that used for cardiopulmonary bypass; we need an output of 100–500 ml/minute. Connections are needed to the vascular access and the dialyser and these are conveniently provided as a pre-packed sterile system of tubes – the blood

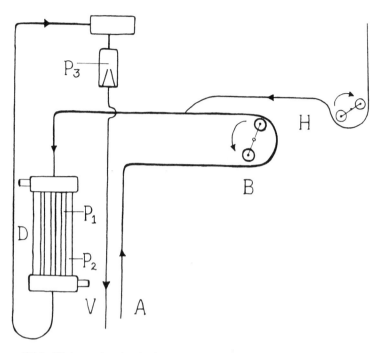

Figure 23.4 Diagram showing basic equipment for haemodialysis. A V, arterial and venous lines; D, hollow fibre dialyser; B H, pumps for blood and heparin; P_1 and P_2, pressure inside and outside the hollow fibre; P_1-P_2 = transmembrane pressure

lines (Figure 23.4). The controls allow the blood flow to be adjusted at will. The pressure of blood in the hollow fibre is measured (Figure 23.4 P1). To remove extracellular fluid from the blood, and hence the interstitial and intracellular fluids, a pressure gradient is created between blood (P_1) and dialysate (P_2). This is done by lowering the dialysate pressure below atmospheric and the value of P_2 is displayed. Additional devices detect unwanted air.

(c) Dialysate. As might be expected from a study of first principles (Chapter 4) the dialysate is very like healthy ECF without protein, nitrogenous waste or amino acids. All that is necessary is to warm a physiological solution to 37°C and circulate this through the dialyser and then to waste. For convenience the dialysate is supplied in concentrated form and diluted by a proportioning system, the 'dialysis fluid monitor'. Should the local supply be of hard water, this is softened by ion exchange. The soft water is next treated by means of reverse osmosis to remove foreign particles, including bacteria and ions such as albumin. This purification means another module named 'reverse osmosis monitor'. This pure water is mixed with the right amount of concentrate, warmed to 37°C in another unit, the dialysis fluid monitor. We have already said the dialysate resembles the normal ECF of which the buffer is bicarbonate. It is therefore logical to use bicarbonate in the dialysate. An alternative is acetate, which is converted via the Krebs cycle to bicarbonate; unfortunately in some ICU patients this process is impaired, so that bicarbonate is the first choice. It is impossible to store bicarbonate on the shelf. This problem is readily overcome by yet another device, the bicarbonate monitor, which proportions two separate concentrates. The final product circulates through the dialyser at about 500 ml per minute and runs to waste. It would be very convenient to have a device which measured the volume of fluid removed by ultra filtration over a given time. Such a 'filtration controlled monitor' is commercially available as another unit. The nurse pre-sets the volume (just like a ventilator) and the machine adjusts the necessary pressure which can be read off. A final item of knowledge. During dialysis the volume of fluid removed from the patient is proportional to the difference between the pressure in the blood and that in the dialysate (Figure 23.4); this is called the trans-membrane pressure (TMP).

(d) Blood outside the body clots in about eight minutes depending on the surfacing contact. Not even the high tech pumping industry can prevent this happening in the extra-corporeal circuit of the artificial kidney, so an anticoagulant is necessary. To minimize the risk of clotting in the circuit or haemorrhage in the patient, the minimum amount of anticoagulant is used, and the agent is infused continuously into the blood leaving the blood pump on its way to the dialyser. Heparin is the most commonly used anticoagulant and is infused by a small peristaltic or syringe pump conveniently fitted to the blood monitor. Prostacyclin is an expensive alternative, but gives a longer filter life and thus may be cheaper in the long term.

(e) Controls. When driving a strange car, the best approach is to sit in the driving seat rather than to study the controls in the maker's manual. The same applies to the equipment for dialysis and filtration; although a teaching video also helps. The most important requirement is the safety of the patient. The essentials can be broken down as follows. The blood: flow in ml/min; arterial and venous pressures; a device to detect and prevent air embolism. Ultra filtration: the volume of ECF removed and the pressure required to achieve this; in addition, we can monitor the pressure difference between the membrane and dialysate, a variable labelled the transmembrane pressure (TMP). The dialysate: observations on the dialysate; the volume, flow in ml/min, temperature, pH, conductivity and presence of any unwanted blood.

(f) Commercial systems. In choosing the hardware the following have to be considered. The capital outlay, the servicing cost and the evaluation made by experts. In the UK there is an independent unit which tests medical equipment and publishes the results, which is of great practical value (Medical Devices Agency). The various pieces of machinery can either be housed in a large unit or left in individual modules, as described here. Similar policies operate in Australia.

(g) The system in use. As with IPPV so with the dialysis. Never start without a plan of action; in this case the dialysis programme. Even more important requirements are described in Chapter 22. Armed with the dialysis programme the treatment follows the scheme of Table 23.1 hopefully avoiding the emergency stops.

(h) Monitoring depends on the clinical and laboratory assessments of the body fluids described in Chapter 4. The apprentice to intensive care can apply these principles to patients with either oliguric or polyuric renal failure. But the facts already given need supplementing. Blood tests are carried out at the start and end of a dialysis to assess the effects on the milieu intérieur. For example the restoration to normal or near normal values of sodium, potassium, calcium and hydrion. The waste nitrogen is monitored by the concentrations of urea and creatinine, but these results will not tell us the amount of nitrogen removed by each dialysis. An estimate of the latter is needed if we wish to construct a rough balance of nitrogen intake and output. To calculate the urea removed from the body fluids (this molecule diffuses freely between the ECF and ICF) we will need the information listed in Table 23.2.

The external balance in renal failure is the last topic in monitoring and is illustrated in our standardized way in Figure 23.5. Consider first the acute oliguric type (B). It is imperative to give a diet high in energy but to reduce water, sodium and potassium to the minimum; the nitrogen intake should be roughly normal. Such a diet invariably exceeds the losses in the urine (B) but the dialysis (vertical shading) restores a balance as shown at 'B'. For the sake of simplicity the diagram shows dialysis throughout the whole day, but in practice haemodialysis will achieve the same result in four hours. The disturbances in electrolyte balance are in complete contrast when there is polyuria or large losses from the gastro-intestinal tract. An example of this pattern is given at C. In such patients the maintenance of electrolyte balance does not require dialysis, but this is necessary to maintain nitrogen balance. In consequence, the dialysis is adjusted so that only small amounts of electrolyte were removed (C'). The next disturbance to consider is that for

Table 23.1   Haemodialysis: the system in use

Dialysis programme (Haemofiltration as well?)	Duration: 4–8 h Select dialyser and dialysate Dialysate: bicarbonate or acetate flow rate Heparin: loading dose, maintenance dose Priming fluid: saline, albumin or blood

Preparation of equipment	Assemble blood and heparin lines
	Heparin infusion
	Prime the circuit
	Pre-set: blood flow rate
	              dialysate flow rate
	              ultrafiltration

Preparation of the patient	Explanation Blood pressure and body weight if possible Insert cannulae or make adjustments to cannulae or Scribner shunt
Start	Blood, dialysate and heparin pumps
Continue	Standard monitoring of patient and machine
Stop	Blood and heparin pumps Disconnect arterial blood line Wash through the circuit to return blood to patient Reconnect shunt or adjust cannulae Body weight
Emergency stop	Blood leak, inadequate blood flow or severe hypotension

nitrogen; these changes are more complex than those for electrolyte. Renal failure, irrespective of the urine output, causes a positive balance for nitrogen. But this is quite different from the positive nitrogen balance of the growing child or the period of convalescence following injury. The former balance is harmful and the latter beneficial. Examining the results shown at B and C, where in both cases the diet contained 10 g of nitrogen, only 1.0 g was excreted in the urine, and the 10.0 g of urea produced in the body remained in the body fluids to give a positive balance. During the day of the

Table 23.2 Data required to calculate the urea removed from the body during a dialysis

The patient	Body weight (kg)
	Blood urea (mmol/l):at start
	at end
	Protein catabolic rate (g.protein/kg body weight/day)
	Duration of dialysis (min)
The machine	Characteristics of the dialyser: area M^2; material
	Ultrafiltration coefficient (ml/mmHg/h)
	Blood flow (Q_b, ml/min)
	Transmembrane pressure (mmHg)
Tables to calculate the urea or nitrogen removed	Supplied by the manufacturer of the dialyser

balance the blood urea rose by 6.0 mol/l. At B and C, the changes in nitrogen balance are shown, brought about by dialysis. The urea and creatinine removed are charted on the negative side and the end-result is an approximate balance, and a corresponding fall in the blood urea. Finally, what happens during the recovery phase of acute renal failure? An example is shown at D. At this stage of the diuretic phase of reversible renal failure, the patient was eating and drinking as he pleased, and dialysis had been stopped. The kidney was capable of maintaining a balance of water, sodium and potassium but the urea clearance remained low. The nitrogen balance (D) was positive and this was due to two factors; the retention of the urea and the increased protein synthesis of convalescence.

IV HAEMOFILTRATION

At last, for the learner, something much simpler than haemodialysis! The arrangements are shown in Figure 23.6 and need only a brief description. (a) The filter is of the hollow fibre type (Figure 23.7) also used in dialysis, but the membrane has quite different properties to allow rapid filtration of blood plasma, retaining the proteins. The filtrate, from 1 to 25 litres a day according to the aim, passes from the filter – neat as it were – into a calibrated container. The amount of fluid removed depends mainly on the blood flow and pressure, itself proportional to the height of the filter above the collector. Polyamide is one of the materials used to make the membrane and the sieve closely resembles the glomerular basement membrane. As

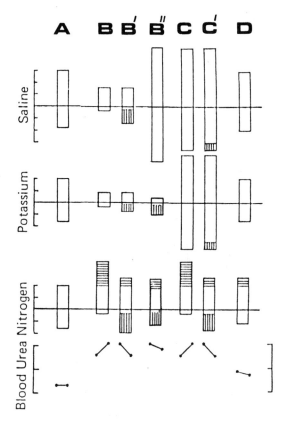

Figure 23.5 Balance data for saline, potassium, nitrogen and the blood urea in health and in renal failure. Intake and output above and below the horizontal line. Horizontal hatching shows positive balance due to retention of urea and vertical hatching shows the removal of urea by dialysis or filtration, A, control; B acute oliguric renal failure; B′ effects of haemodialysis on B; B″ effects of haemofiltration on B; C, acute polyuric renal failure; C′ effects of haemodialysis on C; D, during recovery from acute renal failure

we shall see, the filtration takes place continuously day and night, and the same filter will last 2–10 days before it will become blocked or clotted, when it is replaced. (b) Arterial blood is circulated through a simple circuit, and the choice is to use the patient's own pump or to interpose a roller pump exactly as for dialysis. Likewise the vascular access is that for dialysis. (c) Having a system which will remove large, even huge, volumes of ECF from the body, we now have to put most of it back again, less the nitrogen waste, acids and may be potassium or phosphate. This replacement fluid is shown

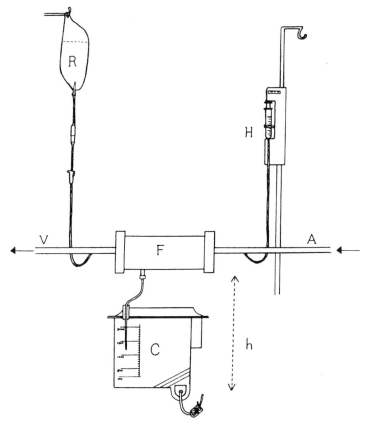

Figure 23.6 Diagram showing basic equipment for haemofiltration. AV, arterial and venous lines; F, hollow fibre; C, container to collect and measure filtrate; R, replacement fluid; H, heparin infusion; h, height of filter above collector

in Figure 23.6 as a big bag and the composition is illustrated by an example in Table 23.3. (d) The aim of heparin therapy is to prevent clotting in the extra-corporeal circuit without causing haemorrhage. This is achieved by giving a relatively small dose i.v. at the start of treatment and by infusing heparin continuously into the arterial blood line, as shown in Figure 23.6. The continuous heparin can be infused by syringe or peristaltic pumps and the dose adjusted according to the HBCT or apTT. (e) Controls. These are readily understood by setting down the aims of the therapy, and this can be done at intervals by a nurse, using the basic equipment of Figure 23.6 or by means of a machine. The amount of fluid removed by filtration will be laid down in the dialysis-filtration programme, itself part of an overall

Table 23.3 An example of replacement fluid used during haemofiltration. Concentrations are given in mmol/l

Sodium	140
Potassium	2
Calcium	2
Magnesium	0.75
Chloride	101
Bicarbonate	45
Osmolarity	292

therapeutic plan. Control of the daily intake is equally vital. This will depend on the state of the metabolic balance, including the nutrition. A striking benefit of haemofiltration is that it is quite safe to give a diet of 3.0 litres of fluid. The replacement fluid can be delivered by gravity from a big bag and monitored by a nurse or pump and measured by another black box as described shortly. It must be stressed here that unlike dialysate the replacement fluid must be sterile and pyrogen-free. (f) The system in use. Filtration is learnt not from a text but by apprenticeship at the bedside. However, some knowledge of the sequence of operation can help the beginner, and this is set out in Table 23.4. (g) Commercial equipment. The reader can conclude from the foregoing that the basic equipment is simple and inexpensive. At the other extreme is a series of five units to purify, pump, and measure (Table 23.5). The choice will depend on the nurse staffing levels, finance, and personal opinion. (h) Monitoring follows the methods described for dialysis. The striking difference is the large intake and output, which is illustrated at B" in Figure 23.5. The input consists of the replacement fluid (Table 23.3) and the i.v. nutrition; an example is given in Table 23.6. The amount of replacement fluid given over 24 h will be specified in the therapeutic plan for the day; the i.v. nutrition is also pre-planned and depends on the rate of catabolism. With such large intakes and outputs there is a risk of severe shifts in the electrolyte concentrations of the ECF. It follows that plasma electrolytes are measured 6 hourly and supplements of K, Ca, PO_4 or Mg are added to the replacement fluid to preserve the milieu intérieur. The output is made up of urine and the filtrate measured in the collecting bag; the volume of the latter is set out in the filtration programme for each day. Both fluids are analysed for Na, K and N_2 and the balance chart can then be completed. In the example shown in Figure 23.5 the amount of ECF removed was approximately similar to the intake. During the 24 h period of filtration the potassium balance was negative – more was removed

Table 23.4 Haemofiltration: the system in use

Filtration programme	Continuous filtration Select size and composition of filter Volume of ECF to be removed Priming fluids; saline, albumin or blood Heparin: loading dose, maintenance dose
Preparation of equipment	Assemble blood and heparin lines Heparin infusion Prime the circuit Pre-set: blood flow, filtration rate height of filter
Preparation of patient	Explanation Blood pressure and body weight if possible Insert cannulae or make adjustments to cannulae or Scribner shunt Loading dose of heparin
Start	Blood and heparin pumps
Continue	Standard monitoring of patient and machine
Stop	Blood and heparin pumps Disconnect arterial blood line Wash through the circuit to return blood to patient Reconnect shunt or adjust cannulae

than taken in. The balance for the nitrogen was positive due to retained urea. This undesirable result is reflected in the small fall in the blood urea.

Dialysis and filtration can be used separately or in combination. At the RPA hospital the following system is chosen for intensive care. A double lumen catheter provides vascular access and the blood is pumped continuously vein-to-vein (CVV). A haemofilter is used and this removes about ten litres of fluid a day, but not enough urea. So dialysate is pumped through the filter (outside the hollow fibres) to achieve urea clearance; effective, simple and safe. So much for the technology. The newcomer to intensive care must be reminded that these treatments will not succeed unless they form part of a therapeutic plan. This plan (Chapter 22) is initially based on

Table 23.5 Equipment for haemofiltration

Vascular access	Cannulae, single or double lumen
	Scribner shunt
Circulation of the blood	Blood lines, blood pump with monitor
Volume of filtrate	Collecting vessel. Pump with monitor
Replacement fluid	'Big bag', gravity fed
Heparin therapy	Heparin lines
	Pump

Table 23.6 Example of intravenous therapy during continuous haemofiltration

Fluid	Volume (ml) in 24 h
Replacement fluid (Table 23.2)	3000
Glucose 50%	500
Aminosol 14	1000
Intralipid 20%	500
Total	5000

Supplements of K, Ca or Mg are given to maintain the plasma concentrations.

the natural history of the disease and then revised daily or more often depending on the findings in the individual patient.

V COMPLICATIONS

Some of these are common to dialysis and filtration; affecting the vascular access, blood circuit or machinery. Others are peculiar to each treatment. The cannulae or shunt may fail to provide satisfactory flow or return. This can be due to vascular spasm or clotting. The remedy is to change the cannula(e) to investigate the shunt as described in the appendix. Enough has already been written on the colonisation or infection of the wound. Air embolism, clotting or pump failure can complicate the extra corporeal circulation. The first two are preventable. Should the system clot, then it is necessary to return to square one! When the machinery or electronics fail then this is the opportunity for the technician to prove his worth.

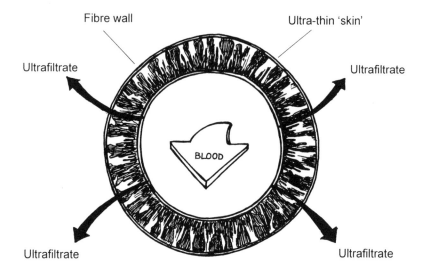

Figure 23.7 Diagram of a hollow fibre used for filtration showing holes and channels

Dialysis has its own problems. A dialyser can leak blood, quickly detected by vigilant observer or electronically. When this happens the flow of blood and dialysate are stopped, the dialyser isolated and then replaced. Haemodialysis can cause varying degrees of hypotension, due to hypovolaemia. The problem is most likely in the septic or toxic patient or when rapid ultra-filtration is employed. It may help to start the dialysis with a low rate of filtration, and an increase after the first hour. At times the hypovolaemia causes a severe reduction in flow making it impossible to continue. The programme is then changed to include filtration.

We are grateful to the staff of Gambro UK for help with this chapter.

APPENDIX: THE TEFLON–SILASTIC SHUNT

The surgery can be carried out under local or regional anaesthesia. The latter has two advantages over the former; (I) narrowing of the vessels due to spasm is reduced and (ii) a restless or confused patient cannot move the arm and this hinder the surgeon. The surgical technique is essentially similar for artery and vein and the cannulation of a radial artery will illustrate the more important technical points. The artery is palpated and is marked out for 5 cm proximal to the anterior retinaculum. Blunt dissection is used to find and separate the artery from its accompanying veins. The distal end of the artery is tied off with silk but the ends of the ligature are left uncut and later tied around one end of the silastic tubing (Figure 23.8). A second proximal ligature is passed around the artery which, when lifted anteriorly by the assistant, will occlude the artery. The arterial section of the shunt is filled with heparinized saline and clamped with a Seattle clip. The radial artery is now incised for about half its diameter and the blood flow controlled by the ligature. A cannula is now carefully introduced into the artery. The vessel tip is slowly passed into the artery and the introducer is removed. The assistant relaxes the proximal ligature and arterial blood will be seen to pulsate in the silastic tube. The proximal ligature is tied and a second ligature passed around the artery to secure the vessel tip in position. The arterial flow can next be tested, but the vessel is again filled with heparinized saline whilst the silastic tube is placed into position. The subcutaneous tissues are undercut to provide a tunnel for the U-bend. A small skin incision is made to allow the step in the silastic tubing to pass through the skin and to lie in its natural position. The wound is closed with interrupted catgut

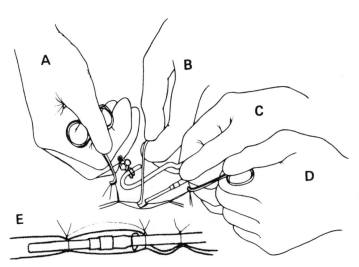

Figure 23.8   Scribner shunt. Insertion of vessel tip into the radial artery. A loop of silk held in hand A occludes the flow; hand D maintains tension on the artery; the shoe-horn and vessel tip are operated by B and C respectively. E, arterial end of shunt in final position (From *Essential Intensive Care*, with permission)

sutures and a continuous nylon skin stitch. The operator next inserts the venous side of the shunt. A forearm vein is located preferably within 10 cm of the arterial side and a medium or large vessel tip is inserted by the same technique. The free ends of the shunt are finally connected by a 2.0 cm length of Teflon and the flow from artery to vein observed. The flow may at first be sluggish, but if the surgical technique was good, then a rapid flow will develop over some hours. Gauze dressings and crêpe bandage are applied, leaving the U-shaped loop of the shunt clear of the bandage. If possible the arm should be elevated in a sling to minimize the subsequent oedema. Over the ensuing few hours the U-shaped loop of the shunt is examined to detect possible clotting at the earliest moment. The examination consists of observing the colour of the blood through the translucent tubing, palpation of the tubing for a pulse and auscultation through a diaphragm stethoscope lightly pressed over the U-tubing.

Complications arising from the Teflon silastic shunt are two in number; clotting and infection, either local, embolic or even bacteraemic. Clotting of the shunt starts in the vein and proceeds upstream to involve the artery. The precipitating causes are poor surgical technique, poor flow due to hypotension or cold, and bacterial infection. Early detection of a clotted shunt holds out the best chances of successful de-clotting. Recognition is achieved by frequent observations of the colour of the blood in the exposed silastic tubing by palpation, and by auscultation. De-clotting of a shunt should be carried out promptly and systematically. The arterial and venous limbs are clamped and separated and gentle suction applied to each in turn with a 5 ml syringe containing heparinized saline previously warmed to body temperature. Suction alone can sometimes clear the arterial limb but if this fails a plastic catheter is fitted to the syringe and threaded along the obstructed limb of the shunt and this is gently irrigated with the heparinized saline. When these preliminary measures fail to restore the blood flow, then the shunt is filled with a solution of urokinase. The tube is clamped and the urokinase is left in position for twenty minutes. Such clot-lysis treatment is often successful at the first or second attempt. When all these measures fail, then the offending vessel must be explored surgically and one or both cannulae re-sited. Clumsy attempts at de-clotting can dislodge a blood clot and thus cause pulmonary or cerebral embolism. In common with accidental or surgical wounds, a shunt can become colonized by bacteria, usually transmitted by the staff. Incidents of infection are reduced by meticulous aseptic and antiseptic techniques and by keeping the skin supple by the daily application of hydrous wool fat BP supplied in small individual packs. The skin wound and apertures are swabbed frequently for bacterial contamination.

24
Intensive care of renal failure: peritoneal dialysis

I	PRINCIPLES
II	TECHNIQUE
III	COMPLICATIONS

In 1923 Gantner reported the first successful peritoneal dialysis, a treatment now widely used in both general ICUs and renal units throughout the world. The earlier methods of PC caused an unacceptably high incidence of complications; these were reduced in frequency and severity by the modifications described by Berlyne *et al.* (1966).

I PRINCIPLES

1. Anatomical

The surface are of the peritoneum is about $2.0 \, m^2$. The membrane covers the intestine and mesentery, both of which are richly supplied with blood vessels. To carry out dialysis the abdominal wall and peritoneum are perforated by a cannula which is directed towards the contents of the pelvis (Figure 24.1). The cannula is held in place by a small metal stabilizer, itself held to the skin with adhesive tape. The trunk is inclined at an angle of 30 to 60° to the horizontal. Dialysate at about 37°C is run into the peritoneal cavity by gravity, from a collapsible plastic bag of the type used for intravenous infusions. The dialysate flows into the peritoneal cavity and distends the abdomen but should not be allowed to collect under the diaphragm. There are two reasons for this. Firstly, fluid will elevate the diaphragm and cause collapse of the underlying lung and consequently reduce the vital capacity by litres. Secondly, the fluid will also pass through apertures in the diaphragm and produce a pleural effusion. The dialysate remains in the peritoneal cavity for 20 min and the peritoneum is then quickly drained into a sterile container. This emptying phase of the cycle takes place by gravity, sometimes aided by a low pressure vacuum. Following drainage a further quantity of dialysate is run into the peritoneal cavity and the cycle thus repeated. An alternative method is to employ two cannulae, one for the entry

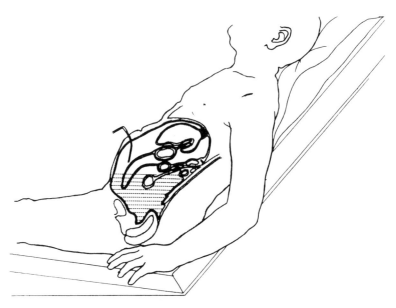

Figure 24.1 Diagram illustrating the anatomy of peritoneal dialysis (From *Essential Intensive Care*, with permission

and exit of fluid respectively. In this way the peritoneal cavity is continuously perfused by dialysate.

2. Physiological

The peritoneal cavity is an inert membrane and the substances which cross the membrane do so by passive transport. The peritoneum is permeable to water, salts, urea, creatinine, water soluble vitamins and less so to the serum proteins. When a dialysate is in contact with the membrane a state of partial equilibrium is reached between the composition of the fluid and that of the interstitial fluid. In the treatment of renal failure the following uni-directional changes commonly take place: (i) Urea leaves the interstitial fluid and therefore the blood and its concentration in the dialysate rises from zero to 13.3 mmol/l (80 mg/100 ml), depending on the level in the blood and the duration of the equilibrium. A total of 25 g of urea can be removed over 24 h, using the rapid cycling method of dialysis. The blood urea falls rather slowly because during dialysis more urea enters the blood from the large intra-cellular compartment. (ii) The dialysate contains a high concentration (76 mmol/l) of glucose (dextrose) and is hence hyperosmolar (about 350 mmol/l). Glucose enters the blood and is metabolized in the normal

Table 24.1 Fluids for peritoneal dialysis

Reference in text	Na	Cl	Calcium	Magnesium	Lactate	Acetate	Glucose
				mmol/l			
A	130	91	1.8	0.75	45	0	76
B	140	101	1.8	0.75	45	0	76
C	140	101	1.8	0.75	45	0	359
D	130	98	1.8	0.75	0	40	76

manner. However, the fluid draws water from the interstitial fluid, blood and intracellular fluid by osmotic action. Peritoneal dialysis can remove excess body water – that is reduce oedema or even dehydrate the body. The amount of fluid can be judged from the negative balance of dialysate and from the fall in weight of the patient. (iii) In renal failure, hyperkalaemia is common but not invariable. When severe, and especially when the Kp rises rapidly, it is essential to quickly reduce the Kp by a concentration gradient of two or more fold. In contrast, when the Kp is normal or low, potassium chloride is added to the dialysate to give a final concentration of 4.0 mmol/l. (iv) An exchange of acids and bases between extracellular and dialysis fluids can correct a metabolic acidosis, itself due to the retention of renal acids and other mechanisms (Chapter 5). Base in the dialysate is in the potential form as lactate or acetate, either being converted in the body to bicarbonate. The latter cannot be used because it is unstable. Should the patient have a lactic acidosis then the dialysate containing lactate cannot correct the acidosis. However, a dialysate containing acetate (Table 24.1) will do so because, as far as is known, pathological processes rarely interfere with its conversion to bicarbonate. When the plasma bicarbonate is reduced, acetate will diffuse across the peritoneal membrane and is then rapidly converted to bicarbonate. Renal acids – naturally absent from the dialysate – are removed at the same time. The acidoses may, in addition, be partly due to the acids formed in excess during the starvation which commonly accompanies renal failure. These acids are also removed during dialysis and their rate of formation is reduced by the increased utilization of glucose obtained from the dialysate. (v) Peritoneal dialysis invariably causes a serious and undesirable loss of plasma protein. The total protein loss averages 0.5–1.0 g/l of dialysate. Albumin, γ-globulin and small proteins such as serum amylase are all lost in the dialysis fluid. The body may not be able to synthesize albumin or γ-globulin to keep pace with the losses in which case hypo-proteinaemia will develop. The loss of γ-globulin can reduce the patient's resistance to infection.

Table 24.2 Materials for peritoneal dialysis. Many of the items* are pre-packed in commercial kits

Skin preparation (0.5% cholorhexidine in 70% ethanol)
Disposable syringes and needles
* Catheter set

Local anaesthetic (1% lignocaine hydrochloride BP with adrenaline)
Knife blade (Swan-Morton No. 11)
Nylon or silk suture on a cutting needle
Scissors and toothed forceps
Adhesive plaster for anchoring the trocar and covering the wound (plastic
    adhesive strapping BPC)
* Drainage bag
Clear plastic dressing (Hibispray, ICI)
* Y-type solution administration set

3. Dialysate

This is commercially available and supplied in 1 litre collapsible containers. To prevent the fluid changing in composition during storage, sodium acetate takes the place of sodium bicarbonate. Separate dialysates containing normal or low concentration of sodium are required; the former will deplete the body sodium. For most cases of renal failure dialysates containing 76 mmol/l (1.36% dextrose) will remove sufficient water by osmotic action. When this strength of fluid fails to produce a negative balance, then a dialysate containing 350 mmol/l (6.3%) of dextrose often succeeds. The composition of the dialysates are given in Table 24.1.

II TECHNIQUE

Two techniques are now described, manual and mechanical.

1. Manual

We use a method described by Boen in 1964, the equipment is listed in Table 24.2 and illustrated in Figure 24.3. The treatment is explained to the patient; pain and fear are allayed by an injection of pethidine and promethazine, 50 mg of each in the same syringe. The bladder is emptied. The trunk is raised to 60° to the horizontal by adjusting the bed, and the skin of the abdomen is prepared as for a laparotomy. A catheter can be placed in almost any site of the anterior abdominal wall. Our first, second, and third choices are shown in Figure 24.2. The skin and abdominal wall

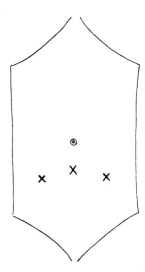

Figure 24.2 Abdominal wall sites for the cannula (From *Essential Intensive Care*, with permission)

are next infiltrated with lignocaine (lignocaine and adrenaline injection, BP) and a few minutes allowed for the drug to take effect, during which time the delivery and drainage tubes are connected up to the dialysis fluid and drainage bag or bottle. A knife blade is now inserted through the needle tract. A catheter is next introduced into the peritoneal cavity. This is done by firm pressure, at the same time twisting the catheter through 90°. If this procedure causes severe pain then more local anaesthetic is injected. The operator can feel the stilette 'give' when the peritoneal cavity has been entered. The stilette is now withdrawn and a small volume of dialysate is quickly run into the catheter to minimize the risk of obstruction due to fibrin. The next stage is to push the catheter further into the abdomen so that its side holes all lie within the peritoneal cavity. The catheter is directed towards the pelvis, preferably to the left. A purse-string suture is made around the catheter and the metal stabilizer fitted. The plastic elbow is momentarily disconnected so that the catheter can be cut, leaving two centimetres protruding above the skin. A dressing of gauze or clear plastic dressing is applied and covered with adhesive strapping. Dialysis is commenced and the details charted.

2. Choice of the dialysate

Four fluids are kept in stock and their composition is shown in Table 24.1. It is usually necessary to add potassium chloride to each litre bag of dialysate to give final concentrations of 2.0, 3.0 and 4.0 mmol/l. All three fluids are hyperosmolar and dialysate 'C' will exert the most powerful osmotic force. The patient with oedema, peripheral, pulmonary or both, is dialysed with fluid 'A'. If this fluid does not cause a negative balance, then dialysate 'C' is used in the sequence of one bag followed by three bags of 'A'. When the blood lactate is elevated or there is a probability of a lactic acidosis then fluid 'D' is used. The dehydrated or hypotensive patient is treated with fluid 'B'. Potassium is added according to the concentration in the patient's plasma. For hyperkalaemia the final concentration is 2.0 mmol/l and when the K_p is normal the dialysate contains 4.0 mmol/l. To reduce the deposition of fibrin around the catheter, 1000 units of heparin are added to each litre bag. This dose does not affect the clotting time of the peripheral blood. We never add antibiotics with the idea of preventing bacterial peritonitis simply because this will not be achieved.

3. Design of the cycle

We use the design of Berlyne *et al.* (1966), referred to as the small-volume, rapid cycle method. By using 1 litre at a time rather than 2, the incidence of pulmonary complications is greatly reduced. The smaller volume reduces the efficiency but this can be compensated by rapid cycling. The programme is as follows: one litre of dialysate is run into the peritoneal cavity over 10 min and remains there for 20 min. The taps are next adjusted to drain the fluid by gravity over the next 30 min. Each cycle lasts 1 h, and excluding complications, 24 cycles take place each day. The fluid in the drainage bag or bottle is transferred to a graduated measuring cylinder and the balance recorded. Each day an aliquot is sent to the laboratory for culture. Although a simple treatment, peritoneal dialysis is very time-consuming.

When the fluid drains slowly and successive cycles show a positive balance, the cause must be investigated systematically. (i) If the patient was dehydrated at the start of treatment, then the positive balance is to be expected and is of benefit to the patient; the dialysis is continued. (ii) If on the other hand the patient had oedema, the positive balance is dangerous. Drainage can sometimes be improved by one of the following: tilting the patient from side to side; gentle pressure on the abdomen; sitting the patient in an armchair; by applying a small vacuum (5 cm, 0.8 kPa water pressure) to the drainage bottle. When these methods fail the balance may be restored by using the high dextrose dialysate ('C' of Table 24.1). When

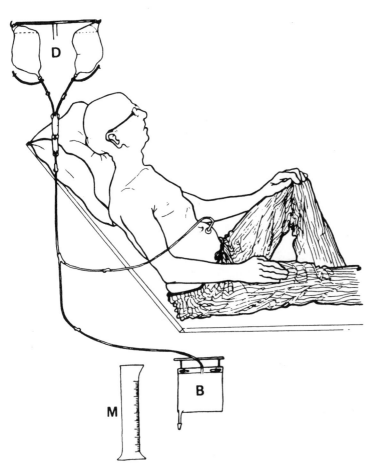

Figure 24.3 Arrangement of equipment for peritoneal dialysis. D, dialysate; B, drainage bag; M, measuring cylinder (From *Essential Intensive Care*, with permission)

after one cycle with a strong osmotic solution, the balance remains positive it is more than likely that deposits of fibrin have made the catheter valvular. The obvious and only remedy is to replace the catheter at the same site. On occasions, the new catheter quickly shows a rapid inflow but slow outflow and the physician should then try a new site in the abdomen. On rare occasions all attempts to induce a negative balance fail, the patient's oedema worsens and the treatment has to be abandoned.

Table 24.3 Equipment for intermittent mechanical peritoneal dialysis

Item	Function
Administration set	Delivery and removal of dialysate
Dialysate	Bags containing 5.0 or 10.0 litres
Peristaltic pump	Pumps the used dialysate from drainage bag to waste
Heater	Warms dialysate to 37.5°C
Monitor	Volume per cycle Inflow time Dwell time Outflow volume and time Cumulative balance Number of cycles
Alarms	Failure to deliver dialysate Poor inflow Poor outflow

4. Mechanical

As described, peritoneal dialysis is very labour intensive and therefore demands a high nurse to patient ratio. Some of the tasks can be automated by means of a machine. The system is housed in the invariable building blocks; the essentials are one or two peristaltic pumps, a heater, a monitor to enable the nurse to programme the system, and alarms (Table 24.3). The dialysate is pumped from a 5.0 or 10.0 litre bag into the reservoir, which is equivalent to the dialysate bag in the manual method. The height of the reservoir above the patient can be altered. The warmed dialysate runs into the peritoneal cavity by gravity or rarely, by means of a pump. Dialysate drains by gravity to a collector and is measured and then pumped to waste. The nurse dials in the programme: volume per cycle, inflow time, dwell time, outflow time. The monitor displays the outflow volume, cumulative balance and the number of cycles. Finally, an administration set is needed to connect the system to the PD cannula. A mechanical system is simple and reliable, but the patient still needs intensive nursing care and a lot more therapy if they are to survive.

III COMPLICATIONS

Peritoneal dialysis is plagued by complications, some serious and invariable, other serious but largely avoidable.

1. Pain

Pain due to puncture of the abdominal wall is prevented by the use of a local anaesthetic and pre-medication. Pain during entry of the fluid varies from trivial discomfort to agony. When it occurs the pain is invariably in the lower abdomen but may be felt in the perineum or penis. The following measures can help to relieve pain during later cycles. Cut the purse-string suture and withdraw the cannula a few centimetres; test for pain by running in dialysate. Should this fail, withdraw about half the cannula and re-insert in a different direction. As a last resort add local anaesthetic to the dialysate (bupivacaine hydrochloride (0.5% 10 ml to a bag).

2. Leakage or perforation

Leakage of dialysate around the cannula is distressing to the patient, renders the balance sheet valueless and may encourage infection of the puncture wound. The cure consists of a new purse-string suture, or if this fails, a new cannula is inserted at a new site. Seepage of fluid along the planes of the abdominal wall and into the genitalia and thighs causes considerable discomfort. The catheter should be checked to ensure that the side perforations all lie within the peritoneal cavity and the purse-string suture is then replaced. Perforation of the bowel has been reported – ironically from a renal unit – but we have never seen this and attribute the disaster to incorrect technique.

3. Positive balance

During oliguria a positive balance will invariably lead to oedema and possibly hypertension. The following steps are recommended. During drainage tip the patient from side to side and exert intermittent gentle pressure on the abdomen. Apply a vacuum (5 cm, 0.5 kPa water pressure) to the drainage bottle. Use a dialysate having a high concentration of dextrose (6.3%, 350 mmol/l). If successful, the strong dialysate is alternated with three cycles of the weaker dialysate. When these steps fail the cannula is changed when it will be found that the fine side perforations are blocked by fibrin.

4. Immobilization

Peritoneal dialysis, unlike intermittent haemodialysis, immobilizes the patient for long periods with the attendant risk of pressure sores or a deep venous thrombosis. Preventive measures are started with the dialysis. The bed is tilted from side to side so that only one-third of the time is spent lying with pressure directly on the sacrum. Active movements of the legs, especially at the ankle, are performed regularly.

5. Pulmonary

Numerous and occasionally fatal pulmonary complications can beset peritoneal dialysis. They are of sufficient importance to contra-indicate PD in a patient with renal failure and chronic lung disease. The complications are as follows: basal collapse caused by elevation of the diaphragm or the retention of mucus due to an ineffective cough; linear atelectasis; pleural effusion, consolidation, respiratory tract infection with purulent sputum or bacterial consolidation (pneumonia). Daily X-rays of the chest and sputum culture are needed for early recognition; it is also helpful to measure the vital capacity once a day with the abdomen empty. The complications can partly be avoided by using a 1-litre rapid cycle, by diligent attention to the posture of the patient and by deep breathing exercises, assisted coughing or by the use of intermittent positive pressure breathing. When deep breathing or coughing cause pain an analgesic is given before starting chest physiotherapy. IPPB is a valuable treatment to prevent or treat atelectasis and to help raise sputum. Hypoxaemia is an indication for using oxygen therapy and is usually corrected by means of 35% oxygen (Chapter 18). Bacterial consolidation requires intensive treatment with oxygen, an intravenous antibiotic and intermittent IPPB. When these measures fail, IPPV through a tracheostomy should be considered.

6. Infection of the wound or peritoneum

The incidence and severity of wound infection can be kept to a minimum by good aseptic technique and by keeping the wound clean and dry. In this way the use of antibiotics is avoided. Culture swabs are taken each time the wound is dressed. In the early days of peritoneal dialysis, peritonitis was a frequent and dangerous complication. The incidence dropped following the introduction of a sterile closed system, prepacked equipment and commercial dialysis fluid. Peritonitis is detected at an early, that is at a preclinical, stage, by daily culture of the dialysate in the draining bag or bottle. Coliforms (*E. coli, Klebsiella* spp.) or staphylococci may be cultured without causing harm to the patient; in this instance antibiotics or antiseptic treatment is withheld. If local signs of peritonitis appear and especially when these signs are associated with the recent development of fever or a worsening of the general condition, a wide spectrum antibiotic is given intravenously in full therapeutic doses. The antibiotic can also be added to the dialysate so that the solution infused contains a therapeutic concentration. The dialysis is continued if it is required to control the uraemia or oedema. When pulmonary complications or peritonitis are clinically serious, then haemodialysis/filtration is substituted.

7. Metabolic

(a) A potentially harmful degree of fluid imbalance can cause hypotension or alternatively oedema; prevention and correction were described earlier. (b) PD invariably removes large quantities of plasma protein; about 20 g of protein and 15 g of amino-acid/day of dialysis. When PD is used for more than 24 h or there are multiple injuries, recent surgery or systemic infections, the loss of protein should be made good by giving infusions of albumin. (c) A deficiency of water soluble vitamins is prevented by giving a daily supplement by mouth or vitamins intravenously. (d) Serious hyperglycaemia occurs from time to time and causes drowsiness or coma. The blood sugar is measured daily and when values of 16.7 mmol/l (300 mg/100ml) or more occur, high sugar dialysis is stopped and insulin is given by continuous intravenous infusion. (e) Hypernatraemia must be detected early, because if severe and prolonged, irreversible brain damage will result. If the Nap rises above 155 mmol/l the concentration is quickly reduced by intravenous therapy and the sodium in the dialysate is lowered to 120 mmol/l.

ACKNOWLEDGEMENTS

We are grateful to the staff of Gambro UK for help with this chapter.

25

Intensive care of renal failure: final part

This chapter briefly describes the training required to treat renal failure, how to put the various pieces together, how to manage some complications, an assessment of the results, and ends with a word on prevention.

I ESSENTIALS

The intensive care of renal failure is learned by apprenticeship to those with training and extensive experience. This apprenticeship is served in the ICU and in a chronic dialysis unit, and is supplemented by a teaching programme and personal study. The nurse-to-patient ratio is 1.3 : 1.0 and the best results will only be obtained when the unit has the appropriate complement of experienced nurses. The service doctors must possess extensive knowledge of the diagnostic problems as well as technical training in dialysis and filtration. But it is equally essential for the service doctors to have years of experience of failure of all the other body systems. The writers do not believe that the patient with renal failure or any other organ failure should be treated by a group of ologists – too many cooks spoiling the broth. But, from time to time, the intensive care medical team will certainly need the expertise of the urological surgeons.

II THERAPEUTIC PLANS

Following resuscitation, the treatment is pre-planned twice a day every day. The overall plan is made up of packages, as previously described, not omitting the relief of pain, ensuring sound sleep, and support of the morale. Dialysis and filtration, alone or together, comprise another package. For each therapy and for each day, a programme is written out with all the technical details and the aims; how much ECF is to be removed, and so on. In one case the electrolyte balance may be achieved by employing continuous arterio-venous haemofiltration (CAVHF). In another patient daily haemodialysis for four hours proves satisfactory in controlling uraemia and fluid balance.

III HOW AND WHEN TO STOP

The first is easy, the second can be difficult. Stopping dialysis/filtration is a simple technical exercise; the clever machines are removed and the vascular access dispensed with. When to stop dialysis/filtration can also be easy. When the renal failure is due to obstructive nephropathy and the obstruction can be relieved, then the supported therapy lasts only a few days. If the failure is reversible ATN, then weeks of dialysis can tide the patient over to a diuretic phase, although dialysis/filtration will be required until the kidney is able to excrete nitrogen as well as electrolytes. In other cases the rescue operation restores the milieu intérieur, but the previously undiagnosed intrinsic renal disease is irreversible. Such patients are assessed for maintenance dialysis and transplantation. This leaves us with a group of patients who cannot recover, although when intensive care was started it was thought that recovery was possible. The prognosis alters because of a new diagnosis – malignant disease for example, or because of irreversible failure of the lungs or persistent heart failure or brain failure. This syndrome of multiple organ failure is most commonly due to bacterial infection. This desperate situation requires a thorough assessment of the whole patient, including the morale; has the patient given up the good fight? An acute physiological assessment (APA) is next incorporated with a chronic health evaluation (CHE) to calculate a score APACHE II (Chapter 19) which will serve as a dependable predictor of the outcome (Maher *et al.*, 1989). Such predictors will tell us the outcome of a group of patients with similar signs, although not in individual patients. The assessment, made with or without the use of outcome scores, must lead to decisive action. Sentimentality or guilt take no part in deciding whether to stop or continue intensive care. Indeed, the renal failure is a minor factor, since the uraemia can be controlled by dialysis/filtration; the brain, heart and lungs, are the organs of chief concern. It is cruel to patient and family and wasteful to persist when the sign points to irreversibility. The ethical action is to stop the intensive therapy and tell both patient and relatives the truth. High technology medicine is replaced by the care of the dying and subsequently of the bereaved.

IV TREATMENT OF COMPLICATIONS

Microbial infection or gastrointestinal haemorrhage complicate the natural history of renal failure, even when the uraemia is well controlled by dialysis/filtration, and adequate nutrition is given. Either can kill the patient, and the renal lesion is reversible. As yet we cannot restore the immune system nor prevent stress ulceration of the stomach. Prevention and early detection are the key measures for dealing with infection. the former depends on the application of the nursing methods devised to contain infectious diseases, but in reverse – the patient is at risk, not the staff; the label 'reversed barrier nursing' is applied, and detailed in Chapter 27. Extensive and daily bacterial monitoring is also essential. Multiple shallow ulcers in the stomach commonly occur in the intensive care patient, but it seems that in only a minority does serious haemorrhage develop; when we do not know. Can serious haemorrhage be prevented? Much more information is required to answer this question, and until this becomes available, treatment is empirical. Two treatments may reduce the incidence of serious haemorrhage, antacid or H_2 inhibitor. Aluminium hydroxide gel 10 ml is syringed down the naso-gastric tube hourly. Alternatively, ranitidine is given i.v. in a dose of 150 mg/day. When to stop either drug is a reasoned guess. A third option is not to give drugs and pray!

V RESULTS

To put it bluntly, the results are awful. Even more depressing, is that the death rate has not fallen during the last thirty years. During this time the financial cost of failure during the prolonged intensive care has risen to over five figures sterling per patient. The valuable break-down of the results is that relating to other organs or systems involved, rather than to the renal lesion itself. When renal failure is the sole problem (obstructive nephropathy, saline depletion), then the death rate is about 8%. Depending on the organisation (or more probable, disorganisation) these patients may or may not be treated in the ICU. The death rate rises alarmingly when other systems fail following emergency operations or intra-abdominal sepsis. The results are similar whether the surgery is on the biliary tract, the bowel, or required for ruptured aortic aneurysms. When two organs have failed the death rate is 50% and if four systems are involved then survival is exceptional.

VI PREVENTION

If the results spell gloom and frustration, prevention has reduced the incidence of acute renal failure, and the results justify some optimism.

Table 25.1 Programmes for the prevention of acute renal failure (From *Essential Intensive Care*, with permission)

---

1. Common to all departments
   Prompt investigation and treatment of shock
   Appropriate fluid therapy and nutrition
   Prompt recognition and treatment of bacteraemia

2. At the site of injury or poisoning and Accident and Emergency Departments
   Prompt resuscitation
   Appropriate transportation

3. Operating theatre and surgical wards
   The right surgery by the right surgeon at the right time on the right patient
   Prophylactic dopamine
   Prophylactic antibiotics; operations on infected urinary or biliary tracts

---

Firstly, a lesson from the horrors of war. the incidence of renal failure in battle casualties fell progressively from one in twenty (World War II) to one in eight hundred (Korean War) and one in eighteen hundred (Vietnam). The improvement was due to improved resuscitation, rapid transportation (the helicopter) which made early surgery possible. The reader will remember the scenes televised during the Falklands conflict of 1982. A wounded combatant was quickly resuscitated on the spot by paramedics, pain was quickly relieved and an i.v. infusion started to prevent serious hypovolaemia and oliguria. Similar good progress has been achieved in civilian practice. Prompt resuscitation of the injured by medical teams or paramedics has greatly reduced the incidence of renal failure due to hypovolaemic shock. Twenty-five years ago the incidence of renal failure was 30%, but this is currently about 10%. What about prevention in the DGH? The essential programmes are shown in Table 25.1. In addition, the ICU has an essential role to play by using educational feedback. When a patient in renal failure is either admitted or assessed by the service staff, then errors and omissions are analysed and the correct management taught again and again.

26

Intensive care of brain failure

Can't thou not minister to a mind diseas'd.

Macbeth

...to think of curing the head alone and not the
rest of the body also, is the height of folly.

Socrates, 430 BC

I   STRATEGY
II   TREATMENT OF SOME CAUSES
III   THE BRAIN DEAD: THE POTENTIAL ORGAN DONOR
IV   STATUS EPILEPTICUS
V   PREVENTION

I STRATEGY

The beginner, after a week or so of attendance or apprenticeship will learn that only a minority of patients in a general ICU are unconscious. The wrong lay impression was formed because patients sedated and given muscle relaxants look unconscious, but may not be. Another early lesson is that those who are unconscious remain in the unit for a few days at most and then recover or die. General ICUs should not give intensive care to those in prolonged irreversible coma because these patients have no future.

1. Impaired consciousness and coma

When the unconscious patient arrives at your hospital two questions must be instantly answered. Is resuscitation required and is resuscitation the right thing for this patient? The same decisions apply to cardiac arrest (Chapter 21). We do not resuscitate the frail, elderly or patients severely disabled by incurable diseases! Resuscitation follows the invariable ABC of airway, breathing and circulation. Easy so far. Often the difficulty is to find a cause and the diagnosis will decide the type of care to be given. Let us start with the vascular causes. A provisional diagnosis of spontaneous subarachnoid haemorrhage under 60 is a signal for immediate transfer to the ICU; when cerebral thrombosis, capsular haemorrhage or embolus is the cause, then intensive care cannot benefit the patient. The patient who does need intensive care will need two or more therapeutic packages. All need high

Table 26.1 Drugs used to relieve delirium

Diazepam	2 to 10 mg i.v.
Midazolam	2 to 10 mg i.v.
Haloperidol	5 to 10 mg i.v.
Chlorpromazine	25 to 50 mg i.m.

Chlormethiazole edisylate solution, 8 mg/ml
Initially 5–15 ml/min, then 0.5 to 1.0 ml/min i.v.
Propofol emulsion 0.3–4 mg/kg/h i.v.

dependency nursing and all need examination of the airway which will decide the method of protection, as described in Chapter 18. A reliable guide is the universal Glasgow Coma Scale – a score of 8 or less means that protection is necessary.

2. Delirium

Delirium can be dealt with quite briefly because the cause (Chapter 10) must be treated rather than the group of symptoms. The prime therapy will be as varied as the cause: folate deficiency, potassium depletion, hypoxia, bacterial toxaemia, brain abscess! Never forget that the delirium can readily be caused by one or more of the drugs on the prescription sheet! We are confident that inadequate sleep will be high on your mental list. Symptomatic treatment may become necessary to induce sleep, damp down hallucinations or make it possible to nurse a patient; a selection of drugs is given in Table 26.1. In extreme instances it becomes impossible to nurse a patient and IPPV is used as a last resort, but only when the primary disease is curable.

II TREATMENT OF SOME CAUSES

1. Hypoxia

If the reader reflects on the hypoxia which starts immediately following cardiac arrest and results in brain death within four minutes, then the conclusion is that the brain failure due to hypoxia must be prevented altogether or treated early and efficiently. Therapy is directed at the respiratory failure, shock, or both, and was described in Chapters 18–20.

Secondary changes, especially acidosis, can require correction. It is essential to list the treatments which cannot be shown to be effective. Hypothermia induced before brain hypoxia occurs reduces damage; but hypothermia induced after the event is useless. Two treatments have been used in an attempt to reduce the swelling of the brain which follows hypoxia, as can happen following trauma; the aim is to prevent ischaemic damage due to the raised intracranial pressure. The osmotic diuretic mannitol or deliberate hyperventilation to induce hypocapnoea, which in turn reduces cerebral blood flow, have their advocates. We use neither because these treatments do not benefit patients with hypoxic brain damage.

2. Acute poisoning

By following the flow chart of Figure 26.1 the right patient reaches the right bed at the right time. A therapeutic plan is then necessary in which the various treatments are listed in their priority. When poisoning impairs consciousness, then respiratory failure is usual, but there may also be shock, cardiac dysrhythmias, renal or liver failure as well. The basis of the plan is to restore and maintain the composition of the ECF until the poison is either metabolized or removed artificially; the treatments are in the main supportive; oxygen therapy, IPPV, inotropes, not forgetting fluid therapy. It is salutory to recall that this supportive therapy originated in Denmark and Sweden in the late 1940s. The Scandinavian method was defined as 'centralization of patients, regular systematic control of the clinical condition and prevention or treatment of possible complications'. The result was that the death rate fell from 30 to 10% and by 1960 to 1%. There could be no clearer vindication of a method which had been stigmatized as therapeutic nihilism. The pharmacology of acute poisoning can be divided into 'antidotes', methods to reduce absorption and those which accelerate removal. These are summarized in Table 26.2.

3. Metabolic

A return to the concept of the milieu intérieur. Many of the disturbances of the body fluids (Chapter 4) cause brain failure and therefore demand prompt and effective therapy (Chapter 16). The multiplicity of the disturbances is best illustrated in diabetic keto-acidosis; when the latter causes delirium or impaired consciousness, the patient should certainly be treated in the ICU. Other common metabolic disturbances are given in Table 26.3. Finally, metabolic disorders like acute porphyria or Wilson's disease can require intensive care. Careful selection is essential before advising intensive care in brain failure due to liver failure (hepatic encephalopathy), otherwise the burdens exceed the benefits.

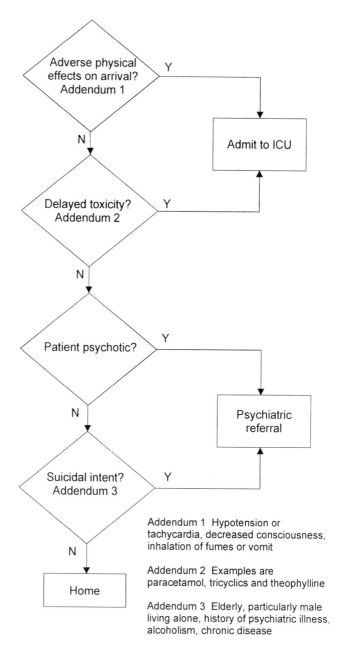

Figure 26.1 Strategy for acute poisoning

Table 26.2 Acute poisoning: antidotes; methods for reducing absorption or accelerating removal

	ANTIDOTES
Benzodiazepines	Flumazenil (not to be used in concomitant tricyclic poisoning)
Narcotics	Naloxone hydrochloride injection
Paracetamol	Acetylcysteine infusion
Insulin	Glucagon injection
β-Blockers	Isoprenaline hydrochloride; dobutamine hydrochloride, glucagon
Organophosphorus agents	Pralidoxime mesylate and atropine
Cyanide	Sodium nitrite injection, sodium thiosulphate injection, dicobalt editate injection
Iron compounds	Desferrioxamine mesylate infusion
Phenothiazines Metoclopramide	Procyclidine hydrochloride
	REDUCING ABSORPTION
Anything ingested	* Induced vomiting
	* Gastric lavage
	Activated charcoal
Insulin	Excision of injection site
Ingested iron compounds	Desferrioxamine mesylate IG
Paraquat	Fuller's earth IG
	ACCELERATING REMOVAL
Carbon monoxide	Hyperbaric oxygen
Salicylate, phenobarbitone	* Forced alkaline diuresis
Amphetamine, pethidine, quinine	* Forced acid diuresis
Lithium, bromide, barbiturates	* Forced neutral diuresis
Lithium, barbiturate, salicylate, bromide, ethanol, methanol, isoniazid	Haemodialysis
Theophylline, paracetamol, paraquat	* Haemoperfusion

* These treatments were widely used from 1960, but now rarely given. Some patients probably benefited and certainly some were harmed. How difficult it is to prove that a treatment does good!

Table 26.3 Restoring the milieu intérieur

Disorder	Therapy
Saline depletion	i.v. saline
Potassium depletion	i.v. potassium chloride
Deficiency of folate vitamins B, trace elements or essential fatty acids	Nutrition!
The ECF; changes in properties or concentrations	
Hyperpyrexia	Cooling the body
Hypothermia	Warming the body
Metabolic acidosis	i.v. bicarbonate
Keto-acidosis	i.v. insulin
Metabolic alkalosis	i.v. potassium
Hyperglycaemia	i.v. insulin
Hypoglycaemia	i.v. glucose, glucagon
Hypernatraemia	i.v. glucose or hypotonic saline
Hyponatraemia	amend fluid therapy, i.v. hypertonic saline
Hypercalcaemia	Forced diuresis, hydrocortisone
Hypocalcaemia	i.v. calcium gluconate

4. Head-injured

In the DGH, a general ICU has an important role to play in determining the right care for the head-injured: 'the right patient in the right bed at the right time'. The twenty-thousand dollar question is 'does this patient require neurosurgery'? During the diagnostic period which must include CT scanning, the unit gives all the supportive care necessary: the upper airway, ventilation, and so on, as described in Chapter 29. In the head injured, when diffuse damage causes prolonged coma, then it is important to acknowledge treatments which cannot be proved to help the patient; these are steroids, barbiturates, prolonged IPPV and diuretics.

5. Meningitis and encephalitis

When one of these conditions causes delirium – impaired consciousness or convulsions – then intensive care should be considered. Antimicrobial therapy should ensure a low death rate from bacterial meningitis. Unfortunately, the figure is 5–20%. Delay in starting treatment is probably the chief reason but inadequate supportive therapy also accounts for some deaths.

Table 26.4 Essentials for organ donation

1.	Criteria for admission of the potential donor, rigidly enforced
2.	Technical skills for the diagnosis of brain death and supportive therapy
3.	The courage and skill to ask *THE* question

The latter cannot occur when the patient is in the general ICU which will ensure intensive monitoring and the support of all the body systems.

III THE BRAIN DEAD: THE POTENTIAL ORGAN DONOR

1. The role of the ICU in organ donation

The techniques and laws relating to organ removal from a heart-bearing donor are well known; public attitude is sympathetic and relatives seldom refuse to give consent for donation; and statistics show that there is a surplus of potential donors. Nevertheless, the supply of viable cadaveric organs falls far short of the need. The fault lies with the medical profession and must be due to lack of knowledge and skills or to inappropriate attitudes of hospital medical staff. Table 26.4 lists the requirements for participation in a transplantation programme. The administration is facilitated by means of a flow diagram (Figure 26.2).

2. Care of the donor

This is an easy technical exercise for any ICU worth its salt. The therapy is threefold: pulmonary gas exchange; the circulation and urine formation. The treatments are described in other parts of this book and for convenience are summarized here in the form of a flow chart (Figure 26.3).

3. Care of the bereaved

Spontaneous subarachnoid haemorrhage or head injury is an unforeseeable tragedy especially when, as usual, the patient is young. The technical exercise of maintaining some body functions is simplicity itself compared to the caring of the relatives. The latter demands the nurse and doctor (yes, the doctor!) who must be trained in both basic counselling techniques and specifically in the care of the bereaved; this caring starts when brain death is diagnosed and continues as long as it is needed, for weeks or months. Training courses are available within the NHS.

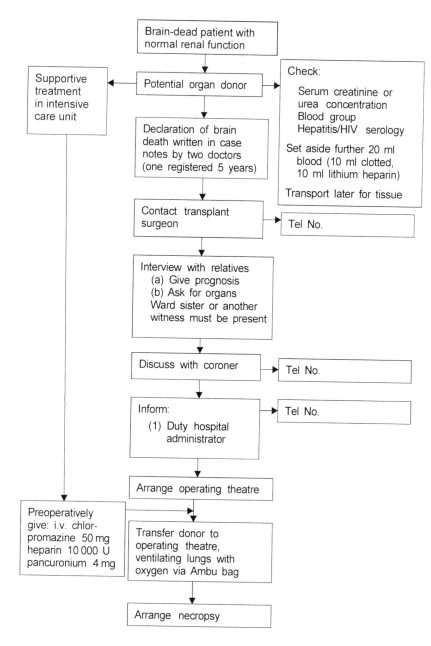

Figure 26.2 Protocol for organ donation (From Luksza, *Br Med J* 1979; 1: 1316–19, with permission)

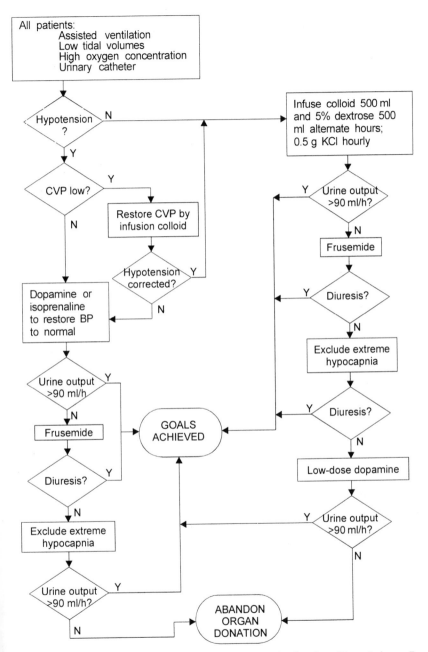

Figure 26.3 Methods to maintain the circulation and urine flow (From Luksza, *Br Med J*, 1979; 1:1316–19, with permission)

IV   STATUS EPILEPTICUS

The intensive care unit helps to reduce the high death rate of this terrible condition. This will not happen unless criteria for intensive care are formulated (by consensus patient management) and are in force. We start with the assumption that the status is due to idiopathic epilepsy and not caused by a glioma or encephalitis. When subsequent events prove an assumption to be wrong, then the rescue is called off. The first assessment in casualty should take only seconds. If either of the following signs are present, then the trachea should be intubated under relaxant: apnoea with central cyanosis or a suspicion that vomit has been inhaled (a nice test for your medical trainee!). Mechanical IPPV is continued in the unit. In the remaining patients the airway is protected; a naso-gastric tube passed and apsirated, 35% oxygen given and the patient admitted to the ICU. Drug therapy then follows the flow chart of Figure 26.4. A common and dangerous error (one which never happens in ones own hospital) is to literally poison the brain with drugs given to stop the fits, in particular the benzodiazapines. Such treatment causes respiratory failure which is not a therapeutic aim. Clearly defined doses must be laid down in the standardized method for status. To return to the patient not having ventilator treatment. This will become necessary when the fits continue non-stop. Continuous epilepsy causes harm and kills chiefly by reason of brain hypoxia, but also because the explosive cell activity (easily seen on EEG) damages individual neurones. IPPV was first used to treat status in Liverpool in 1958 and is life-saving. Pulmonary gas exchange is restored and maintained. IPPV is continued (controlled with pancuronium and phenoperidine), together with therapeutic, but not toxic, doses of one or two anti-convulsants until the electrical storm subsides. How can fits be observed when the patient cannot convulse? Simple. The relaxant can be interrupted for a few hours and any convulsions noted.

Alternatively, a portable EEG (at last, we have found a valuable use for this machine!) will easily monitor the grand mal discharges. When the convulsions cease, in days or a week the IPPV is stopped, weaning is easy. The foregoing summarizes the methods at Whiston. At the Royal Prince Alfred hospital the drug therapy is different. The IPPV is again controlled by muscle relaxant and anticonvulsants given i.v. It will take 24–48 hours to achieve therapeutic levels and during this time thiopentone is given to suppress the grand mal discharges. This drug is given as an infusion in a dose of 1–2 mg/kg/h.

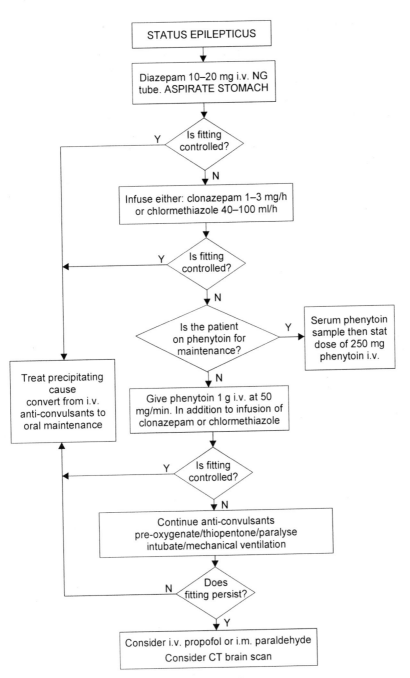

Figure 26.4 Intensive therapy of status epilepticus

V PREVENTION

Was prevention ever more important than cure! A valuable exercise for the beginner is to list, from their own experience, patients in whom early treatment would have prevented brain failure. You will end up with the contents page of a textbook! It is important to stress the early treatment of respiratory failure, shock or head injury. Here the educational value of intensive care is at its most valuable. Feedback will ensure expert resuscitation outside and inside the hospital, training of A & E staff and effective use of the recovery room.

27

Prevention and intensive care of infections

I	PREVENTION OF HOSPITAL ACQUIRED INFECTION
II	TREATMENT OF PRIMARY INFECTIONS
III	TREATMENT OF SECONDARY INFECTIONS

I PREVENTION OF HOSPITAL ACQUIRED INFECTION

About half of the patients admitted to a general ICU face a high risk of secondary infection. The reasons are the impaired defences (systemic and local), a stay of weeks and the numerous sources of bacteria and fungi. Preventive measures are therefore essential and the commonest aim is to prevent infection reaching the patient by a system of protective isolation or reversed barrier nursing. In a few instances, e.g. meningocolcaemia, the patient is a source of infection and isolation is necessary to prevent spread. But the same problem will exist when secondary infection develops in the injured or surgical patient; they too are a source of infection. There now follows a review of the preventive practices, most of which date to the fever hospitals of a hundred years ago! But these well tried methods are doomed to failure unless they are strictly enforced by the nursing officer and service doctor.

1. The patient

The preventive measures should be tailored to suit the needs and these can be divided into two groups. Patients in the first group only need standard ward practices; examples would be acute myocardial infarction and asthma not requiring IPPV. In such conditions the host defences are not severely impaired and the risks of secondary infection are low. The patients in the second group (trauma, surgery) face a high risk of developing a secondary infection and every effort at prevention should be made. As already stated, most of this prevention is based on the sound principles of nursing in the infectious diseases hospital, a barrier must be maintained to prevent the spread of infection. But these procedures can be modified as new knowledge is gained. Indeed, important advances in microbiology were made in the ICU; the patient was found to be an important source of infection to himself!

367

Table 27.1 Sources and transmission of hospital acquired infection

Patient	Nostrils, mouth, pharynx
	Skin
	Sputum, gastric aspirate, faeces
	Wounds, drains, burns
Staff	Nostrils, expired air (talking, coughing)
	Skin, fingers, hand cream
	Clothing
Immediate environment	Air, dust
	Walls, floors, trolleys
	Bed linen
	Handbasins, taps, lotions, soaps
	Shaving equipment, toothbrushes
	Thermometers
Equipment	Suction apparatus
	Ventilators, anaesthetic machines
	Dialysers, filters
	Catheters
Nutrition	Beverages, ice-cubes, food
	Intragastric feeds
	i.v. infusions

The sources of self-colonization and secondary infection were dealt with in Chapter 15 and by using Table 27.1 the beginner can revise their knowledge. How, during illness, do the colonic bacteria reach the lung? This background knowledge can be used to design preventive measures to reduce the colonization and infection as shown in the same table. Such programmes are described later or in other chapters but a useful summary of current practice is given in Table 27.2.

2. Staff and visitors

Infection due to microbes transmitted by the staff currently dominates the scene. This is because infection due to germs brought in by visitors is rare, and by 1970 infection from the patient's environment (Section 3) was virtually eliminated so we cannot blame the ventilators, humidifiers and handbasins! The chief source of the infecting organisms are the long-stay ICU patients; they have become carriers of the 'hospital' flora. How are the bugs transmitted? On the fingers of the staff! The beginner will soon remember which bacteria are causing secondary infection and it must be emphasized that all these familiar bugs can be carried on the hands: *Klebsiella* spp., *Enterobacter* spp., *Acinetobacter* spp., *S. aureus*, *P. aeruginosa*. It follows that frequent hand washing is the most single important

Table 27.2 Recommendations of the Centers for Diseases Control for ICU (Atlanta, USA) (From Daschner 1985, with permission)

1. Handwashing
   Personnel should wash their hands between all patient contacts and when otherwise indicated. Sinks should be provided at convenient locations throughout the ICU and in each of its isolation rooms or alcoves to encourage handwashing. Gloves should be worn for high-risk patient contacts. Antiseptics when indicated should be easily accessible for handwashing.

2. Isolation facilities
   Appropriate isolation facilities should be available in an ICU if infected patients requiring isolation are admitted to these units.

3. Spacing patients
   Sufficient space should be provided around each patient for equipment and the passage of personnel to decrease the chance of infection transmission by direct contact.

4. Supervision and in-service training
   Supervision and in-service training should be done in ICUs to ensure that proper handwashing is performed, that disposable equipment is not reused and that reusable devices are properly cleaned and sterilized.

preventive measure, even though good practice will reduce but not eliminate the transmission. The hands are washed with an alcoholic solution containing chlorhexidine or providone iodine, before and after every procedure and dried on a good quality disposable paper towel. Success depends on self discipline, good training and the right numbers of nurses and not too many doctors! Much research has confirmed this and also shown that the medical staff are, time and again, the chief sinners. And so it was in the 1840s when Ignaz Philipp Semmelweiss working in the Vienna Maternity Hospital 'insisted that students coming from the dissecting rooms or postmortem theatre washed their hands in a solution of chloride of lime. Immediately, the mortality in the wards under his care fell from 18% to 3% and then to 1%' (Guthrie, 1958).

The next problem is to reduce the infection transmitted by exhaled air and clothing. Face masks are worn when talking to patients but only those at a high risk of secondary infection. The other indications are given in Table 27.3. To reduce the bacterial contamination of the patient or bed from clothing, aprons rather than gowns are worn because these are more effective.

Table 27.3 Indications for wearing a face mask

Vascular cannulation, preparing and giving infusion or injections

Oral or endotracheal suction

Introducing or changing drainage systems; urinary, chest or peritoneum

Wound care

Taking blood or bacteriological samples

3. Environment

This huge and controversial subject will be reduced to the essentials. The newcomer to intensive care should start by observing the contents of a treatment room with the astuteness of Dr Conan Doyle's famous detective. Just every item can be a source of bacteria or fungi and a microbiologist would soon confirm this. From the handbasin to the bed linen, water in a flower vase, the patient's iced beverage. Three facts should be grasped. The microbes isolated are only pathogenic to the susceptible patient and you can already identify this group. Secondly, the germ population can be reduced but never eliminated by simple but labour-intensive hygiene, standardized into packages. Lastly, bacterial monitoring can be safely reduced to the minimum, thus saving money on unnecessary ritual.

We next briefly consider the worthwhile methods of reducing the likelihood of secondary infection (a) The air. Airborne infection has to have a source: staff, expired gas from a ventilator, and many more. When all these are contained how best to reduce the microbial population? The choice is simple: natural ventilation or special and expensive air conditioning – that used in offices or hotels is worse than none. It is, therefore, reasonable to settle for natural ventilation. In hot climates air conditioning has definite advantages provided safeguards are taken. In offices and homes some air is recirculated, but this will not do for intensive care or operating theatres. Imagine removing air from a sluice to the vicinity of patient with impaired resistance to infection. The correct method is to exhaust all the air to the exterior of the building. The 'ultimate' air conditioning is called laminar flow, but like the ultimate driving machine, is not justified on cost. (b) The fixtures. Walls, floors, handbasins, kitchens, sluice, can be grouped together. Frequent and thorough cleaning is the essential requirement to reduce the microbial contamination. Disinfections are of secondary value and cannot be used as a substitute for hygiene. Success will therefore depend on a team of cleaners who, by proper training, recognize their essential service and on strict management. Handbasins require additional comment. A perforated disc to create a spray is a potential source of contamination of the hands and should not be fitted. The sink trap is a notorious source of bacteria which can contaminate the hands during washing. A heating element fitted to the trap can be used to boil a phenol solution in the trap, a method used each day. (c) The bed. Clean sheets every day, like the best hotels! The quality of a fresh laundry is the responsibility of the manager who maintains a liaison with the microbiologist. Contaminated linen is dealt with according to the standardized hospital practice, by methods proved effective by the infectious diseases hospital (Ayliffe, 1990). A vacated bed and mattress is washed down. (d) Patient hygiene. The various items required are allocated to each patient and on discharge are discarded or sterilized. This principle applies to washing bowls, cloths and toilet soap. Oral hygiene with sterile water follow regular practice, but unfortunately does not reduce colonization. (e) Fluid therapy and nutrition. Let us start with the materials for i.v. and i.g. therapy. The pharmacy service will ensure that infusions and injections are sterile and a good nursing team will make certain that these are not contaminated. So far so good, but it should be recalled that the commonest cause of bacteraemia in the hospital patient is an indwelling i.v. line of any type. The bacteraemia arises from a colonized puncture site or the fluid infused. It is therefore no surprise that numerous trials have tried to find the best protective dressings. In the end any technique is bound to fail unless hygiene is near perfect. The beginner might think that enteral nutrition must be safe; wrong. Beverages, tube feeds, even ice cubes may be contaminated and bacteria or fungi then colonize the oropharynx, stomach and gut.

There are two practical problems. Starting with safe materials it is necessary to make sure that these remain safe. Nutritious drinks and tube feeds are discarded after twelve hours and during use they are stored at 4°C in a sterile container fitted with a lid. A short digression on refrigerators. The domestic 'fridge' is unsuited to use in a hospital kitchen because the temperature fluctuations allow too much bacterial growth. The second problem is that of starting off with a sterile feed but this is contaminated by the bacteria growing in the patient's stomach (Chapters 15 and 17). This dangerous complication is inevitable when a pump is used to give the nutrients unless the machine is set to prevent contraflow. (f) Urethral catheters and drainage tubes. The student of general intensive care will already be familiar with the management of prolonged catheterization of the urethra with closed drainage. The essentials are: sterile, pre-packed equipment and the wearing of polythene gloves. This leaves the additional use of antiseptics to further prevent infection. Even healthy subjects excrete bacteria in the urine and retrograde flow is prevented by one-way valves. Antimicrobials installed in the bladder clearly have been tried extensively.

Table 27.4 Sterilization or disinfection of equipment

Ventilator	Cleaned at end of patient use. Patient circuit cleaned and sterilized. New bacterial filter Patient hoses and connections changed every 48 h Humidifier cleaned and autoclaved at end of individual use; when in service, use sterile water
Suction apparatus	Changed daily, cleaned and autoclaved
Suction catheters	Pre-packed sterile, used once
Dialyser of haemofilter: Hardware	cleaned
Patient circuit, Dialyser or filter	Pre-packed sterile
Endoscopes*	Washed in detergent. Disinfected in 2% alkaline gluteraldehyde. Rinse channel and wipe insertion tube with 70% alcohol

*British Thoracic Association (1988)

Since these fail to prevent secondary infection they can be omitted. Policies are also required for chest drains and peritoneal dialysis. (g) Equipment. The good news for the beginner is that the thirty year nightmare of infection carried by equipment is over. With present day machinery, properly maintained and correctly used, such secondary sepsis can be prevented. This section can therefore be quite brief. The first essential is that there is no substitute for cleanliness. Suction equipment, ventilators, dialysers must be cleaned thoroughly by technical staff permanently allocated to the job. Some components are disposable and already sterile; others are clean and then sterilized by heat. The gases supplying a ventilator pass through bacterial filters as does the expired gas, at one time a potent source of cross infection. The use (and misuse) of suction apparatus requires emphasis. Particular standards of endotracheal suction is the top priority (Chapter 18). The other requirements are easier; filters are fitted to the suction line; overflow from the collecting vessels must be prevented. Table 27.4 summarizes the sterilization of equipment, but never forget the cleaning.

Table 27.5 Prophylactic antibiotics during intensive care

Problems	Disease to be prevented	Antimicrobials
Penetrating wound or compound fracture of the skull	Meningitis	Cefotaxime
Endoscopy or surgery and infection of the urinary tract	Bacteraemia or bacterial toxaemia	Cefotaxime
Surgery on infected biliary tract	Bacteraemia or bacterial toxaemia	Cefotaxime
Inhalation of nasopharyngeal bacteria	Pulmonary infection	S.D.D.*
Paralytic ileus. Bacterial colonization of the stomach and nasopharynx	Pulmonary infection	S.D.D.*
Oropharyngeal carriage of yeasts	Pulmonary infection or fungaemia	2% amphoteracin B paste or suspension

*S.D.D.; Selective decontamination of the digestive tract; see text.

4. Prophylactic antibiotics

'Kills all known germs' as the TV advertisement says. As a general principle the prophylactic use of antimicrobials has caused more harm than good, and the burdens exceed the benefits. Should the beginner be interested in recent history then we recommend the study by Price and Sleight (1970) as an example. Head-injured patients with a tracheostomy were given antibiotics prophylactically. The high incidence of infection with Gram negative bacteria was dramatically reduced when the treatment was abandoned! In only one application are we on sure ground; when the urine is infected and endoscopy or surgery is planned, then an antimicrobial is essential. Other indications are listed in Table 27.5. Some trials claim success for prophylaxis following trauma. One such scheme called selective decontamination of the digestive tract (SDD) has been tested out by controlled trials. The early oropharyngeal colonists were reduced by giving i.v. cefotaxime. The greatly expanded gram negative aerobic colonists and yeasts in the oropharynx and gut are reduced by a combination of antimicrobials applied as a gel to the oropharynx and also put down the naso-gastric tube. Action in the gut does not commence for four days. The drug scheme is polymyxin E, tobramycin and amphotericin B (van Saene *et al.*, 1991). This method of prophylaxis has been widely adopted but is not used by authors McWilliam and Coakley.

II TREATMENT OF PRIMARY INFECTIONS

In any general ICU the primary infections will consist of those which are endemic and on the sporadic occurrence of epidemics or smaller outbreaks in the local community. These principles are best illustrated by examples. In the UK generalized tetanus is almost unknown, but this is common in Africa. Outbreaks in the UK of Legionnaires' disease have a death rate of 25%. A future epidemic of influenza will probably overwhelm the ICU beds. Any general hospital should keep the staff informed on trends in infectious diseases; in the UK there are monthly bulletins. Firstly, wherever we work, the passenger on a jet aircraft can spring surprises, sometimes ending tragically. Malaria kills ten patients a year in the UK and in Australia the annual deaths vary from none to three.

Before summarizing the intensive care of primary infections, the vital (literally vital) role of early diagnosis should be emphasized. The learner should compare the problem with the golden hour following major injury (Chapter 29). Unless bacterial pneumonia or meningitis are diagnosed early, then intensive care can never lead to good results. Early diagnosis will depend on high standards of primary medical care, partly maintained by the educational feedback from the ICU. Thus, when late referral to the unit is the chief factor in the death of the patient, then the case is discussed at joint medical meetings so that hopefully the same error will not be repeated.

Admission criteria will help to get the right patient treated at the right time and avoid fruitless rescue operations. The therapy is made up of the now customary packages, arranged according to a changing priority; examples appear later in this chapter. Antimicrobials are essential but will not succeed without the other therapies. The initial choice is decided by a series of antibiotic policies and the i.v. drugs are started as soon as bacteriological samples have been taken. Clinical monitoring of the body systems and bacteriological monitoring will decide whether the drugs have to be changed. In general, the dose of an antibiotic is calculated according to body weight, but with gentamicin and tobramycin it is essential to measure the blood concentrations of the drug to ensure effective peak levels and avoid harmful trough levels. This is done by taking a blood sample half to one hour after an intravenous dose – the peak concentration – and a second sample just prior to the injection – the trough concentration.

Table 27.6 Pneumonia: laboratory tests at the initial examination

Sputum or bronchial aspirate	Gram stain and culture
	Pneumococcal antigen
Blood	Culture
	Pneumococcal antigen
	Mycoplasma IgM
	Full blood count
	Tests for DIC
	Electrolytes and urea
	Legionella titres

1. Primary pneumonia

The newcomer to intensive care might think that pneumonia in the previously fit adult would no longer be a killer – how wrong! It should not be, but in fact the disease kills three times more adults in a year than does asthma. The writers believe, but have no proof, that many of these deaths are avoidable. The term primary is used to separate this form of pneumonia from pulmonary consolidation secondary to trauma and surgery and that developing in the immune incompetent patient.

(a) The patient. An early diagnosis depends on intuition as much as a painstaking history and this is of far more value than the signs in the chest. Symptoms of bacterial infection, perhaps pleural pain, and an increased breathing pattern are valuable pointers. It is important to recall that the chest radiograph will show consolidation only when the latter is well established; homogeneous opacity with air bronchogram. The differential diagnosis is beyond the brief of this book – years of experience cannot be crystallized into a few lines!* Laboratory tests listed in Table 27.6 are carried out as a matter of urgency and antibiotic therapy started immediately, before the results are to hand. It is clearly logical to obtain secretions from as near the consolidation as possible by invasive sampling. The following have been tried out: trans-tracheal puncture, fibreoptic bronchoscopy and percutaneous lung puncture. With a previously healthy subject and pathogens (Table 27.7) sensitive to antimicrobials then the treatment should guarantee a minimal death rate; not so. Respiratory failure, shock, renal failure and so on cause a shameful slaughter not as yet much improved by intensive care.

---

* The best textbook of medicine in the English language – the Oxford – now weighs 11 kg.

Table 27.7 Pathogens causing primary pneumonia

S. pneumoniae
H. influenzae
M. catarrhalis
S. aureus
Influenza A virus
L. pneumophila
M. pneumoniae

Some of the answers to the high death rate are known; delay in diagnosis or delay in starting antibiotics; delay in admission to the ICU. In our opinion lack of clinical judgement is the real culprit.

(b) Criteria for intensive care. The first essential is to err on the safe side and admit a patient who may or may not deteriorate, rather than leave them in a ward where the deterioration can pass unnoticed, or is observed but no action is taken. Predicting the course in the individual depends on intuition – the eye of experience – rather than the chest radiograph or blood gases. The more obvious indications for intensive care are: respiratory fatigue, brain failure, shock, or oliguria. The factors which diminish the chances of recovery are age, a white cell count of below 4.0 or above 30×10^9/l, a serum albumen less than 35 g/l.

(c) Intensive therapy. Although the primary disease is confined to one or both lungs, with or without bacteraemia, the novice to intensive care will realise that the whole patient requires obsessional monitoring and care. The principles are summarized in Table 27.8 but it is necessary to supplement the chapter on IPPV. The beginner may be surprised and dismayed to find that IPPV can fail to maintain gas exchange, despite the previously healthy state of the lungs and despite the fact that the pneumonia is rarely widespread. The V/Q balance is severely disturbed. This means that a high F_1O_2% is necessary. The pneumonic lung is also very stiff, resulting in high tracheal pressures which in turn cause hypotension. Just the case for using PEEP? This can improve the PaO_2 but may further drop the cardiac output to dangerous levels. This desperate situation led to the trial of alternative methods of IPPV, which are experimental rather than desperate! When the disease affected one lung, then it was logical to try differential lung ventilation which is old hat in thoracic anaesthesia. Each lung is ventilated separately and in theory the 'good' lung should be more then sufficient to maintain life. An alternative is the relatively new technique of very high

Table 27.8 Primary pneumonia: summary of therapy

Body system	Treatment	Chapter reference
Respiratory	Oxygen, physiotherapy, humidification, IPPB, IPPV	18, 19
Circulatory	Inotropic agents, i.v. polygeline	20
Body fluids, nutrition	Liquid diet or i.v. nutrition, insulin	16, 17
Renal	Low dose dopamine, dialysis, haemofiltration	22–25
Coagulation	Heparin, clotting factors	28

frequency ventilation.* The principle is to ventilate the lung at a frequency of about 150. The advantages are that the P_{aw} remains much lower than during standard IPPV, thus avoiding the harmful effects on the circulation. Unfortunately, for our patients these newer techniques have not yet proved their worth.

It is salutary to remember that patients recovered from primary pneumonia before antibiotics were clinically available. But the patients considered here will not survive with antibiotics alone. The essentials are to start early and give the best drugs. Our antibiotic policy is shown as an algorithm in Figure 27.1.

2. Meningitis and encephalitis

As with primary pneumonia so with primary meningitis. Isolated causes occur in a healthy community as do small sporadic outbreaks. When the disease kills then the community is rightly angered and surprised. Diagnosis depends on the following groups of symptoms: those of meningeal irritations; the manifestations of infection; the signs (hopefully minimal) of brain failure (Chapter 10); laboratory tests on the CSF and blood (Table 27.9). The early diagnosis hinges on intuition as much as science and the differential diagnosis would easily fill this book! The pathogens causing meningitis in

---

* 'High frequency ventilation is still a fascinating technique in search of application'. Trier Mörch, 1990.

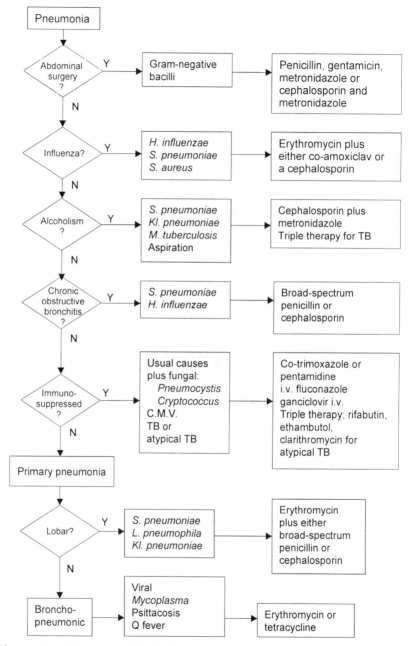

Figure 27.1 Choosing antibiotics for pneumonia. This algorithm will need to be updated using guidelines published by the British Thoracic Society

Table 27.9 Tests on blood and cerebrospinal fluid in meningitis and encephalitis

	BACTERIAL MENINGITIS
A. Blood tests	Blood cultures; often positive Infectious mononucleosis test of value when the blood shows a lymphocytosis
B. Tests on CSF	(i) Routine. (a) When gram-stain is diagnostic the special tests may be unnecessary. (b) Bacterial cultures. Routinely for aerobes. In a case of brain abscess, anaerobic culture as well. (c) White cell count is needed to distinguish bacterial from non-bacterial meningitis. (d) Glucose and protein
	(ii) Special tests. (a) Counter immuno-electrophoresis may give an early diagnosis in *S. pneumoniae, H. influenzae* type 6, and *N. meningitidis*. (b) Latex particle agglutination test, a rapid method for encapsulated micro-organisms. (c) Limulus lysate assay may help to detect endotoxin produced by Gram-negative bacteria. (d) Cytology required for brain tumor or obscure meningitis. (e) India ink preparation for chronic meningitis or the immuno-compromised
	NON-BACTERIAL MENINGITIS AND ENCEPHALITIS
A. Routine	To isolate a virus, take samples of saliva, faeces and CSF Acute and convalescent samples of serum for retrospective diagnosis
B. Herpes simplex suspect	(i) Brain biopsy for definite diagnosis Serology not diagnostic

the adult are given in Table 27.10. Medical and nursing staff must be alert to the cerebral presentation of malaria and this includes the UK.

The criteria for intensive care is an easy one – all patients. Not quite correct, because in extreme old age with coma or apnoea intensive therapy would not be justified. At the other end of the severity scale is the apparently well patient who mistakenly is not thought to be ill enough. This might be the policy of a doctor with a blinkered mechanistic view. The aim of intensive care in these patients is to make sure that they survive with minimal disability and this can only be achieved if complications are anticipated and expertly managed. The therapeutic plan for each patient on each day is formulated. Since the systematic reader is nearing the end of this book, they can test

Table 27.10 Causes of meningitis and encephalitis in the adult

Bacteria	Primary meningitis
	N. meningitidis
	S. pneumoniae
	H. influenzae
	L. monocytogenes
	M. tuberculosis
	Meningitis from otitis media or mastoiditis
	S. pyogenes
	S. aureus
Spirochaete	*Leptospira* spp.
Protozoa	*Plasmodium* spp. (*?falciparum* only)
Viruses	Herpes spp.

themselves by listing the treatment for an imaginary case and then arranging these in priority – triage.

The antibiotic treatment needs to be started as quickly as possible. Two milestones are worth recalling. During the years 1936–1944 the sulphonamides reduced the death rate of meningococcal meningitis from 50 to 20%. Monitoring the dose was possible from 1939 by measuring the sulphonamide concentrations in the blood and CSF. The mortality from pneumococcal meningitis remained at 90% until treatment with penicillin was described by Cairns and his colleagues in Oxford in 1944; the death rate then fell to 20%. The current drugs are listed in Table 27.11 and the diagnosis and management of organ failure is dealt with in other chapters as shown in Table 27.15.

3. Bacterial endocarditis

A few patients with this disease require intensive care. Three factors will decide selection; the acuteness of the disease, the severity of the infection or organ failure and the existence (or likely absence) of high dependency areas in the medical wards. The obvious aim is to get on top of the infection as quickly as possible, in which case the patient can continue the treatment in an intermediate care ward. The natural history can be grouped as acute or subacute; the former invariably needs intensive care. Just a word on diagnosis. This depends on a knowledge of the natural histories, remembering that the course of subacute endocarditis has changed greatly over the past forty years. Blood cultures are the mainstay of both diagnosis and antibiotic treatment. At least four samples are taken (doctor wears gloves and face mask!) at ten minute intervals. Further cultures are essential during

Table 27.11 Intravenous antibiotic policy for bacterial meningitis and brain abscess

A. BACTERIAL MENINGITIS

Organism unknown, i.e. blind therapy	Cefotaxime 2 g 8-hourly
Neisseria meningitidis	Benzyl-penicillin 2 meg units 4-hourly or cefotaxime 2 g 8-hourly Penicillin allergy: chloramphenicol 1 g 8-hourly **Duration of therapy 7 days**
Streptococcus pneumoniae	Cefotaxime 2 g 8-hourly Penicillin allergy: erythromycin 1 g 6-hourly or chloramphenicol 1 g 8-hourly **Duration of therapy 14 days**
Haemophilus influenzae	Cefotaxime 2 g 8-hourly Penicillin allergy: chloramphenicol 1 g 8-hourly **Duration of therapy 10 days**
Listeria monocytogenes	Ampicillin 2 g 6-hourly Penicillin allergy: erythromicin 1 g 6-hourly
Staphylococcus aureus	Flucloxacillin 2 g 6-hourly plus sodium fusidate 500 mg 8-hourly Penicillin allergy: vancomycin 500 mg 6-hourly – **monitor levels**

B. BRAIN ABSCESS

Pathogens are likely to be a mixture of aerobes and anaerobes

Initial blind therapy	Cefotaxime 2 g 8-hourly plus metronidazole 500 mg 8-hourly

treatment to monitor progress and to determine the serum bactericidal activity and minimal bactericidal concentration. A guide to antibiotic treatment therapy is given in Table 27.12.

4. Tetanus

A little knowledge on severe tetanus should help the beginner, whether or not cases are ever seen. The pathophysiology is due to the powerful exotoxin

Table 27.12   Guidelines for intravenous antibiotic treatment of bacterial endocarditis

Organism	Antibiotics
ACUTE	
Organism unknown	Flucloxacillin 1 g 6-hourly
	Benzyl-penicillin 5 mega units 6-hourly
	Gentamicin 5 mg/kg daily in divided doses
Staph. aureus	As above without benzyl-penicillin
SUB-ACUTE	
e.g. *Strep. viridans,*	Benzyl-penicillin 10–20 mega units daily
bovis, mutans	depending on sensitivity of organism
	Gentamicin 80 mg 12-hourly (as synergist)
Strep. faecalis	Ampicillin 2 g 6-hourly
	Gentamicin 80 mg 12-hourly (as synergist)

– a change from endotoxin – of *Cl. tetani*. In the adult patient the pathogens gain access to the body through a wound, sometimes quite trivial and not always found. The effects of the toxin on the brain stem, spinal cord and sympathetic nervous system are summarized in Table 27.13. The disease processes continue for 2–4 weeks but are reversible.

The treatment of life-threatening tetanus was a milestone in the evolution of intensive care. Whether or not the beginner sees severe tetanus, the essentials of treatment provide valuable lessons. The irony is that the disease is very rare in those countries with readily available ICUs. A bit of history first. The horrendous muscle spasms were treated with analgesics and sedatives and the patient was nursed in almost solitary confinement to avoid stimuli which triggered off the agonizing spasms and also caused terror. Intensive care changed radically following the introduction of the muscle relaxant tubocurarine into clinical practice in 1942. The combination of intensive care nursing, sedation, muscle relaxants, tracheostomy and IPPV would abolish the spasms, maintain gas exchange and metabolism until the body defences reversed the pathological changes in 2–4 weeks. The first successes were reported from Leeds in 1961 (See Edmondson *et al.*, 1982) and the methods were adopted by other regional tetanus units and then by the general ICU.

The criteria for admission have been published (Edmondson *et al.*, 1982) and it is essential to know that deterioration can occur in minutes, but cannot be predicted; the ICU motto is to be prepared! The overall treatment

Table 27.13 Patho-physiology of severe tetanus (From Edmondson *et al,*
1982)

	PRIMARY
Wound	Any severity, but absent in 40% of cases
Brain stem	'Lock jaw', trismus, dysphagia, stridor
Spinal cord	Stiffness, pain, spasms, apnoea, exhaustion, crush fractures, abdominal pain
Sympathetic nervous system	Labile hypertension, vasoconstriction, sweating, salivation, pyrexia, gastrointestinal stasis Tachycardia common. Dysrhythmias occasional. Episodes of hypotension, bradycardia or arrest
	SECONDARY
Body fluids	Large deficits of saline (6–8 litres per day)
Lung	Ineffective cough, inhalation of foreign material, absorption collapse, infection, respiratory failure
Brain	Agonizing pain, terror
Skeletal muscle	Exhaustion and fatigue
Gut	Constipation
Kidney	Renal failure

programme is given in Table 27.14. Keeping the lungs healthy by endotracheal suction and physiotherapy, replacing the large fluid losses are now
familiar territory. After the application of controlled IPPV, life was still
threatened by new problems. Heart rates of 200 and ectopics are usual and
may need drug treatment. Less common is unexpected extreme bradycardia
or arrest. This can be set off by endotracheal suction and this may be avoided
by anaesthesia with nitrous oxide. A challenging exercise in high technology
medicine should save life and restore the patient to full health; the benefits
indeed exceed the burdens. But there is an obvious sting in the tail. Tetanus
is safely, easily and cheaply preventable. Moreover the ICU can help in
prophylaxis. When a community becomes lax about immunization then a
little propaganda can work wonders. Thus, the Swedish people were jolted
out of their apathy by the showing on television of the generalized spasms;
the agonizing cry of the patient struck terror into the viewers.

Table 27.14 Treatment of generalized tetanus

Problems	Treatment	Chapter Ref.
Wound	Excision of necrotic material, removal of foreign body; leave open for a week	
Infection by *Cl. tetani*	Penicillin for a week Immunoglobulin injection BP	
Immunity	**Passive** – one dose of immunoglobulin 250 IU. Further dose if heavy contamination, wounds over 12 hours old, patient over 90 kg. **Active** – toxoid	
Muscle spasms	Benzodiazepines, analgesics, IPPV with muscle relaxants	19
Upper airway	Tracheostomy with or without IPPV	18
Sympathetic overactivity	Analgesia and sedation: intermittent 50% nitrous oxide with oxygen. β blockers	
Body fluids and nutrition	Maintain metabolic balance i.g. or i.v. nutrition	16 17

III TREATMENT OF SECONDARY INFECTIONS

A secondary infection following trauma or surgery invariably prolongs the illness and may kill the patient. Therefore, a condition which was given the right care at the right time, and from which recovery was expected, ends in death. This depressing outcome certainly does not occur because of ineffective antibiotics; indeed some secondary infection is due to antibiotics. The explanation has already been given (Chapters 12, 14 and 15). To get the best results we therefore depend on prevention as described in Section 1. The bacteria and fungi which can cause secondary infection are listed in Table 27.16. We now follow with the essential features at four sites in the body.

1. Respiratory tract and lung

A good starting point is to record that the infection can come from above (nasopharynx) or below, through the diaphragm. The reader could test

Table 27.15 Organ failure in primary infections: chapter reference

Organ or system	Diagnosis	Treatment
Respiratory failure	6	18, 19
Shock and heart failure	7	20
Renal failure	9	22–25
Brain failure	10	26
Metabolic failure	12	17
Coagulopathy	13	28

Table 27.16 Micro-organisms causing secondary infection

Site	Bacteria	Fungi
Respiratory tract and lung*	E. coli, Kl. pneumoniae, Ps. aeruginosa, S. aureus, Enterobacteria spp., Proteus spp., Serratia spp., Acinetobacter spp	Candida spp., Aspergillus spp.
Intra-abdominal	E. coli, Kl. aerogenes, Proteus spp., Bacteroides spp., St. spp., Cl. welchii	Candida spp.
Biliary tract	E. coli, St. faecalis, Bacteroides spp., Cl. welchii, Salmonella spp.	
Urinary tract	E. coli, Proteus spp.	Candida spp.
Wounds, blood	Enterobacteria Pseudomonads Yeasts Enterococci Coagulase negative staphylococci	

*Based on a large multi-centre study by Ruiz-Santana *et al.* (1987)

Table 27.17 Indications for antibiotics in Gram negative infections during IPPV (from Atherton *et al.*, 1977 with permission)

1.	Gram negative bacilli in stained films of the tracheal aspirate and radiological evidence of consolidation or absorption collapse
2.	(a) Core temperature of 38.5°C or more
	(b) White blood cell count of 11.0×10^9/l or above
	(c) Blood glucose level of 11.2 mmol/l (200 mg/100 ml) or above
3.	Laparotomy

his/her knowledge by listing the predisposing factors; those in the respiratory tract and lung and those involving body defences. The diagnosis hinges on the clinical signs, the chest radiograph and microbiology. During spontaneous respiration, the breathing pattern and signs of retained secretions are key observations (Chapter 6). During IPPV the mechanical properties of the lung, clinical signs of increased secretions (the chest physiotherapist often scores here); purulent tracheal aspirate and a worsening of gas exchange all point to infection. Unfortunately, the systemic signs are less dependable because we are usually dealing with the post-surgical or injured. But the temperature chart and white cell count are still essential monitoring as we shall see later. When a chest radiograph shows absorption collapse or consolidation (homogeneous shadowing with air bronchogram) an infection is assumed to be the cause until proved wrong. Daily microbiological examination of the sputum or tracheal aspirate are essential for diagnosis and treatment. The results of Gram staining will give a clue to the pathogens (Table 27.16) pending their isolation by culture. The critical step in diagnosis has now been reached. Are the bacteria (or fungi) colonists or invaders? The decision is based on all the evidence outlined above, together with quantitative bacteriology. The signs of infection are a leucocyte count greater than 25 organisms per high power field or a bacterial count of more than 10^5 organisms per ml of the sample.

The therapeutic plan consists of the now familiar packages. Examples are intensive chest physiotherapy with analgesia; oxygen therapy, starting IPPV because of exhaustion and lack of sleep and antimicrobials. The latter are necessary but by themselves will not get the patient better; choosing the correct drug is guided by an algorithm (Figure 27.1). The indications for starting antibiotics should be worked out by consensus and published. Our own are given in Table 27.17. The drugs are given i.v. in doses according to body weight. For gentamicin and tobramycin, the dose is adjusted according to the blood levels. Bacterial monitoring already in progress is

Table 27.18 A guide to the origin and cause of bacteraemia

Site	Pathogen	
	Community acquired	*Hospital acquired*
Boils, carbuncles, osteomyelitis	*S. aureus*	*S. aureus*
Burns, i.v. lines	*S.* spp.	staphylococci, enterobacteriae, pseudomonads
Mastoiditis, pneumonia cellulitis	*S. pyogenes* pneumococci	Enterobacteriae, pseudomonads
Urinary tract	*E. coli, S. faecalis*	Enterobacteriae, pseudomonads, enterococci
Genital tract, appendix, colon, gallbladder	Gram negative bacteria, *S. faecalis,* *Bacteroides* spp., *C.* spp.	Enterobacteriae pseudomonads *Bacteroides* spp. *C.* spp.

continued and alarm bells sounded when superinfection by bacteria or fungi appears. Errors are easily made and invariably increase the morbidity and mortality; starting too late or too early and continuing drugs too long can spell disaster.

2. Intra-abdominal

At least we know where the bugs come from! Bruising or perforation of the colon are the result of trauma or primary colonic disease, diverticular, neoplastic, inflammatory bowel disease and so on. Peritoneal dialysis can be complicated by peritonitis, largely avoidable. It is no surprise that peritonitis arising from the colon is caused by a mixture of bacteria (Table 27.16) clearly relevant to antibiotic treatment.

Before even contemplating resuscitation or intensive care, predictions are quickly made of both short- and long-term outcome. Such procedures are incorporated in the criteria for intensive care already published for the hospital. The existing diseases and age (CHE) of the APACHE scheme (Chapter 19) influence the decisions, but the crucial question is can immediate surgery cure? Intensive care of the system failures, shock, respiratory or renal failure are quite unjustified unless the leaking bowel or abscesses can be dealt with immediately. No patient is too ill for surgery!

A combination of antimicrobials are given blind, according to the con sensus policy. These can be altered by the results of specimens taken a laparotomy. Even with appropriate patient selection, the cause of th disease during intensive care will not invariably be favourable. The bod systems are monitored and treatment given as described in the precedin chapters. The worst APACHE score within the first 24 hours will provide predicated risk of death, which coupled with clinical judgement, will allow an answer to other essential questions. It is justified to continue intensiv care? Is the intensive therapy of a further system failure justified?

3. Biliary tract

The life threatening problems are cholangitis with bacteraemia or bacteria toxaemia. These are secondary to chronic cholecystitis with or withou gallstones. The likely pathogens are shown in Table 27.16. A diagnosis i clinical and after taking blood cultures antimicrobials are given i.v.

4. Urinary tract

The newcomer to intensive care will already have experience of the chroni diseases, obstruction, or calculi. Severe pyelonephritis with bacteraemia o toxaemia can maim or kill by causing failure of one or more body systems Diagnosis is essentially clinical, confirmed by finding pathological bacteri uria – more than 10^5 bacteria/ml of urine. The likely pathogens are listed i Table 27.16 together with the antimicrobial therapy. Finally, we woul emphasize the importance of prophylactic antibiotics given before an during surgery on an infected urinary tract.

Dr HKF van Saene assisted with this chapter.

28
The blood

Restoring and maintaining the chemistry of the blood was described in Chapters 16–25 leaving a few diverse therapies to this brief chapter.

I BLOOD TRANSFUSIONS

The supply of blood for transfusion is, in both countries, organized on a regional basis and administered centrally by the Health Departments in the UK by the Red Cross in Australia. Banked blood is given to restore the capacity to carry oxygen and to replace volume lost by haemorrhage; the content of platelets and white cells are negligible. The products available from the two services are given in Table 28.1. Banked blood for haemorrhage is given by a peripheral or central line and when possible the blood is warmed to 37°C. The transfusion is monitored by measuring the central venous pressure, arterial blood pressure and skin temperature (Chapter 20). Massive blood transfusions, that is more than five in 24 h, are hazardous but nearly always avoidable by the right surgery at the right time by the right surgeon. The changes in the patient's blood resulting from a massive transfusion are variable and reflect the severity and duration of accompanying shock. It follows that for each patient the changes will be diagnosed by measurement and cannot be predicted. A recurring pattern would be thrombocytopenia, a depletion of some clotting factors and a fall in plasma ionized calcium; the latter is due to the citrate used as an anticoagulant. The important clinical issue is haemorrhage. Since the primary haemorrhage has an obvious cause, then further bleeding due to a transfusion coagulopathy is easily missed. Regular haematological measurements are the order of the day (or night!) so that the coagulopathy can be quickly corrected. Three treatments are available; platelet concentrates, clotting factors and calcium. Here is a standardized scheme which assumes that if surgery is

Table 28.1 Blood products used during intensive care

Citrated whole blood

Red cell concentrate

Red cell concentrate diluted with nutrient

Platelet concentrate

Fresh frozen plasma (FFP)

Cryoprecipitate

Dried factors VII, VIII, IX and XIII

Stabilized plasma protein solution (SPPS)

Albumin solutions: 4.5, 5, 20 and 25%

required to stop bleeding it will be prompt and expert. (a) Platelets are infused to maintain a count of about 30×10^9/l. Should bleeding due to coagulopathy continue, then infusions are given to bring the count up to 80 $\times 10^9$/l. (b) Fresh frozen plasma is used to correct a deficiency of clotting factors and to then maintain safe concentrations. This coagulopathy is readily diagnosed and monitored by measuring the prothrombin time and expressing this as a ratio of patient to healthy control; the Prothrombin International Normalized Ratio (INR). When the INR exceeds 2.0 or is less than 2.0 but the bleeding continues, then 2 or 3 units of FFP are infused and the INR again measured. (c) Calcium is given i.v. as the chloride or gluconate, with or without laboratory measurements. The ionized calcium in the plasma can be measured in about ten minutes and calcium given i.v. to maintain a normal concentration of 1.3 mmol/l. The alternative is to give calcium 'blind' whenever blood is transfused at a rate faster than 100 ml/min; the dose is 500 mg of calcium chloride or 3 g of gluconate per unit of blood. The second indication for blood transfusion is anaemia which develops following injury or sepsis. This is due to a metabolic failure – deficient synthesis of haemoglobin – and occurs despite appropriate nutrition including all the haematinics. Oxygen transport is so vital to the ICU patient that the concentration of haemoglobin must be maintained above a critical level. But what is this critical concentration? The true answer is unknown, although armchair science abounds! Our practice is to transfuse blood at intervals to maintain the haemoglobin above 10.0 g/dl.

II INFUSIONS OF PROTEIN

Deficient protein synthesis and accelerated catabolism affect the plasma protein, immunoglobulins and much else. A third pathological process is at work especially during bacterial toxaemia or widespread hypoxia. This is capillary leak, not only of electrolyte but of plasma protein. In health the osmotic force exerted by the plasma albumin maintains the delicate balance between the pressure in the capillaries and that of interstitial fluid. This balance is crucial in the lung; a fall in the plasma osmotic pressure means that ECF can more readily pass into the alveoli; pulmonary oedema is one of the intensive care nightmares. The aim of treatment therefore is to maintain the plasma proteins (back to the milieu intérieur again) and to keep the serum albumin above 30 g/l. Unfortunately, since we can neither accelerate synthesis nor stop capillary leak, we are left with infusions of protein, listed in Table 28.1.

III BLOOD THERAPY OF DISSEMINATED INTRA-VASCULAR COAGULATION

Three blood products, together with heparin are part of the therapeutic plan for disseminated intra-vascular coagulation (DIC, Chapter 13). The other therapeutic packages depend on the systems involved; IPPV or dialysis for example. The DIC which can follow injury or infection differs greatly from the obstetric type and the blood therapy of each is described separately. The coagulopathies which can follow cardio-pulmonary bypass or burns are outside the scope of this book.

1. DIC of trauma or infection

Tissue damage, shock, or infection trigger off the consumption of clotting factors and platelets (consumptive coagulopathy) which is easily diagnosed by blood tests. This process may in turn be related to widespread thrombosis in the capillary circulation (DIC) causing failure of one or more organs; the latter is nearly impossible to diagnose because the organ failure can be directly caused by the trauma or infection which also set of the DIC! Testing the value of treatment is further compounded by the fact that the consumptive coagulopathy, and possibly the DIC, is often self-curing. This digression is necessary for the novice to grasp that the blood therapy needs viewing with scepticism. There are no agreed quantitative criteria for diagnosis and none for therapy.

Removing the precipitating factors is more important than the blood therapy, so no excuse is needed for listing them: shock, acidosis, infection, devitalized tissue or manipulation of injured limbs. The blood therapy consists of giving clotting factors with or without heparin. (a) When there is haemorrhage due to consumption, the PTT and the aPTT will be prolonged, even the WBCT likewise. These signs are indications when transfusing clotting factors as FFP, two units to start with and the tests are repeated. (b) The second line of blood therapy is heparin. The actions of heparin in health and disease led to an attractive hypothesis; this agent would prevent intravascular coagulation in the capillaries. The idea was enthusiastically put into practice for some twenty years but proof of benefit by controlled trial was lacking. Anecdotes suggested that heparin arrested the consumption of platelets and clotting factors but it seems that 'nature healed and doctor took the credit'. Heparin is therefore not routinely given but we have included a brief description of the method. The drug is given as a continuous i.v. infusion using a mechanical pump. During DIC the dose cannot be predicted and the therapy is monitored by twice daily measurements of the WBCT or aPTT. The former can be carried out at the bedside; only a glass tube and a water bath at 37°C are required. The aPTT is measured in the hospital laboratory, which must know the sensitivity of its reagent and hence establish the therapeutic range. The most practical procedure is to start with an infusion rate of 750–1000 units per hour and adjust the dose according to the test. Using the WBCT, this should be prolonged to between two and three times the normal (8–10 minutes). The required prolongation of the aPTT varies according to the reagent; an example would be 1.3–1.5 fold. The beginner to clotology must be aware of the pitfalls in the interpretation of blood tests during heparin therapy. A good policy is to keep the monitoring as simple as possible. Favourable trends are a rise in the platelet count and of less value a fall in the fibrin degradation products (FDP). The heparin therapy lasts weeks rather than days.

2. DIC of obstetrics

This is rare and, like all rare conditions, likely to be missed. When diagnosis is delayed or treatment inadequate, then life threatening respiratory and renal failure ensue. With the exception of the mildest cases the patient needs all the resources of a general ICU, including intra-vascular monitoring. The strategy is to remove the cause, correct the haemorrhage and coagulopathy and treat the failure of any other systems. Since the DIC is triggered off by the foetus, the pregnancy has to be terminated, preferably by the genital delivery, if not by Caesarean section; the latter cannot be done until the blood is made coaguable.

The blood therapy must be given according to the circulatory and haematological findings, and not in a haphazard manner. The blood products required are three in number; citrated whole blood, platelet concentrate and FFP, the latter providing all clotting factors. The blood transfusion is monitored by measuring the pulmonary artery pressure, (PAP) and pulmonary artery wedge pressure, (PAWP) using the Swan-Ganz technique (Chapter 7). The reason for this is that the CVP will not guarantee that the patient is not over-transfused (pulmonary oedema), or under-transfused (oliguric renal failure). The coagulopathy is monitored 4-hourly by measuring the following: platelets, fibrinogen, PT and aPTT. Heparin was formerly given as for the DIC of trauma or sepsis, but its use is now restricted to the rare event of a retained dead foetus. The early recognition of ARDS depends on the breathing pattern (Chapter 6) finding hypoxaemia and, of less value, the chest X-ray. The diagnosis cannot be made unless the team can be certain that the patient has not been over-transfused – hence the measurements of the PAWP. The coagulopathy of obstetrics is self-limiting when the cause has been removed. The exception is when secondary uterine infection occurs. The overall aim is the survival of the mother without physical disability; the wounds of the psyche may never heal but can be ameliorated by counselling, started as early as possible.

IV ANTICOAGULANTS FOR THROMBOEMBOLISM

From the rare to the almost universal disturbance, the hypercoagulable state and its lethal consequence, pulmonary embolism. In elective surgery, both morbidity and mortality can be reduced by preventive treatment. This consists of low dosage heparin, started before the operation and continued afterwards. The scheme is simplicity itself. Subcutaneous heparin, 5000 units at intervals of 8 or 12 hours; laboratory control is unnecessary. Can this therapy help the intensive care patient? It is likely that low dose heparin would reduce the incidence of deep venous thrombosis and pulmonary embolism but this has not been proved by trial. Unfortunately, this treatment cannot be started before the onset of the illness. We give low dose heparin to the long-haul intensive care patients; examples are crushed chest and the Guillain-Barré syndrome. When a deep venous thrombosis is diagnosed clinically, then this is treated by continuous i.v. heparin, controlled by measurements of the HBCT or aPTT. Pulmonary embolism occurring in an intermediate care ward or A & E department requires admission to the ICU when there is shock.

Table 28.2 Thrombolytic therapy for acute myocardial infarction: two alternative schemes (Royal Prince Alfred hospital)

Streptokinase:
Loading dose; 250 000 units of streptokinase, diluted in glucose or saline are given i.v. over 10 min. This is followed by an infusion of 1.25 million units over 50 min. Thus the total dose is 1.5 million units.

Tissue-type Plasminogen Activator (TPA):
The initial dose is a bolus of 10 mg diluted in water. This is followed by an infusion of TPA diluted in 1.0 mg/ml. In the first hour 50 mg are given and then 20 mg/h for 2 h. Thus, the total dose is 100 mg.
There are similar therapeutic plans for pulmonary embolism and thrombotic strokes.

V THROMBOLYTIC THERAPY

When a thrombus occludes a vein or artery the idea of dissolving the clot and restoring blood flow has great merits. Numerous trials in pulmonary embolism which threatened life did not lead to the widespread use of this treatment. Benefits do result from thrombolysis in acute myocardial infarction when the treatment is started within four hours of the onset; two schemes are given in Table 28.2.

ACKNOWLEDGEMENTS

We are grateful to Dr B. J. Bain and Dr A. J. N. Shepherd for their help with this Chapter.

29

Intensive care of the injured

A society that does not care for its injured has
no right to call itself civilised.

Henry Miller

The sedated patient lies quietly in bed and his
shallow paradoxical movements escape critical notice.
But death steps in suddenly, peacefully, naturally
and unnecessarily.

N. R. Barrett, 1960

I	**PRIMARY CARE**
II	**HEAD INJURIES**
III	**CHEST INJURIES**
IV	**ABDOMINAL INJURIES, INCLUDING THE PELVIS**
V	**THE REVISED TRAUMA SCORE**

I PRIMARY CARE

Blankets and sweetened tea – nothing could be worse! If the primary care given to the injured civilian, inside or outside the home, was of a uniform high standard then the intensive care which follows would benefit many more patients. Stated the other way round, intensive care cannot retrieve the damage caused by delay in starting treatment or make good for errors or omissions. Primary care is very simple and can be given by paramedics or qualified nurses or doctors. The two critical factors are a prompt start – within the golden hour as the Yanks have it – and the resuscitation should be given before transportation to hospital. We offer not excuse for summarizing the primary care of the injured. The essentials come first – A, B, C; A is for airway, B is for breathing, C for circulation. These topics have been dealt with in preceding chapters and the remaining treatments are listed in Table 29.1. But the appropriate use of the ET tube must again be emphasized. This is readily done by a teaching quote from Malcolm Wright: "It is fallacious to think that intubation is not needed because the patient resists this procedure".

Finally, a word on the major civilian disaster. Obviously more personnel are required to carry out primary care, extricate the trapped and transport the survivors. It is equally important that the person in charge of the primary

Table 29.1 Primary care of the severely injured

Rususcitation	
Airway	Brook airway or ET tube
Breathing	Ambu bag, oxygen
Circulation	Drip set, polygeline
Pain	i.v. morphine; record dose on label or skin
External haemorrhage	Pressure bandages
Limb fractures suspect	Immobilize with splints
Impaired consciousness	A and B of above Assume cervical spine injury and immobilize the neck
Burns	i.v. fluid therapy Airway protection for burns of the respiratory tract
Drug list	Morphine i.v. ketamine for on-site amputation Diazepam for hysteria in the non-injured

care is ble to speak by radio-telephone to the area hospitals. In the UK, where distances are short, the patients likely to need intensive care can be allocated to two or three hospitals, so that not more than five such patients are sent to any one ICU. Those with spinal injuries or burns should reach specialist centres as soon as possible following resuscitation.

II HEAD INJURIES

I. Strategy

General intensive care in the DGH can only be effective (long term survival with independence) when integrated with every department of the hospital. This applies to the head-injured, but, in addition, neurosurgery may be necessary. Although the criteria for this are clear-cut, the organization often fails, resulting in avoidable morbidity and mortality. Without an effective liaison between neurosurgical unit and general ICU the patients' suffer and the medical staff indulge in acrimonious mud slinging. The ultimate hypocrisy was a paper published by neurosurgeons blaming the district ICUs for not referring the patients at the right time; this from a centre which found every reason not to admit! No such problems exist at the RPA hospital which has a regional neurosurgical unit. The problems created by the transfer of patients is therefore avoided and continuity of medical care is assured by the three staff specialists of intensive care. The strategy is straight forward and given in Figure 29.1. At the site of the accident the resuscitation will have ensured a clear airway and prevent hypoxia – what is called the second insult. In the unconscious, the brain can be damaged further by shock, hypercapnia, over-transfusion and head-down tilt. A word on pain. This should be relieved whatever the severity of the head injury; unconscious patients still feel pain!

The hospital assessment is quick and easy. The conscious patient with normal cognition has X-rays of the skull (but not by a portable machine). When no fracture is found then the patient can be taken home. In contrast, when there is a fracture the patient is admitted, even in the absence of signs. This is because there is a high risk of an expanding intracranial haematoma. The observations can be made in any ward staffed by nursed trained to use the G.C.S. Turning next to those with brain failure – impaired consciousness, delirium or convulsions – the question is asked and quickly answered: is the patient likely to benefit from intensive care or are they too ill to benefit? An elderly person with significant previous disability and a GCS of three is not for intensive care. The doctor carrying out the assessment will have the criteria for intensive care at hand and fruitless debate and long telephone calls are thus unnecessary.

2. Intensive care

When a patient fulfils the criteria for intensive care, then the next essential is a CT scan to determine whether or not there is an intracranial haematoma. When one or more is found it is then decided if urgent removal is likely to result in improvement. Surgery or no surgery, intensive care is continued and the numerous therapeutic packages are planned: long term airway care, nutrition and so on. The neurological monitoring comprises the GCS and the pupils. Monitoring the intracranial pressure (ICP) has been tried because we know that a raised pressure is harmful and lowering the pressure might be beneficial. However, ICP monitoring presents a problem of patient selection, not yet resolved. What we need to know is which patients will benefit.

3. Additional treatment

Preserving the milieu intérieur (Chapters 16, 17) and neurosurgery are the corner-stones of therapy. But the feeling of therapeutic frustration has born additional therapies, all hazardous, some dangerous. The osmotic diuretic

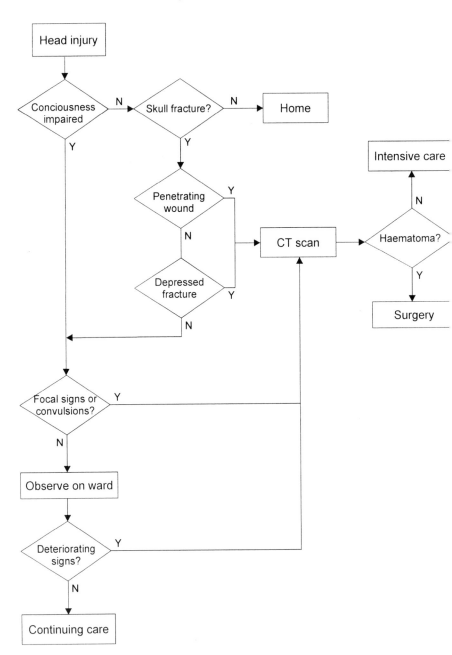

Figure 29.1 Strategy for the head-injured

Table 29.2 Initial classification of closed chest injuries (After Moore, 1977)

Grade I	Mild	can ventilate can cough
Grade II	Moderate	can ventilate cannot cough
Grade III	Severe	cannot ventilate cannot cough

manitol can reduce the ICP. A single dose of 500 ml of 20% given over 24 hours is safe, but should not be repeated. Other treatments given are: IPPV to induce hypocapnia with the aim of reducing brain swelling, steroids (the pharmacological last rites), induced hypothermia, and, lastly, induced barbiturate coma. These treatments, while potentially beneficial in small numbers of patients with head injury, have not been shown to be so in large series of patients with head injuries of varying severity. This conclusion is supported by substantial observations summarized in a Rock Carling lecture (Jennett, 1984).

III CHEST INJURIES

1. Strategy

Resuscitation, started at the site of the accident, is continued in the A & E department. In the UK and Australia about 10% of the patients have penetrating wounds and require transfer to a thoracic surgical unit, but not before one or more chest drains have been inserted. As described later, a few patients with non-penetrating injuries will need thoracic surgery at a later stage when additional lesions are diagnosed. The next task is to place the injuries into one of three grades (Table 29.2); this only takes a minute or so. We are now in a position to make the second major management decision: is IPPV needed immediately? A patient in grade III certainly needs tracheal intubation and IPPV, manual if necessary until transferred to the ICU. But there are other indications for immediate IPPV, equally important. These can be grouped as thoracic and extra-thoracic and are listed in Table 29.3. A graded patient has now arrived in the ICU and we would emphasize that the time spent in the A & E should be less than one hour; delay harms or kills.

Table 29.3 Indication for IPPV (After Wright, 1982)

A   Thoracic
 1   Flail chest with serious paradoxical movement (Grade III)
 2   Lung contusions causing respiratory failure
 3   Bleeding from the airway
 4   Absent or weak cough (Grades II and III)
 5   Imminent general anaesthesia

B   Extrathoracic
 1   Coma or impaired consciousness
 2   Delirium
 3   Vomiting
 4   Serious injuries to the abdomen, pelvis or limbs
 5   Imminent general anaesthesia

2. Pneumothorax and haemothorax

It is not surprising that the penetrating wound of the thorax should cause a pneumothorax, but this also commonly follows a closed injury. The pneumothorax can usually be attributed to a rib fracture, but on occasion, no fracture can be seen on X-ray. In addition to a lung puncture allowing air to enter the pleural sac, the air may also appear in the tissues of the chest wall and mediastinum. Surgical emphysema is obvious clinically and may spread alarmingly in the fascial planes and under the skin to involve the abdominal wall, and head and neck. A pneumothorax following a chest injury may on the one hand prove an immediate threat to life, or pass unnoticed until the first radiograph is examined. It follows that the treatment of a pneumothorax occupies a variable place in the priority list. Two examples may illustrate the point. (a) A patient with extreme breathlessness shows no paradox, but one side of the chest moves less than the opposite side and the breath sounds are faint. If the blood pressure is normal a radiograph of the chest is taken before starting treatment. When the blood pressure is low a tension pneumothorax is probable and the affected side should be quickly explored with a cannula inserted into the second or third rib space anteriorly. If air under tension can be heard to escape through the needle, the diagnosis was correct. The cannula is removed and the pleural cavity drained by means of a rubber or plastic catheter fitted with an underwater seal. (b) In the second case, severe crushing injuries required IPPV to correct severe hypoxaemia and to stabilize the chest. A radiograph showed multiple rib fractures, homogeneous shadowing in the mid and lower zones of the lung and a small pneumothorax; these signs were unilateral. Although the pneumothorax is a relatively unimportant cause of the severe hypoxaemia, nevertheless the affected pleural cavity should be drained until the lung is fully expanded. The drain should be inserted through the second or third rib space in the mid-clavicular line. Following blunt dissection through the chest wall, a cannula is inserted into the pleural space. A catheter is next introduced and connected to the customary underwater seal. The latter are usually made up in the ICU preparation room and kept at the ready. An alternative is to purchase a stock of commercial sets. Sterile water is used to make the seal and the height of the water must not exceed 5.0 cm above the lower end of the drain tube. Also, it must be possible to read the volume of fluid (water plus exudate) in the bottle. An important feature of the system is that the tubing connecting the catheter to the bottle should be elastic so that compression between finger and thumb (or a pair of rollers) will propel fluid from the pleural space to the bottle. When the air has been drained, the fluid level will show a respiratory swing but air will no longer bubble. At this time a radiograph is taken to confirm that the lung has expanded. The drainage system will require observation and milking of the tube at hourly intervals; obsessional observation is the order of the day. A blocked drainage tube requires immediate attention. The management of a pneumothorax has deliberately been laboured because errors and omissions can easily kill the patient.

There are two reasons why it is essential to drain a haemothorax (or two). The fluid will reduce ventilatory capacity (and cause long term burdens) and it is vital to make certain that the haemorrhage stops. The equipment is that used for a pneumothorax. One or two drains are inserted in the posterior auxiliary line below the inferior angle of the scapula. Should the haemorrhage continue, further blood transfusions will not seal the torn blood vessel – only a thoracic surgeon can do this.

3. Management according to grade

The dominant cause of morbidity in chest wall injuries is pain, and its relief is the fulcrum upon which overall management rests. Pain causes shallow breathing and inhibits effective coughing; absorption collapse results. Powerful analgesics will control pain but there comes a point when the side-effects are dangerous; ventilation is reduced*, cough suppressed and

---

* Self-assessment for the trainee doctor. How would you demonstrate to nurses or medical students that a single dose of morphine or pethidine affects ventilation?

Table 29.4 Clinical features and therapy according to grade (After Wright, 1982)

Clinical features	Grade I	Grade II	Grade III
Chest wall injury	minor flail	obvious flail	severe flail
Lung injury	minimal	contused	contused
Other injury	moderate limb damage	extensive limb damage	laparotomy visceral injury
General condition	stable	unstable	unstable
Gastrointestinal function	mobile gut	ileus	ileus
Head injury	absent	minor	significant
Patient co-operation	good	poor	absent
Spinal injury	absent	usually absent	often present
Pre-existing lung disease	absent	present	present
Mode of treatment			
Airway support	not required	may need tracheostomy	will need tracheostomy
Ventilator	not needed	not needed	always used
Mobility	ambulant if feasible	bed fast	bed fast
Physiotherapy	active	active	passive
Analgesia	simple oral	narcotics	narcotics
Regional block	intercostal	intercostal, thoracic extradural	thoracic extradural

somnolence prevents co-operation with essential nursing and physiotherapy. When this point is reached, then IPPV is essential.

Grade 1. The clinical findings and management are summarized in Table 29.4. The essentials are three in number: the control of pain by mild analgesics, regional anaesthesia and Entonox; early mobilization and, lastly, chest physiotherapy. The first task is to explain the plan to the patient, without whose determination and co-operation the treatment is bound to fail. Paracetamol or aspirin are given two hourly. Narcotics are used sparingly in the day time and liberally at night. Intercostal block is induced with bupivacaine and Entonox is inhaled during chest physiotherapy. To facilitate mobilization, all unnecessary cannulae catheters are removed. The patient is instructed to move about the bed, sit up, stand and subsequently walk a few steps. The final essential is chest physiotherapy, given by a team of specialists three times a day, every day. This vital treatment is to prevent, as well as treat, retained secretions and absorption collapse. Two mechanical aids are valuable adjects. A patient triggered ventilator will provide large tidal volumes and help to prevent collapse; this passive IPPB causes less pain than does voluntary deep breathing. In addition, we have long used an incentive spirometer. This simple device (Triflo-II, Cheseborough Ponds, Inc. US) enables both patient and therapist to hear and see full ventilatory capacity.

This therapeutic plan lasts weeks, when the chest wall becomes stable, the lung fields are as clear as they ever will be and the patient can cough effectively. It must not be thought that the treatment is second quality or a cheap alternative to IPPV. Indeed the plan is as labour intensive as IPPV and few hospitals can give the treatment outside their ICU.

Grade II. Damage to the thoracic cage and lung are more severe and there are serious problems outside the chest (Table 29.5). Even so, IPPV is not immediately essential, but may become necessary within forty-eight hours. During this critical period the pathophysiology of both thoracic cage and lung can increase leading to worsening respiratory failure. The therapeutic plan consists of continuous oxygen therapy, continuous i.v. morphine (2–4 mg/kg/hour), chest physiotherapy and possibly a tracheostomy to keep the airways clear. Pain relief – prevention is better – in this and the next grade of chest injury is achieved by continuous extradural anaesthesia. In addition to this respiratory package, much additional monitoring and therapy are essential; a metabolic balance and intravenous nutrition to list just two. When the signs – chiefly those gained at the bedside – indicate worsening, then IPPV is started without hesitation or recrimination. In those not requiring IPPV the healing process takes two to three weeks.

Grade III. IPPV is started as soon as possible because of one or more flail segments. The patient can neither ventilate nor cough. In this grade there are frequently extra thoracic problems which also threaten life (Table 29.4). Tracheostomy is carried out within 12 hours and an appropriate ventilatory programme is carried through (Section 4). Extensive monitoring is essential together with intravenous nutrition and low dose dopamine.

Table 29.5 Ventilator therapy of crushed chest; summary of treatment and monitoring

Stage of treatment	Treatment	Monitoring
Resuscitation	Relief of pain Intravenous infusions Anaesthesia/manual IPPV with O_2 Chest drainage	BP and CVP every few minutes. Oximetry Skin temperature Hourly urine volume, chest X-ray, ECG
First 48 h of mechanical IPPV	Controlled IPPV Tracheostomy Chest drainage Endotracheal suction IV nutrition Physiotherapy	Continuous BP, pulse. Oximetry Ventilator readings Blood gases once or twice daily Chest X-ray daily and immediately after tracheostomy Metabolic balance for water, sodium and potassium WCC, Hb, urea, sugar Bacterial monitoring of nose, throat and tracheal aspirate
Subsequent mechanical IPPV	Controlled IPPV Later IMV or triggered IPPV Endotracheal suction Physiotherapy Tube feeding Treatment of the complications, e.g. antibiotics or diuretics Pleural aspiration	As above

4. Ventilatory programme

Before describing the method, the beginner should know how the method enables the stove-in chest to heal with minimal long-term deformity. To understand this application of IPPV it is only necessary to recall that the indrawing (paradoxical movement) of the flail segment occurs because inspiration is negative (sub-atmospheric) pressure breathing (Chapter 19). Hence, when IPPV – that is positive pressure breathing – is substituted for spontaneous breathing, the flail segment will no longer paradox but will move with the adjoining chest wall. All the ribs will move in the normal manner and the adjoining ends of the fractured ribs will remain in rough apposition forming strong calluses within 10 to 13 days. IPPV therefore restores the proper movements of the thoracic wall by a process of 'internal pneumatic stabilization' as the originators so aptly termed their method. The first case record of this use of controlled IPPV was published in 1955 and this classic in the annals of intensive therapy still repays study. The summary merits repetition here: 'The most striking benefits of this mechanical hyperventilation treatment were: correction of all paradoxical motion of the chest; removal of all hypoxia and hypercapnia; absence of pulmonary oedema; hyperventilation analgesia requiring less sedation; no serious deviations in blood chemistry with prolonged mild respiratory alkalosis; prompt return of blood chemistry and physiological responses to normal with cessation of hyperventilation; no late ill-effects; and, of course, the survival of this patient with a seemingly hopeless prognosis' (Avery, Mörch, Head and Benson, 1955).

In Chapter 19 it was explained that, although ventilator treatment depends on the principle of IPPV, the technique is varied considerably according to the disease. This is true even when the same machine is used in the different diseases. When treating the crushed chest low frequencies and large tidal volumes gives excellent results. On rare occasions artificial respiration must be started within minutes of the first assessment; more commonly IPPV is started after a more thorough and more leisurely period of observation. In this instance an intravenous infusion has been set up, pain relieved and the patient is breathing oxygen from a mask (Chapter 18). The patient is dogmatically reassured and the future treatment outlined. Anaesthesia is next induced and a rapid sequence induction is mandatory. Two points should be recalled, to use the minimum dose and to show patience, because the arm-to-brain time may be prolonged, thus delaying the onset of anaesthesia. The anaesthesia is quickly followed by the muscle relaxant suxamethonium (1.0 mg/kg) and the trachea intubated with a low pressure ET tube, an assistant exerting pressure on the cricoid cartilage. Manual IPPV is started with oxygen and the trachea aspirated. Ventilation is increased progressively, an assistant closely observing the blood pressure and pulse volume. Pancuronium 4 or 6 mg is given to continue total muscle paralysis. Mechanical IPPV is next started. Our hundred years combined experience dictates the use of a front-line ventilator; by this is meant a machine which is safe, reliable, well-tried and easy to use. Examples are the Servovent (Siemens) and the Erica (Datex-Engstrom). For one of these the V_T is pre-set to 10–12 ml/kg, frequency of 12 and an F_1O_2 of 50. The clinician now closely checks the chest movement for equal expansion – the flail segment will no longer show paradox. The circulation and urine flow are also observed. If IPPV leads to hypotension, the V_T is quickly reduced to 8 ml/kg. The CVP is next read taking into account the effects of IPPV. If low or normal, colloid is infused until the blood pressure is restored. The V_T is again increased to 10–12 ml/kg. Chest drains are next inserted unless these are already in place. We will invariably insert a drain on the injured side(s) even in the absence of a pneumothorax. The reason for this is that there is a significant chance of a tension pneumothorax occurring after starting IPPV and this can kill before it is recognized. A haemothorax is also drained. A further chest radiograph is taken and the following points are noted: position of the lower end of the E-T tube; pneumothorax, absorption collapse position of the CVP catheter and chest drains. Adjustments or new measures are made according to the findings. After about one hour of mechanical IPPV the blood gases are measured. One would hope to find a high pH (respiratory alkalosis) moderate hypocapnia and a normal or high PaO_2. Should this favourable result occur then the ventilator settings are left alone, except when the PaO_2 is above normal in which case the F_IO_2 is reduced to 30%. If on the other hand the $PaCO_2$ is normal or high, then the tidal volume is increased and the blood gases analysed after 15 min. Hypoxaemia during IPPV with 50% oxygen is a depressing sign and demands urgent investigation of the lung and circulation. The beginner in intensive care will need a check list, concentrating firstly on the treatable conditions rather than haematomas, which only nature can heal. Look for and then treat retained secretions, pneumothorax, haemothorax and pulmonary oedema. Then concentrate on the signs of a low cardiac output and select the correct therapy, infusions of colloid, dopamine or both (Chapter 7). When these measures are not applicable or have failed, then the F_IO_2 can be increased to 70 and/or PEEP tried. Try is the right word; the PaO_2 will certainly rise but the PEEP may cause harmful hypotension. If the circulation can tolerate 10 cm of PEEP but the PaO_2 is below 7.0 kPa (53 mmHg) then increase the PEEP in increments of 5 cm.

Having successfully negotiated the first few hours of IPPV attention can be diverted to plan the other aspects of intensive care; monitoring, sedation, physiotherapy, fluid therapy and nutrition. After 8–12 h of IPPV the V_T is adjusted to keep the $PaCO_2$ in the range of 4.0–5.0 kPa. To achieve this aim the $\dot{V}_E$ will be in the range of 15–20 litres depending on the body weight and the metabolic rate. The latter will have increased during the 8–12 h following the injury and accordingly the total ventilation will have to be increased. The V_T is increased in steps every 10 min and the blood gases are measured when the $\dot{V}_E$ is 15–20 litres.

We have now reached day two of IPPV and a tracheostomy is performed. Following this step the use of a muscle relaxant is drastically curtailed. The dose and frequency of the drug is reduced and it may be possible to limit the relaxant to occasional use. This is a big step forward, because communication with the patient is greatly improved. Sedation is continued with phenoperidine or papaveretum. Whilst on the topic of sedation it should be emphasized that sleep is a real problem. Prolonged natural sleep is impossible during ventilator treatment. Unfortunately, there is no universally satisfactory hypnotic and trial and error is needed. We try one of the following, often ringing the changes; phenoperidine, morphine and papaveretum.

The ventilator treatment is now on a set course of some 5–20 days and both the observations and treatments follow a predetermined plan summarized in Table 29.5. Treating the crushed chest is a classical example of intensive care and therapy. At least one specifically-trained nurse is with the patient at all times; every facet of the care requires obsessional attention; to the patients fears, discomforts and distress; the care of the largely helpless but conscious being; IPPV and tracheostomy care; metabolic balance. A time and motion study showed that there was something to do for the patient for 50 min of each hour, round the clock. When all goes according to plan, most of the observations and most of the treatment are given by the nursing team. Two points are singled out for consideration. It is clearly undesirable to allow the flail segments to paradox frequently and this will occur during coughing or fighting the respirator. In consequence these are avoided as much as possible by the use of phenoperidine and if necessary a relaxant also. In the absence of an expulsive cough, bronchial secretions will accumulate and are removed by a combination of postural drainage, chest physiotherapy and bagging and suction. At least twice a day the bed is tilted head down and after an hour in this position the nurses and physiotherapist clear the major bronchi. When the secretions are thick and tenacious, intratracheal saline is injected (5 ml aliquots) during the bagging and suction. The second point concerns the positioning of the patient. By day 3, the trunk should be inclined to about 30° to the horizontal except during the periods of drainage or during sleep. This posture often avoids fighting the respirator and always improves morale. If however, intensive treatment with muscle relaxant is required, the patient is kept in the flat posture. By the fifth day, unless contraindicated by injuries to bones or joints, the IPPV is continued with the patient sitting in an armchair for an hour or so. Radio or television are arranged if the patient so wishes. The clinician reviews the patient at each of the regular unit rounds; 0900, 1200, 2230 hours. The first task of the assessment is the reassurance of the patient and enquiries regarding pain and sleep. There follows a systematic examination of the body systems, the chest drains and the respirator. The medical team now withdraw from the patient's room or area to consider the data obtained during the preceding period. The main contents of this check list are given in Table 29.5. When ventilator treatment of the crushed chest proceeds without serious set-backs a stage is reached when the chest drains can be removed and at a later date the IPPV can be stopped. Indications for the removal of a chest drain are: the lung has expanded and remained so for 72 h and the drain shows a respiratory swing but there is no blow; when a haemothorax has been largely drained and bleeding is slight; a blocked drain is useless and replaced when necessary.

Ventilator treatment is first changed from the controlled type to IMV or patient triggered and then discontinued altogether. From the fifth day onwards the chest wall is examined daily during spontaneous respiration. Clearly, prior to this examination muscle relaxant and sedative are stopped. The observations concentrate on the pattern of breathing, the degree of paradox and whether cyanosis develops. Controlled IPPV is stopped when (a) a breathing pattern is normal or increased but the patient can alter the pattern at will and can take deep slow breaths. (b) A cough will expel secretion to the tracheostomy. (c) Paradox is absent. (d) Hypoxaemia is moderate (6.5–9.0 kPa) and can readily by controlled by 30–50% oxygen. (e) Opacities in the lung fields due to oedema or infection are absent or are resolving. When these conditions are fulfilled, weaning from the respirator is carried out and takes 25–48 hours. The first task is to tell the patient that the treatment is nearing the end and then explain the change in treatment. The clinician decides whether to use patient triggered IPPV or IMV to wean the patient. Fortunately, present day ventilators will perform any respiratory tricks required! Whichever technique is used, the golden rule is that the patient may never become exhausted during weaning. The myth of the patient who becomes emotionally dependant on the ventilator is exactly that – a myth. The weaning programme should follow the guidelines given in Chapter 19. When breathing spontaneously a tracheostomy collar is fitted to the neck and the collar supplied with a moist mixture of 30–50% oxygen in air. If all goes well with the weaning process then the cuffed tracheostomy tube is replaced by a tube fitted with a valve which enables the patient to speak and cough into the mouth.

5. Other problems

These are rare, varied and can kill the patient; some are difficult to diagnose and nearly all require thoracic surgery – at the right time. Contusions of the heart lead to a picture like acute myocardial infarction, with or without shock; the diagnosis depends on routine ECGs. Other injuries to the aorta, diaphragm etc. are summarized in Table 29.6 and detailed in more advanced texts.

Spinal injuries are outside the scope of this book and the reader is referred to the review by Davis (1982). A few facts are essential to the general ICU. Injuries of the upper ribs, especially when accompanied by fractures of the clavicle or scapula, should prompt a careful search for cervical spine injury, as the force causing these fractures may also break the neck. Fractures of the middle ribs may divert attention from the very real possibility of a thoracic spine injury. It cannot be overstated how easy it is to overlook such an injury, as bleeding into the mediastinum may obscure the bony injury. Occasionally a degree of chest wall paradox may be seen which cannot be wholly explained by the chest injury. The possibility of paralysis of part of the chest wall as a result of spinal injury should be borne in mind. In particular, the paradox is very striking when the paralysis is unilateral – the whole chest wall on that side appears flail.

Finally, the beginner should be aware of injuries to the larynx, readily missed when attention is focused on the thorax and abdomen. Suspicion should be aroused by bruising about the neck, loss of normal laryngeal outline on palpation and extensive surgical emphysema. Laryngeal damage warrants immediate assessment by direct laryngoscopy by an experienced surgeon. Examination using a Mackintosh intubating laryngoscope is not satisfactory as it does not give an adequate view of laryngeal structures.

Charting the patient's progress depends on the principles contained in the preceding chapters. But, as with head injuries, clinical impressions should be supplemented by using predictions of outcome based on measurement. The best general performance indicator for intensive care is undoubtedly the APACHE II system and this was described in Appendix 19.2.

IV   ABDOMINAL INJURIES INCLUDING THE PELVIS

Penetrating wounds need surgery as soon as resuscitation is underway. Non-penetrating injuries provide treacherous ground and delay in the recognition of a lesion needing surgery can maim or kill. Yet the early pathophysiology is easy; continuing haemorrhage or perforation of the gut. The role of the ICU is to recognize these, or the probability of such a lesion, as soon as possible and organize an operation. Plain X-rays of the abdomen are taken routinely and examined for free gas. Then, peritoneal lavage is used to detect intra-peritoneal blood; the technique is that of peritoneal dialysis (Chapter 24). To start with the easier of the two potentially fatal conditions, continuing haemorrhage. Following resuscitation, recognition of serious haemorrhage is readily done by observing the CVP, which will fall

Table 29.6 Chest injury: indications for thoracic surgery

Problem	Pointers to diagnosis	Surgical procedure
Penetrating wounds		
Lung	Continuing haemorrhage after resuscitation	Explore and repair
Heart	Tamponade, wide mediastinum	Relief of tamponade and repair
Diaphragm, spleen or kidney		Repair diaphragm, remove spleen, repair or remove kidney
Non-penetrating		
Bronchial tear	Bilateral blowing pneumothorax and surgical emphysema; bronchoscopy	Repair
Haemorrhage from lung or intercostal artery	Haemothorax which persists following resuscitation	Explore, find the site and repair
Diaphragmatic tear	Chest X-ray 'stomach in chest', X-ray screening; induce pneumoperitoneum	Explore above and below the torn diaphragm and repair
Aortic tear with pseudoaneurysm	Wide mediastinum, may need angiography or CT scanning	Repair using cardiopulmonary bypass
Oesophageal rupture	Wide mediastinum, pneumothorax empyema, gastrograffin swallow	Repair within 12 h

Table 29.7 Abdominal and pelvic injuries requiring surgery

Problem	Surgery
Penetrating wound	Exploration, repair, excision, prophylactic antibiotics
Haemorrhage	
torn spleen	Splenectomy
torn liver	Repair or resection
contused liver	
torn mesenteric vessel	Repair
retroperitoneal	
Contused or torn bladder	Repair
Urine leak from kidney	Repair
Avulsed kidney	Nephrectomy

long before the arterial pressure (Chapter 20). Urgent laparotomy is the action needed. The common lesions revealed are given in Table 29.7. A final rule on the care of the closed abdominal injury. A laparotomy must never be delayed because of concern that following this operation then IPPV may be necessary. When IPPV is necessary, then use it!

Injuries to the bladder or kidney are investigated on the grounds of suspicion. Haematuria or renal tenderness need a plan of action; cystoscopy and then an i.v. urogram, done in the ICU when transfer to X-ray is thought to be hazardous. Extravasation of urine or avulsion of the kidney can occur without haematuria and the policy should be that on the least suspicion of an injured urinary tract, an i.v. urogram is done.

V THE REVISED TRAUMA SCORE

It helps with patient care and its organization to grade the severity of injuries, as described for the thoracic type. Fortunately, we have the Glasgow Coma Scale and this has been incorporated in a comprehensive system called the Revised Trauma Score (RTS). Such systems are useless unless they have been tested out on large numbers of patients and they are simple to use without the aid of a computer! The RTS is based on data from 30 000 patients and the arithmetic takes about 15 seconds, just the thing for widespread application. To use the RTS the systolic blood pressure and respiratory frequency are each given a value (Table 29.8) and the sum of these is used to plan the strategy. For example, it may be made a rule that a patient with

Table 29.8 The Revised Trauma Score (From Rowlands, 1988)

Glasgow Coma Scale	Systolic BP	Respiratory rate	Coded value	Sum of coded values	Probability of survival
13–15	>89	10–29	4	12	0.995
9–12	76–89	>29	3	11	0.969
6–8	50–75	6–9	2	10	0.879
4–5	1–49	1–5	1	9	0.766
3	0	0	0	8	0.667
			7	0.636	
			6	0.630	
			5	0.455	
			4	0.333	
			2	0.286	
			1	0.250	
			0	0.037	

a value of less than 12 is transferred to a trauma centre (Rowlands, 1989). The Glasgow Coma Scale is used in parallel.

References and further reading

Chapter 1

1. British Medical Association. *Intensive Care*. Planning Report No. 1, 1967;18
2. Crocket GS, Barr A. An intensive care unit: two years' experience in a provincial hospital. *Br Med J* 1965;2:1173–5
3. English National Board for Nursing, Midwifery and Health Visiting. General intensive care nursing. Course No. 100, 1990
4. Haldeman JC. *Elements of Progressive Patient Care*. 1959, US Department of Health, Education and Welfare, Washington
5. Ibsen B. Intensive therapy: background and therapy. *Int Anaesthesiol Clin*, 1966;4:277–94
6. Intensive care in the UK. *Anaesthesia* 1989;44:528–31, Reprinted and obtainable from the King's Fund Centre for London, Camden Town, London, NW1 7NF
7. Jennett B. *High Technology Medicine: Benefits and Burdens*. 2nd edn. 1986;317, Oxford University Press
8. Lancet. *A unit for intensive patient care*. 1964;1:657
9. Le Gall J-R. *La Réanimation*. 1982;126 Presses Universitiés de France
10. Starzl TE. Ethical problems in organ transplantation. *Ann Intern Med* 1967;67:suppl 7:32–6
11. The Cost of Life. Symposium No. 9, *Proc Roy Soc Med* 1967;60:1195–246

Further reading

1. Black DAK. *An Anthology of False Antitheses*. 1984;74. Nuffield Provincial Hospitals Trust

Chapter 2

1. Bates DV. Organisation of intensive care units; results in cases of respiratory failure. *Anaesthesiology* 1964;25:199–204
2. British Medical Association. *Intensive Care*. Planning Report No. 1, 1–18
3. Cohen H. Our hospital systems. *Nursing Times*. 1946; February 16:124–7
4. Crocket GS, Barr A. An intensive care unit: two years' experience in a provincial hospital. *Br Med J* 1965;2:1173–5
5. Jones ES. The organisation and administration of intensive patient care. *Postgrad Med J* 1967;43:339–44
6. Jones ES. Intensive therapy. *Proc Roy Soc Med* 1967;60:1203–7
7. Safar P, ed. *Respiratory Therapy*. 1965;370, Blackwell Scientific Publications
8. World Health Organization. *Seminar on Nursing in Intensive Care*. 1971;94, Copenhagen

Further reading

1.   Intensive care in the UK, *Anaesthesia* 1989;44:428–31. Reprinted (1989) and obtainable from the King's Fund Centre for London, Camden Town, London, NW1 7NF

Chapter 3

1.   Jennett B. *High Technology Medicine: Benefits and Burdens.* 2nd edn. 1986;317. Oxford University Press

Chapter 4

1.   Black DAK. *Essentials of Fluid Balance.* 4th edn. 1969;182. Blackwell Scientific Publications
2.   Bold AM, Wilding P. *Clinical Chemistry.* 1975;48. Blackwell Scientific
3.   Jones ES, Sechiari GP. Method for providing metabolic balance during intensive patient care. *Lancet* 1963;1:19–20
4.   Peaston MJT. Maintenance of metabolism during intensive patient care. *Postgrad Med J* 1967;43:317–38

Further reading

1.   Chernecky CC, Berger BJ. *Laboratory Tests and Diagnostic Procedures.* 2nd edn. 1997;1082. WB Saunders
2.*   Elkington JR, Danowski TF. *The Body Fluids.* 1955;626, Baillière, Tindall and Cox
3.   Gabriel R. *Renal Medicine.* 3rd edn. 1988;322, Baillière-Tindall
4.*   Moore FJ. *Metabolic Care of the Surgical Patient.* 1959, WB Saunders
     *Well worth a visit to the library to examine these masterpieces

Chapter 5

1.*   Nahas CG. Current concepts of acid-base measurements. *Ann NY Acad Sci* 1966;133:1–274
     *Fascinating history and discussion

Further reading

1.   Holmes O. *Human Acid-Base Physiology.* 1993;208, Chapman and Hall

Chapter 6

1.   Campbell EJM. Respiratory failure. *Br Med J* 1965;1:1451–60
2.   Harris EA *et al.* The normal alveolar-arterial oxygen-tension gradient in man. *Clin Sci Mod Med* 1974;46:89–104

Further reading

1. Hlastala MP, Berger AJ. *Physiology of Respiration.* 1st edn. 1996;306. Oxford University Press
2.* Sykes MK *et al. Respiratory Failure.* 2nd edn. 1981;336. Blackwell Scientific
3. Sykes MK *et al. Principles of Clinical Measurement and Monitoring in Anaesthesia and Intensive Care.* 3rd edn. 1991;384. Blackwell Scientific
4. West JB. *Respiratory Physiology.* 5th edn. 1997;224. Williams and Wilkins
   *Out of print, but available in the library

Chapter 7

1. American College of Chest Physicians Society of Critical Care Medicine, Consensus Conference: Definitions for sepsis and organ failure and guidelines for the use of innovative therapies in sepsis. *Crit Care Med* 1992;20:864–74
2. Macaulay MB, Wright JF. Transvenous cardiac pacing, experience of percutaneous supravalvicular approach. *Br Med J* 1970;4:207–9
3. McGowan GK, Walters G. The value of measuring central venous pressure in shock. *Br J Surg* 1963;50:821–6
4. Miller GAH. *Invasive Investigation of the Heart.* 1989;512, Chapters 6 and 21 are especially relevant. Blackwell Scientific Publications
5. Peter SJW. *A Manual of Central Venous Catheterisation and Parenteral Nutrition.* 1983;288, Butterworth-Heinemann
6. Sykes MK. Venous pressure as an indication of adequacy of transfusion. *Ann Roy Coll Surg* 1963;33:185–97

Chapter 8

1. Gilston A, Resnekov L. *Cardio-respiratory Resuscitation.* 1971, Heinemann

Further reading

1. Bennett DH. *Cardiac Arrhythmias.* 4th edn. 1997;224, Butterworth-Heinemann
2. Hampton JR. *The ECG Made Easy.* 5th edn. 1997;130. Churchill-Livingstone
3. Hampton JR. *The ECG in Practice.* 3rd edn. 1997;310. Churchill-Livingstone

Chapter 9

1. Kerr DNS. From a lecture subsequently published as: *Insufficienza renale acuta, in dell'Enciclopedia Medica Italiana 197.* 1987;13:487–522. We hope your Italian is better than ours!
2. Robson JS. *Acute renal failure in Intensive Care – Proceedings of the Eighth Pfizer International Symposium.* 1975;144–57, Churchill Livingstone
3. Wrong O. Management of the acute uraemic emergency. *Br Med Bull* 1972;27:97–102

Further reading

1.   Cameron JS. Acute renal failure in the intensive care unit today. *Intensive Care Med* 1986;12:64–70
2.   Cameron JS. Acute renal failure thirty years on. *Q J Med* 1990;74:1–2
3.   Turney JH *et al*. The evolution of acute renal failure, 1956-88. *Q J Med* 1990;74:83–104
4.   Davson AM *et al.*, eds. *Concise Oxford Textbook of Clinical Nephrology*. 2nd edn. 1997;2512. Oxford University Press

Chapter 10

1.   Luksza AR. Brain-dead renal donor; selection, care and administration. *Br Med J*;1:1316–19
2.   Teasdale G, Jennett B. Assessment of coma and impaired consciousness. *Lancet* 1974;2:81–3

Further reading

1.   Pallis C. *ABC of Brain Stem Death*. 2nd edn. 1996;55, British Medical Association

Chapter 11

1.   de Dombal FT. Measures of disease activity. In *Current Management of Inflammatory Diseases*. TM Bayliss, ed., 1988;1–7, BC Decker
2.   Myren J. *et al*. The OMGE multinational inflammatory bowel disease survey 1976–1982. *Scand J Gastro* 1982;19:1–27
3.   Truelove SC, Witts LJ. Cortisone in ulcerative colitis. *Br Med J* 1954;2:375–8

Further reading

1.   Bouchier IAD *et al. Textbook of Gastroenterology*. 2nd edn. 1993;1400. Baillière-Tindall
2.   Hawker F. Liver dysfunction in critical illness. *Anaesth Intensive Care* 1991;19:165–81
3.*   Morson BC *et al. Gastrointestinal Pathology*. 3rd edn. 1990;758, Blackwell Scientific Publications

      *Lovely pictures

Chapter 12

1.   Cuthbertson DP. Alterations in metabolism following injury. *Injury* 1980;11:175–89,286–303

Further reading

1.   Alberti GKMM. Diabetic emergencies. *Br Med Bull* 1989;45:242–63

2.* Moore FD, Brennan MF. Surgery injury: body composition, protein metabolism and neuroendocrinology. In *Manual of Surgical Nutrition, American College of Surgeons*. 1975, W B Saunders
3. Watkins PJ *et al*. *Diabetes and its Management*. 5th edn. 1996;320, Blackwell Scientific Publications

   *A classic; out of print but available in the library

Chapter 13

1. Bain B. Coagulopathies. In *Intensive Care*. ES Jones, ed., 1982;78–113, Kluwer Academic Publishers

Chapter 15

1. American College of Chest Physicians/Society of Critical Care Medicine, Consensus Conference: Definitions for sepsis and organ failure and guidelines for the use of innovative therapies for sepsis. *Crit Care Med* 1992:864–74

Further reading

1. Ayliffe GAJ *et al*. *Hospital Acquired Infection*. 2nd edn., 1990;152, Butterworth-Heineman
2. Smith GRA, Easmon CSF. Bacterial Diseases. In *Topley and Wilson's Principles of Bacteriology, Virology and Immunity*. 1991;vol 3:746, Edward Arnold
3. Wenzel RP. *Prevention and Control of Nosocomial Infections*. 3rd edn., 1997;1200, Williams and Wilkins

Chapter 17

1. Drummond JC, Wilbraham A. *The Englishman's Food*. 1939;126, Jonathan Cape
2. Gett PM *et al*. Pulmonary oedema associated with sodium retention during ventilator treatment. *Br J Anaesth* 1971;43:460–70
3. Grant A, Todd E. *Enteral and Parenteral Nutrition*. 2nd edn. 1987;278, Blackwell Scientific Publications
4. McWilliam DB. The practical management of glucose-insulin infusions in the intensive care patient. *Intensive Care Med* 1980;6:133–5

Further Reading

1. Grant and Todd above, by far the best small book
2. Payne-James J *et al*. *Artificial Nutritional Support in Clinical Practice*. 1994;600, Edward Arnold

Equipment

In the UK, The Medical Devices Agency (Hannibal House, Elephant and Castle, London, SE1 6TQ) publish a continuing series of reports or reviews giving the evaluation of syringe pumps, volumetric infusion pumps and enteral feeding pumps.

Chapter 18

1.   Barach AL *et al.* Positive pressure respiration and its application to the treatment of acute pulmonary oedema. *Ann Intern Med* 1938;12:754–85
2.   Guidelines for Resuscitation. 1994;64. European Resuscitation Council. Available from Resuscitation Council, 9 Fitzroy Square, London, W1P 5AH
3.   Harris EA *et al.* The normal alveolar-arterial oxygen-gradient in man. *Clin Sci Mol Med* 1974;45:89–104
4.   Spoerel WE *et al.* Transtracheal ventilation. *Br J Anaesth* 1971;43:932–9
5.   Webber BA, Pryor JA. *Physiotherapy for Respiratory and Cardiac Problems.* 1993;461, Churchill-Livingstone

Further reading

1.   Edwards JD *et al. Oxygen Transport. Principles and Practice.* 1993;250, WB Saunders

Equipment

In the UK, The Medical Devices Agency (Hannibal House, Elephant and Castle, London, SE1 6TQ) publish a continuing series of reports or reviews giving the evaluation of humidifiers

Chapter 19

1.   Avery EE *et al.* Severe crushing injuries of the chest; a new method of treatment with continuous mechanical hyperventilation by means of intermittent positive endotracheal insufflation. *Q Bull Northwestern Univ Med School* 1959;39:301–3 (This is one of the epics of intensive care and well worth asking a medical reference library to get you a copy)
2.   Knaus WA, Zimmerman E. Prediction of outcome from critical illness. In *Recent Advances in Critical Care Medicine.* I McLedingham, ed., 1988;1–13, Churchill-Livingstone
3.   Mushin WW. *Automatic Ventilation of the Lungs.* 3rd edn. 1980;904, Blackwell Scientific Publications
4.   Smith PEM, Gordon IJ. An indicator to predict outcome in adult respiratory distress syndrome. *Intensive Care Med* 1986;12:86–9

Further reading

1. The use of I.P.P.V. in the treatment of chest injuries, Guillain-Barré syndrome, tetanus and botulism is dealt with in *Intensive Care*. ES Jones, ed., 1982;464, Kluwer Academic Publishers
2. Henderson A, Wright M. Status asthmaticus: experience of 100 consecutive admissions to an intensive care unit. *Clin Intensive Care* 1992;3:148–52. When you can better these results, please write and tell us
3. Kirby RJ et al., eds. *Clinical Applications of Ventilatory Support*. 1990;546, Churchill-Livingstone
4. Webber BA, Pryor JA. *Physiotherapy for Respiratory and Cardiac problems*. 1993;461, Churchill-Livingstone
   The maker's manuals can be a useful source of information. To take one example: for the Engstom Elvira (Datex-Engstrom) ventilation modes are well described in 19 pages of the user's manual.

Equipment

In the UK, The Medical Devices Agency (Hannibal House, Elephant and Castle, London, SE1 6TQ) publish a continuing series of reports or reviews giving the evaluation of ventilators and humidifiers.

Chapter 20

1. Edwards JD et al. *Oxygen Transport. Principles and Practice*. 1993;250, WB Saunders
2. Herkes RG, Bihari DJ. Management of shock. In *Care of the Critically Ill*. J Tinker, WM Zapol, eds., 1991;259–84, Springer-Verlag

Equipment

In the UK, The Medical Devices Agency (Hannibal House, Elephant and Castle, London, SE1 6TQ) publish a continuing series of reports or reviews giving the evaluation of patient monitors, ECG monitors, syringe pumps and volumetric infusion pumps.

Chapter 21

1. Don Michael TA et al. Mouth to lung airway for cardiac resuscitation. *Lancet*, 1968;2:1329
2. Fenwick P, Fenwick E. *The Truth is the Light*. 1995;278, Headline
3. Levy DE et al. Prognosis in non-traumatic coma. *Ann Int Med* 1981;98:293–301

Further reading

1. Bristow A et al. *Resuscitation and Training*. 1990;228, Farrand Press

2.   Evans TR. *ABC of Resuscitation*. 3rd edn., 1995;82, British Medical Association
3.   Guidelines for Resuscitation. 1994;64. European Resuscitation Council. Available from the Resuscitation Council, 9 Fitzroy Square, London, W1P 5AH
4.   Hampton JR. *The ECG in Practice*. 3rd edn. 1997;310, Churchill-Livingstone
5.   Mackintosh AF *et al.* Hospital resuscitation from ventricular fibrillation in Brighton. *Br Med J* 1979;1:511–13

Equipment

In the UK, The Medical Devices Agency (Hannibal House, Elephant and Castle, London, SE1 6TQ) publish a continuing series of reports or reviews giving the evaluation of patient monitors, ECG monitors, resuscitators and defibrillators

Chapter 22

1.   Jacobs C *et al.*, eds. *Replacement of Renal Function by Dialysis*. 4th edn. 1996;1252, Kluwer Academic Publishers

Chapter 23

1.   Briggs JD *et al. Renal Dialysis*. 1994;488, Chapman and Hall
2.   Lopot F. *Urea Kinetic Modelling*. 1990;184, EDTNA. One of several practical books from EDTNA
3.   Jacobs C *et al. Replacement of Renal Function by Dialysis*. 4th edn. 1996;1252, Kluwer Academic Publishers
4.   Sells, RA, Scott MR. *A Colour Atlas of Vascular Access Surgery*. 1990;160, Wolfe

Association

Join the European Dialysis and Transplant Association/European Renal Care Association (EDTNA/ERCA) c/o Leicester General Hospital, Leicester, LE5 4PW

Equipment

In the UK, The Medical Devices Agency (Hannibal House, Elephant and Castle, London, SE1 6TQ) publish a continuing series of reports or reviews giving the evaluation of equipment for haemodialysis and water treatment

Chapter 24

1. Berlyne GM *et al.* Pulmonary complications of peritoneal dialysis. *Lancet* 1966;2:75–8
2. Boen ST. *Peritoneal Dialysis in Clinical Medicine*. 1964, Charles C Thomas

Further reading

1. Mion C. Continuous peritoneal dialysis. In *Replacement of Renal Function by Dialysis*. C Jacobs *et al.*, eds., 4th edn. 1996;562–602, Kluwer Academic Publishers

Equipment

In the UK, The Medical Devices Agency (Hannibal House, Elephant and Castle, London, SE1 6TQ) publish a continuing series of reports or reviews giving the evaluation of equipment for peritoneal dialysis.

Chapter 25

1. Maher JH *et al.* Prognosis of critically ill patients with acute renal failure: APACHE II score and other predictive factors. *Q J Med* 1989;72:83–104

Further reading

1. Cameron JS. Acute renal failure thirty years on. *Q J Med* 1990;74:1–2
2. Turney JH *et al.* The evolution of acute renal failure 1956–1988. *Q J Med* 1990;74:83–104

Chapter 26

1. Luksza AR. The brain dead kidney donor: from death to donation. In *Intensive Care*, ES Jones, ed., 1982;215–31, Kluwer Academic Publishers

Further reading

1. Proudfood AT. *Acute Poisoning, Diagnosis and Management*. 2nd edn. 1993;320, Butterworth-Heinemann

For References

Martindale; *The Extra Pharmacopoeia*. 30th edn. 1993;1500, Pharmaceutical Press

Chapter 27

1. Atherton ST *et al.* Antibiotic policy for gram-negative infections following thoracic and other injuries. *Thorax* 1976;32:596–600

2.   Aycliffe GAJ. *Hospital Acquired Infection.* 1990;140, Butterworth
3.   Daschner FD. Useful and useless hygienic techniques in intensive care units. *Intensive Care Med* 1985;11:280–3
4.   Edmondson RS *et al.* Tetanus. In *Intensive Care*, ES Jones, ed., 1982;366–87, Kluwer Academic Publishers
5.   Guthrie DA. *History of Medicine.* 1958;319, Thomas Nelson
6.   Price DA, Sleigh JD. Control of infection due to *Kl. aerogenes* in a neurosurgical unit by withdrawal of antibiotics. *Lancet* 1970;2:1213–15
7.   Ruiz-Santana S *et al.* ICU pneumonia: a multi-institutional study. *Crit Care Med* 1987;15:930–2
8.   van Saene HKF *et al.* Selective decontamination of the digestive tract in the ICU: current status and future prospects. *Crit Care Med* 1991;19:1485–90

Further reading

1.   Lowbury EJL, Ayliffe AJ, Geddes AM. *Control of Hospital Infection.* 3rd edn. 1992;400, Chapman and Hall

Chapter 28

1.   Bain B. Coagulopathies. In *Intensive Care.* ES Jones, ed., 1982;98–9, Kluwer Academic Publishers
2.   Baldwin RWM, Hanson GC. *The Critically Ill Obstetric Patient.* 2nd edn. 1990;569, Farrand Press
3.   Napier JAF. *Handbook of Blood Transfusion Therapy.* 2nd edn. 1995;498, Wiley

Chapter 29

1.   A Group of Neurosurgeons. Guidelines for initial management after head injury. *Br Med J* 1984;288:983–5
2.   Avery EA *et al.* Severe crushing injuries of the chest: a new method of treatment. *Q B Northwestern Univ Med School* 1955;38:301–3
3.   Davies WB. Spinal cord injuries. In *Intensive Care.* ES Jones, ed., 1982;253–81, Kluwer Academic Publishers
4.   Jennett WB. *Head Injuries.* Ibid 192–214
5.   Knaus WA, Zimmerman E. Prediction of outcome from critical illness. In *Recent Advances in Critical Care Medicine.* I McLedingham, ed., 1988;1–13, Churchill-Livingstone
6.   Moore BP. Trauma to the chest. In *Trauma to the Chest.* WG Williams, RE Smith, eds., 1977;1–7, John Wright
7.   Rowlands BJ. Management of major trauma. In *Recent Advances in Surgery.* RCG Russell, ed., 1988;1–17, Churchill-Livingstone
8.   Rowlands BJ. Management of abdominal trauma. In *Progress in Surgery*, vol 3, I Taylor, ed., 1989;320, Churchill-Livingstone
9.   Wright DM. Chest injuries. In *Intensive Care.* ES Jonesed, 1982;232–51, Kluwer Academic Publishers
10.   Mollan RAB, Rowlands BJ. *Modern Trauma Management.* 1994;464, Butterworth-Heineman

Index

abdomen, 409–11
  distension, mechanical
    consequences, 162
  infections within, 385, 387–8
  injuries, 190, 409–11
abscess, brain, antibiotics, 381
absorption, poisons, prevention, 358
absorption collapse (atelectasis), 91,
    113
  in IPPV, 282–3
acetate in peritoneal dialysate, 341
acid–base balance, 67–83, 211–14
  disturbances, 57, 67–83, 211–14
    prevention, 211–12
    terminology, 72–3
    treatment, 212–14
  physiology applied to, 67–72
acidosis, 57, 73
  definition, 73
  diabetic, see ketoacidosis
  diagnosis, 81, 82
  harmful effects, 73, 74
  metabolic, see metabolic acidosis
  respiratory, see respiratory acidosis
acute physiological assessment (in
    APACHE), 289, 290
  in renal failure, 352
Addison's disease
  admission criteria, 35
  treatment, 300
admission criteria, 31–6
  GI haemorrhage, 34, 165
  infections, 376, 379, 382
adrenaline in shock, 296, 297
adrenocortical insufficiency, primary,
    see Addison's disease
adult respiratory distress syndrome,
    see respiratory distress syndrome
age and APACHE score, 289, 291
airborne infection hazard, 370
air-conditioning, 29
airway
  management, 231–2
    in cardiac arrest, 304

upper, 231–2
obstruction
  in endotracheal suction, 240
  generalized, 91
  mechanical, upper, 231–2
pressure
  continuous positive, 250
  peak, see peak airway pressure
albumin infusions, 391
alkalosis, 57, 73
  definition, 73
  diagnosis, 81, 82–3
  harmful effects, 73, 74
  metabolic, see metabolic alkalosis
  respiratory, see respiratory alkalosis
alveolar/arterial pressure gradient
  calculation, 105–7, 244
  values in healthy subjects, 108, 245
alveolar CO_2 tension, 87, 107
alveolar O_2, calculation, 105–6, 244
alveolar ventilation, 85–6, 86–7
  assessment, 88, 101
anaemia, 390
analgesics in IPPV, 267–8
anaphylactic shock, 300
antibiotics, prophylactic, 373–4
  in IPPV, 286
antibiotics, therapeutic
  broad spectrum, adverse effects, 196
  in IPPV, 287
  primary infections, 374
    endocarditis, 382
    meningitis/brain abscess, 381
    pneumonia, 378
  in renal failure, 319
  secondary respiratory infections, 386
anticoagulants
  for disseminated intravascular
    coagulation, 392
  in haemodialysis/filtration, 327, 332
  for thromboembolism, 393
anticonvulsants in status epilepticus,
    364, 365
antidotes to poisons, 358